Oral Pathology
for the
Dental Hygienist

SECOND EDITION

OLGA A. C. IBSEN, RDH, MS

Adjunct Professor
University of New Haven
West Haven, Connecticut

•

Adjunct Associate Professor
University of Bridgeport
Bridgeport, Connecticut

•

Adjunct Associate Professor
State University of New York
Farmingdale, New York

•

Formerly, Associate Professor of Clinical
Dentistry and Supervisor of Dental Radiology
School of Dental and Oral Surgery
Columbia University
New York, New York

•

JOAN ANDERSEN PHELAN, DDS

Chief, Dental Service
Department of Veterans Affairs Medical Center
Northport, New York

•

Associate Professor
Department of Oral Biology and Pathology
School of Dental Medicine
State University of New York at Stony Brook
Stony Brook, New York

•

Associate Professor of Clinical Dentistry
School of Dental and Oral Surgery
Columbia University
New York, New York

•

W.B. SAUNDERS COMPANY
A Division of Harcourt Brace & Company

Philadelphia   London   Toronto   Montreal   Sydney   Tokyo

W.B. SAUNDERS COMPANY
A Division of Harcourt Brace & Company

The Curtis Center
Independence Square West
Philadelphia, Pennsylvania 19106

Library of Congress Cataloging-in-Publication Data

Ibsen, Olga A. C.
Oral pathology for the dental hygienist / Olga A.C. Ibsen,
Joan Andersen Phelan. —Ed. 2.

   p.   cm.

Includes bibliographical references and index.

ISBN 0–7216–6051–7

1. Mouth—Diseases.   2. Dental hygienists.   I. Phelan, Joan
   Andersen.   II. WU 140 I14o 1996.   III. Title.
   [DNLM: 1. Mouth Diseases—pathology.   2. Tooth
   Diseases—pathology.   3. Dental Hygienists.]

RK307.I27 1996   617.5′22—dc20

DNLM/DLC   95–30945

Oral Pathology for the Dental Hygienist, second edition   ISBN 0–7216–6051–7

Printed in the United States of America

Last digit is the print number: 9   8   7   6   5   4   3   2   1

Contributors

Anthony J. Casino, DDS
Associate Professor, Department of Oral and Maxillofacial Surgery, School of Dental Medicine, State University of New York at Stony Brook; Chief, Division of Oral and Maxillofacial Surgery, University Medical Center at Stony Brook; Chief, Section of Oral and Maxillofacial Surgery, Department of Veterans Affairs Medical Center, Northport, New York
Temporomandibular Disorders and Dental Implants

Margaret J. Fehrenbach, RDH, MS
Instructor, Pierce College, Tacoma; Former Instructor, Shoreline Community College, Seattle, Washington
Inflammation and Repair; Immunity

Paul D. Freedman, DDS
Director, Section of Oral Pathology, The New York Hospital Medical Center of Queens, and Director, Oral Pathology Laboratory, Flushing, New York
Neoplasia

Joen Iannucci Haring, DDS, MS
Associate Professor of Clinical Dentistry, The Ohio State University College of Dentistry, Columbus, Ohio
Developmental Disorders

Olga A. C. Ibsen, RDH, MS
Adjunct Professor, University of New Haven, West Haven, Connecticut; Adjunct Associate Professor, University of Bridgeport, Bridgeport, Connecticut; Adjunct Associate Professor, State University of New York, Farmingdale, New York; Formerly, Associate Professor of Clinical Dentistry and Supervisor of Dental Radiology, School of Dental and Oral Surgery, Columbia University, New York, New York
Introduction to Preliminary Diagnosis of Oral Lesions; Developmental Disorders; Oral Manifestations of Systemic Diseases

Anne Cale Jones, DDS
Associate Professor, Department of Oral Diagnostic Sciences, University of Florida College of Dentistry, Gainesville, Florida
Neoplasia

Ulla E. Lemborn, RDH, MS
Professor and Clinic Director, Department of Dental Hygiene, West Los Angeles College, Culver City; Lecturer, Section of Periodontics, School of Dentistry, University of California, Los Angeles, California
Inflammation and Repair; Immunity

Joan Andersen Phelan, DDS
Chief, Dental Service, Department of Veterans Affairs Medical Center, Northport; Associate Professor, Department of Oral Biology and Pathology, School of Dental Medicine, State University of New York at Stony Brook; Associate Professor of Clinical Dentistry, School of Dental and Oral Surgery, Columbia University, New York, New York
Inflammation and Repair; Immunity; Neoplasia; Oral Manifestations of Systemic Diseases

Heddie O. Sedano, DDS, Dr Odont
Lecturer, University of California, Los Angeles, School of Dentistry, Los Angeles, California; Professor Emeritus, University of Minnesota School of Dentistry, Minneapolis, Minnesota
Genetics

Richard S. Truhlar, DDS
Assistant Clinical Professor, Department of Periodontics, School of Dental Medicine, State University of New York at Stony Brook; Periodontist, Department of Veterans Affairs Medical Center, Northport, New York
Temporomandibular Disorders and Dental Implants

Anthony T. Vernillo, DDS, PhD
Associate Professor of Basic Sciences (Oral Medicine and Pathology), and Associate Coordinator, Teaching Programs for Oral Medicine and Pathology, New York University College of Dentistry, New York; Member, Board of Trustees, Brooklyn AIDS Task Force (BATF), Brooklyn, New York
Oral Manifestations of Systemic Diseases

Preface

The second edition of *Oral Pathology for the Dental Hygienist* begins with a full-color atlas illustrating common oral lesions. We are delighted to have been able to add this feature to the text and believe that it will provide the practitioner and the student with a valuable resource and eliminate the need for purchasing an additional text.

We received enthusiastic responses from teachers of oral pathology to the format of the first edition. Therefore, the overall management of the material covered in the text is the same as in the first edition, with the chapters introduced by the general pathology topic and followed by discussions of the oral conditions or diseases related to that topic. High-quality black and white illustrations enhance the material discussed. We believe that color illustrations are important aids in the identification of lesions; therefore, within the text, the reader is referred to the Color Plates in addition to the black and white illustrations.

Responses to Chapter 1 in the first edition were also very positive. It is within the scope of responsibility of the dental hygienist to identify and accurately describe abnormal oral findings. This chapter provides a description of diagnostic processes as well as the terms used to describe findings in the oral hard and soft tissues.

Each chapter has been updated with new material, additional vocabulary, objectives, test questions, and references. Our goal was to be as comprehensive as possible while maintaining the format of the first edition, which journal reviews indicated facilitated both teaching and learning. A new chapter has been added covering the topics of temporomandibular disorders and dental implants.

Practicing dental hygienists have an important role in oral health care in identifying and describing abnormal oral findings. Teaching these skills begins early in dental hygiene education. We hope that dental hygiene educators will use the color atlas section to enhance the teaching of these skills to first-year dental hygiene students and then will use the text for the oral pathology course. This will provide a progression from one course to another and reinforce this material. In addition to assisting the student in becoming more confident in the subject area, the student will be better prepared for clinical board examinations and, ultimately, better prepared to provide optimal oral health care.

OLGA A. C. IBSEN, RDH, MS
JOAN ANDERSEN PHELAN, DDS

Acknowledgments

Many wonderful individuals contributed to the success of the first edition of *Oral Pathology for the Dental Hygienist* and to the development of this second edition. First of all, without our outstanding editors at W. B. Saunders Company, Shirley Kuhn and Selma Ozmat, we would still be meeting deadlines. They have continuously guided, nagged, supported, and cajoled us. Without them, the second edition would not yet be a reality.

Our husbands, Lawrence and Jerry, assisted and supported us in innumerable ways. We extend special thanks and appreciation to them.

A special thanks also to Dr. William C. Forbes, from Dover-Foxcroft, Maine, who teaches oral pathology at the School of Dental Hygiene of the University of Maine. Without solicitation, he provided us with an excellent critique of the first edition and suggestions for the second edition. We sincerely appreciate all the time he spent in helping us to meet the needs of students and faculty. We are most grateful to him.

We also wish to acknowledge our oral pathology teachers: Drs. Melvin Blake, Ernest Baden, Leon Eisenbud, Paul Freedman, Stanley Kerpel, Harry Lumerman, Michael Marder, James Sciubba, Philip Silverstein, Marshal Solomon, David Zegarelli, and Edward V. Zegarelli. Olga A. C. Ibsen extends sincere appreciation to individuals with whom she has worked in clinical practice who have encouraged, shared, and supported her efforts: Drs. Christopher Duffy, Irving Kittay, George Laskey, Joseph A. Pianpiano, and Bertram Weissman. In addition, she wishes to acknowledge two very special people who influenced her personal and professional life: her dad, the late Dr. Joseph A. Cuttita, and her godfather, Dr. Edward V. Zegarelli.

Finally, we both thank the many contributors to this text, whether they provided one slide, a segment of a chapter, or an entire chapter. We could not have done this without you.

Thank you all for your assistance in the development of the second edition of *Oral Pathology for the Dental Hygienist.*

OLGA A. C. IBSEN, RDH, MS
JOAN ANDERSEN PHELAN, DDS

Contents

3   *Immunity*   125

MARGARET J. FEHRENBACH   ULLA E. LEMBORN   JOAN A. PHELAN

Color Plates

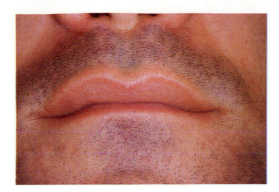

Color Plate 1. **Normal lips.** The vermilion is uniform in color, and the interface between the skin and the vermilion is distinct.

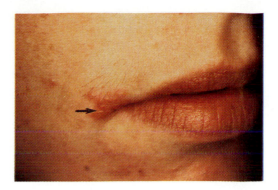

Color Plate 4. **Herpes labialis.** This cluster of vesicles on the right commissure is an example of herpes labialis *(arrow)*, the most common type of recurrent herpes simplex infection occurring in the oral region.

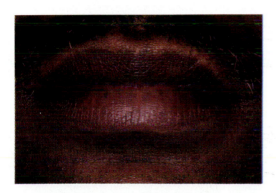

Color Plate 2. **Normal lips.** Melanin pigmentation is increased in the normal vermilion of the lips of this African-American patient.

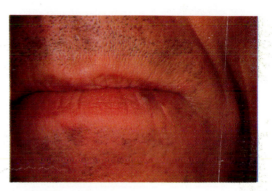

Color Plate 5. **Hemangioma.** The vascular nature of this lesion is clearly evident by its reddish-purple color. This is a benign lesion composed of small blood vessels.

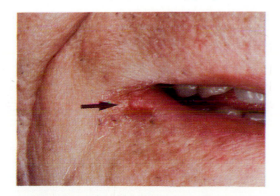

Color Plate 3. **Angular cheilitis.** This ulcerated, erythematous area of the right commissure is an example of angular cheilitis. This condition is often bilateral and occasionally crusted. It is commonly associated with candidiasis.

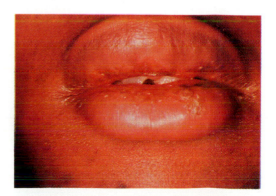

Color Plate 6. **Angioedema.** This diffuse swelling of the lips is due to edema, which results from an increased vascular permeability in deep tissues. Angioedema may be due to an allergic reaction or an inherited deficiency in a component of complement. (Courtesy of Dr. Edward V. Zegarelli.)

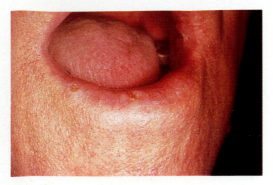

Color Plate 7. **Squamous cell carcinoma.** Squamous cell carcinoma in this location is associated with sun exposure and tends to be more common in individuals with fair skin. The prognosis for squamous cell carcinoma of the lips and skin is much better than that for intraoral squamous cell carcinoma. (Courtesy of Dr. Edward V. Zegarelli.)

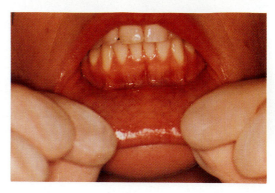

Color Plate 10. **Normal labial mucosa.** Normal labial mucosa appears uniformly pink in color. Palpation reveals a nodular texture caused by the numerous minor salivary glands located within the connective tissue.

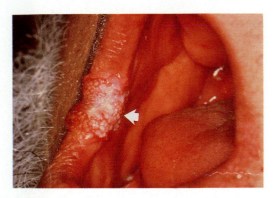

Color Plate 8. **Verrucous carcinoma.** This tumor has an exophytic papillary appearance. The white appearance is due to surface keratin. This type of carcinoma is composed of squamous epithelium, which proliferates in an exophytic manner rather than infiltrating underlying tissues and metastasizing to other locations. Verrucous carcinoma has a better prognosis than infiltrating squamous cell carcinoma.

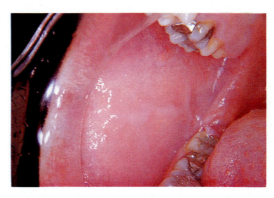

Color Plate 11. **Normal buccal mucosa.** Normal buccal mucosa appears uniformly pink in color and exhibits a smooth surface texture.

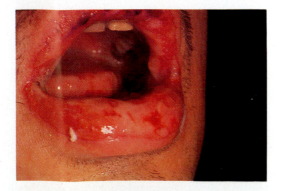

Color Plate 9. **Erythema multiforme.** Bleeding and crusted lips are a frequent and characteristic feature of erythema multiforme when it affects the oral mucosa. (Courtesy of Dr. Edward V. Zegarelli.)

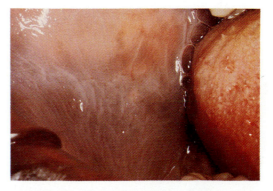

Color Plate 12. **Leukoedema.** This condition is characterized by a generalized white, opalescent quality of the buccal mucosa. It is considered normal, and the white, opalescent appearance disappears when the mucosa is stretched.

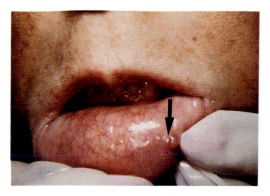

Color Plate 13. **Mucocele.** Although this lesion is most commonly seen on the lower lip, it may occur in any oral mucosal location where minor salivary glands are located. It occurs as a result of trauma to a minor salivary gland duct. The secretion of the gland spills into the adjacent connective tissue, forming a pool of saliva in the tissue. When near the surface, as illustrated here, a fluid-filled, blister-like lesion results.

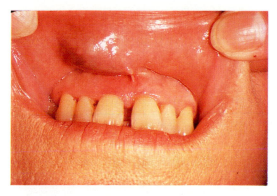

Color Plate 16. **Salivary gland tumor (pleomorphic adenoma).** This benign salivary gland tumor is presenting as a mass on the upper lip. The overlying mucosa appears normal. Salivary gland tumors are more commonly seen on the upper lip than the lower lip; mucoceles are more common on the lower lip. (Courtesy of Dr. Edward V. Zegarelli.)

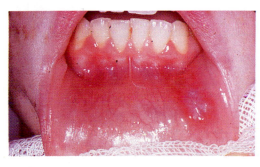

Color Plate 14. **Ulcerated mucocele.** This mucocele is broken, probably as a result of surface trauma. The overlying epithelium is ulcerated.

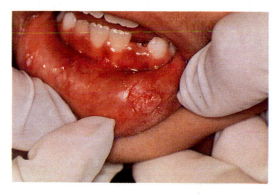

Color Plate 17. **Condyloma acuminatum.** This papillary lesion is caused by one of the human papillomaviruses and is considered a sexually transmitted disease. Accurate diagnosis requires special testing to identify the specific type of human papillomavirus in the epithelium of the lesion. In this illustration the lesion is occurring in a child, which is strongly suggestive of sexual abuse.

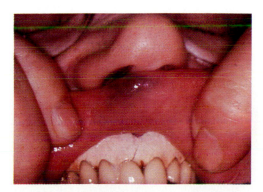

Color Plate 15. **Hematoma.** This blood-filled lesion resulted from trauma to the area during periodontal surgery. Trauma caused damage to blood vessels, allowing extravasation of blood into the tissue. (Courtesy of Dr. Edward V. Zegarelli.)

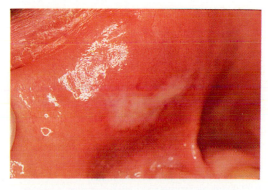

Color Plate 18. **Chemical burn.** This painful, necrotic lesion of the labial mucosa was caused by contact with a caustic substance during endodontic treatment.

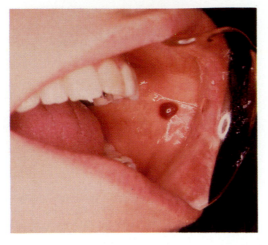

Color Plate 19. **Hematoma.** This hematoma was caused by a cheek bite.

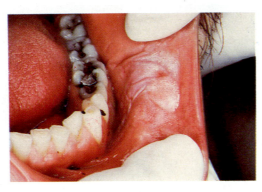

Color Plate 20. **Tobacco chewer's white lesion.** This rough-textured, corrugated white lesion is located where this patient holds smokeless tobacco.

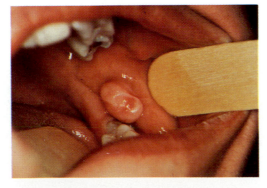

Color Plate 21. **Fibroma.** This exophytic lesion is composed of dense fibrous connective tissue surfaced by epithelium. A small area of surface ulceration occurred as a result of trauma during mastication. When fibromas are located on the buccal mucosa, they are often seen at the occlusal plane.

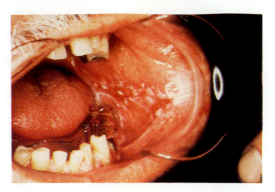

Color Plate 22. **Lichen planus (erosive type).** This lesion on the buccal mucosa is an example of erosive lichen planus. It is characterized by fine lace-like white lines and erythematous, superficially ulcerated mucosa.

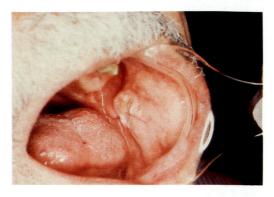

Color Plate 23. **Traumatic ulcer (granuloma).** This ulcerated lesion on the buccal mucosa was caused by chronic trauma to the area. This type of traumatic ulcer is sometimes called a traumatic granuloma. The lesion healed once the trauma was discontinued. This lesion may clinically resemble squamous cell carcinoma, and therefore a biopsy is often necessary to confirm the diagnosis.

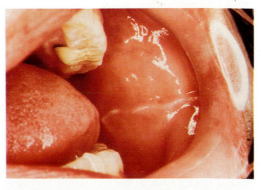

Color Plate 24. **Linea alba.** This elevated white line on the buccal mucosa is a linea alba. It extends anteroposteriorly along the occlusal plane.

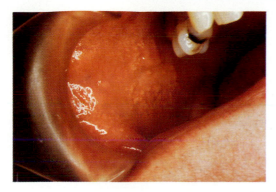

Color Plate 25. **Fordyce's granules.** These yellow granular-appearing structures, seen here on the buccal mucosa, are clusters of sebaceous glands. They are commonly seen on the oral mucosa in this location but may occur in other locations as well. Fordyce's granules are considered a variant of normal.

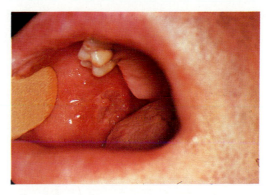

Color Plate 28. **Major aphthous ulcer.** This type of ulcer is larger than a centimeter in diameter and takes longer to heal than a minor aphthous ulcer. Major aphthous ulcers often heal with scarring and are more common in the posterior oral cavity than are minor aphthous ulcers. A biopsy may be necessary to confirm the diagnosis by ruling out other types of ulcers. (Courtesy of Dr. Edward V. Zegarelli.)

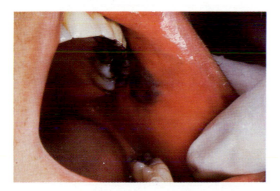

Color Plate 26. **Hemangioma.** This deep-purple lesion on the buccal mucosa is a benign lesion composed of small blood vessels. Hemangiomas are often congenital.

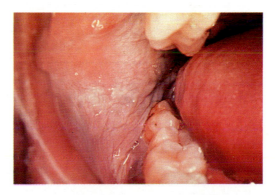

Color Plate 29. **Aspirin burn.** This painful, necrotic lesion of the buccal mucosa occurred because, instead of swallowing an aspirin tablet, the patient placed it on the mucosa.

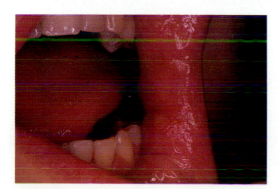

Color Plate 27. **Minor aphthous ulcer.** This type of ulcer is characterized by its size (<1 cm) and its round or oval appearance surrounded by a halo of erythema. Minor aphthous ulcers occur on mucosa that is not keratinized—the labial and buccal mucosa, floor of the mouth, ventral and lateral tongue, and soft palate. They heal within 7 to 10 days.

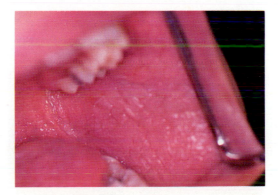

Color Plate 30. **White sponge nevus.** This is an inherited lesion that is transmitted autosomal dominantly. In this patient the unusual appearance of the mucosa was also seen on the labial mucosa and soft palate. The folded appearance of the mucosa can appear much whiter in some patients. (Courtesy of Dr. Louis Mandel).

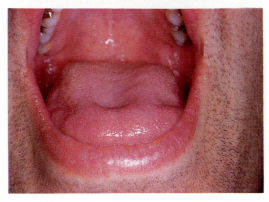

Color Plate 31. **Normal dorsal tongue.** The dorsal surface of the tongue is covered by filiform and fungiform papillae. The color is uniformly light pink.

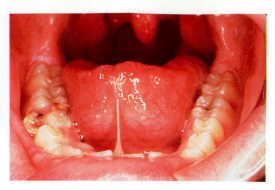

Color Plate 34. **Ankyloglossia.** This condition, also known as tongue-tie, is characterized by adhesion of the tongue to the floor of the mouth. A short lingual frenum is attached near the tip of the tongue.

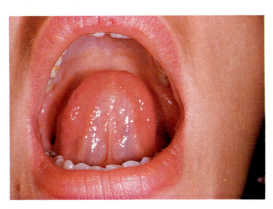

Color Plate 32. **Normal ventral tongue.** The mucosa of the ventral tongue is nonkeratinized and deep pink in color.

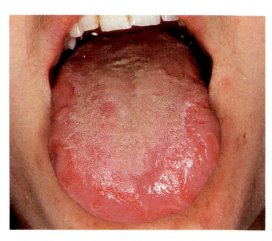

Color Plate 35. **Geographic tongue.** The dorsal and lateral borders of the tongue are affected in this patient. The red patches occur because of the lack of filiform papillae in these areas. These patches are surrounded by an irregular white or yellowish border. When the filiform papillae regenerate, the area returns to normal. This condition is also called migratory glossitis.

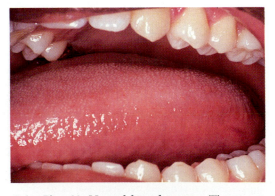

Color Plate 33. **Normal lateral tongue.** The mucosa of the lateral tongue is nonkeratinized and deeper pink in color than the dorsal tongue. Horizontal ridges of tissue seen at the posterior aspect of the lateral tongue are rudimentary foliate papillae.

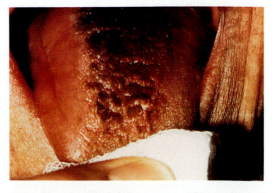

Color Plate 36. **Black hairy tongue.** This condition is characterized by elongation and black discoloration of the filiform papillae on the dorsal surface of the tongue. The black color is due to pigment produced by chromogenic bacteria.

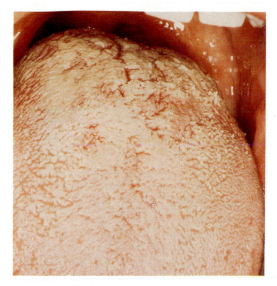

Color Plate 37. **White hairy tongue.** This condition is due to elongation of the filiform papillae on the dorsal tongue.

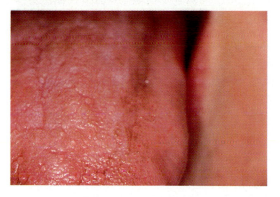

Color Plate 38. **Tongue discoloration in a wine taster.** This discoloration on the dorsolateral area of the tongue was present only when this patient was working as a wine taster. Discoloration of the tongue can occur as a result of different types of exogenous pigment.

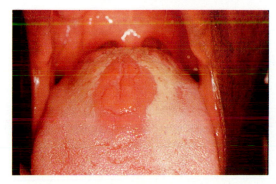

Color Plate 39. **Median rhomboid glossitis.** This condition appears as an erythematous area in the midline of the posterior dorsal tongue. The area is devoid of filiform papillae and is sometimes rhomboid shaped. This lesion has been associated with *Candida albicans.* (Courtesy of Dr. Edward V. Zegarelli.)

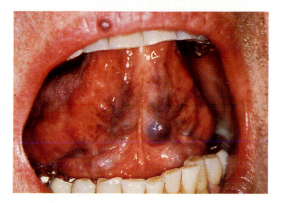

Color Plate 40. **Lingual varicosities.** These are prominent veins that are seen on the ventral surface of the tongue. Varicosities may be observed elsewhere in the oral cavity. Also note the varix on the upper lip. (Courtesy of Dr. David Zegarelli.)

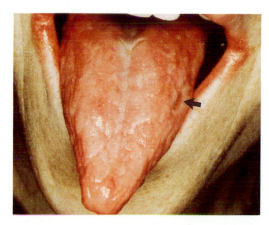

Color Plate 41. **Pernicious anemia.** This atrophic tongue, completely devoid of papillae, is seen in a patient with pernicious anemia. An ulcer is seen on the left lateral border *(arrow)*. Also note the presence of bilateral angular cheilitis, which, though most often associated with candidiasis, may also be associated with anemia.

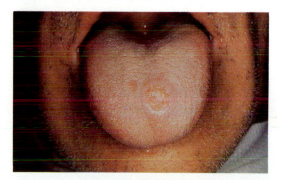

Color Plate 42. **Syphilis (chancre).** This discrete ulcer with raised borders is a chancre, which is associated with the first stage of syphilis and occurs at the site of inoculation. The lesion is teeming with organisms and is highly infectious. (Courtesy of Dr. Norman Trieger.)

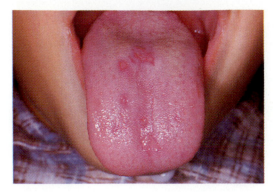

Color Plate 43. **Primary herpetic gingivostomatitis.** This condition is characterized by gingivitis, multiple tiny painful mucosal ulcerations, lymphadenopathy, and low-grade fever. The characteristic tiny oral mucosal ulcerations are seen here on the tongue. (Courtesy of Dr. Edward V. Zegarelli.)

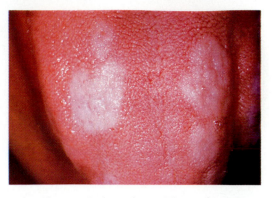

Color Plate 46. **Lichen planus.** These white, plaque-like lesions of the tongue are a form of lichen planus. Biopsy of these lesions may be needed to confirm the diagnosis. Characteristic white linear lesions were present on the buccal mucosa in this patient. (Courtesy of Dr. Edward V. Zegarelli.)

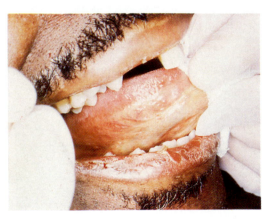

Color Plate 44. **Jaundice (hepatitis).** In this patient with severe alcoholic hepatitis, the ventral surface of the tongue exhibits pallor and a yellowish color. (Courtesy of Dr. Fariba Younai.)

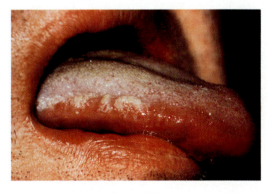

Color Plate 47. **Hairy leukoplakia.** This irregular white lesion is caused by the Epstein-Barr virus. It is characterized by vertical linear corrugations and is seen almost exclusively on the lateral aspect of the tongue. It was first identified and described in patients infected with HIV and has subsequently also been described in patients not infected with HIV.

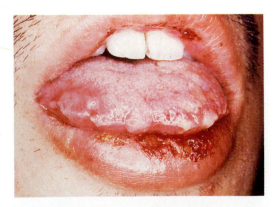

Color Plate 45. **Erythema multiforme.** Lesions are seen here on the tongue and lips. Oral lesions of erythema multiforme include bleeding, crusting, ulceration of the lips, and ulceration and erythema of the involved mucosal tissues. Lesions may occur on the skin as well as on oral tissues.

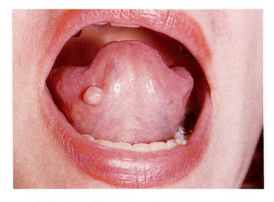

Color Plate 48. **Fibroma.** This benign lesion, which occurs as a result of trauma, is not a true neoplasm. It is a reactive hyperplasia of fibrous connective tissue. Although the fibroma may occur anywhere in the oral cavity, the most common sites are the buccal mucosa, labial mucosa, and lateral tongue.

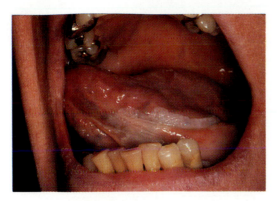

Color Plate 49. **Leukoplakia (epithelial dysplasia).** This white lesion on the lateral and ventral tongue required a biopsy to determine the diagnosis. Histologic examination of this lesion revealed epithelial dysplasia.

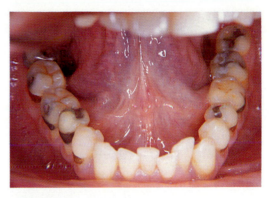

Color Plate 52. **Normal floor of the mouth.** The normal appearance of the floor of the mouth is illustrated. The lingual frenum attaches the tongue to the floor of the mouth. The bilateral nodular appearance is due to the sublingual salivary glands.

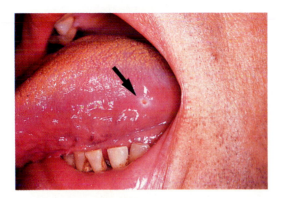

Color Plate 50. **Squamous cell carcinoma.** A biopsy and histologic examination of this small lesion (*arrow*) identified it as a squamous cell carcinoma. If the lesion is completely removed, the prognosis is good because of the lesion's small size. The lateral aspect of the tongue is one of the intraoral locations at increased risk for squamous cell carcinoma. (Courtesy of Dr. Edward V. Zegarelli.)

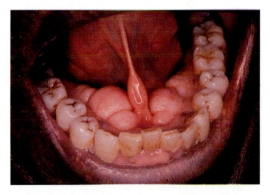

Color Plate 53. **Torus mandibularis.** These bilateral, exophytic, bony, hard nodules on the lingual aspect of the mandible are mandiblular tori. (Courtesy of Dr. Edward V. Zegarelli.)

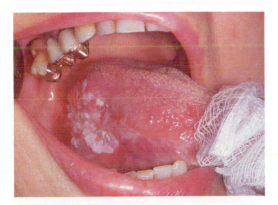

Color Plate 51. **Squamous cell carcinoma.** This large lesion exhibits exophytic areas, white areas, and ulcerated areas. Because of the lesion's large size, the prognosis would be expected to be poorer than for the lesion illustrated in Color Plate 50. (Courtesy of Dr. Edward V. Zegarelli.)

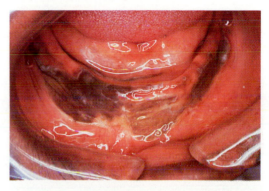

Color Plate 54. **Skin graft.** This African-American patient underwent a vestibuloplasty to deepen the mandibular labial sulcus. The brown pigmented area is a skin graft from the patient's hip.

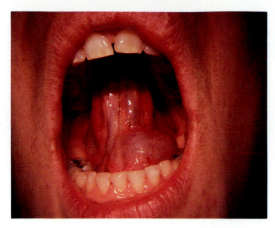

Color Plate 55. **Ranula.** This unilateral swelling on the left floor of the mouth is a ranula. A ranula occurs as a result of mucus extravasation associated with a break in one of the ducts of the sublingual gland or the submandibular gland.

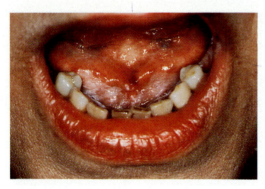

Color Plate 56. **Leukoplakia.** This white lesion of unknown cause located on the floor of the mouth requires a biopsy to determine the diagnosis. Histologic examination of this lesion revealed epithelial dysplasia.

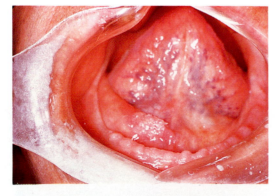

Color Plate 57. **Squamous cell carcinoma.** Biopsy and histologic examination of this rough-surfaced, exophytic, white lesion on the floor of the mouth revealed squamous cell carcinoma. The floor of the mouth is one of the oral mucosal locations at increased risk for squamous cell carcinoma. (Courtesy of Dr. Edward V. Zegarelli.)

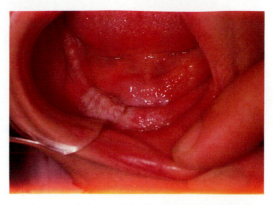

Color Plate 58. **Squamous cell carcinoma.** This rough-surfaced, white lesion on the mandibular alveolar ridge is a squamous cell carcinoma. (Courtesy of Dr. Edward V. Zegarelli.)

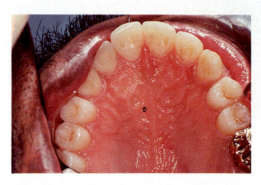

Color Plate 59. **Normal hard palate.** The hard palate is surfaced by keratinized stratified squamous epithelium. It is uniformly light pink in color. The normal palatal rugae are the ridges seen on the anterior hard palate.

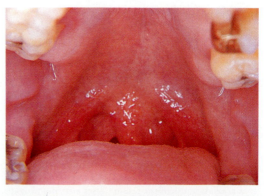

Color Plate 60. **Normal soft palate.** The soft palate and uvula are darker pink than the hard palate because the mucosa is normally nonkeratinized.

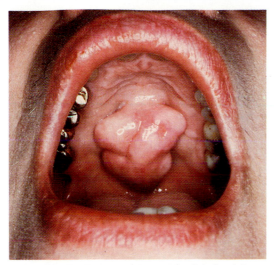

Color Plate 61. **Torus palatinus.** This lobulated, bony, hard protuberance in the midline of the hard palate is a torus palatinus. The tissue covering the bone is usually thin, and ulceration can result from mild trauma. It is a hereditary condition found more frequently in women.

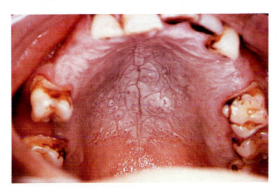

Color Plate 62. **Nicotine stomatitis.** This benign lesion on the palate is associated with pipe smoking in this patient. Increased keratinization results in a white appearance of the palate. Minor salivary glands become raised owing to inflammation, and the orifices of the glands appear as red dots on the raised glands. (Courtesy of Dr. Edward V. Zegarelli.)

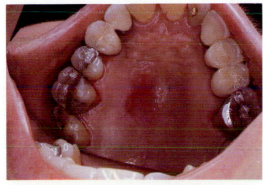

Color Plate 63. **Thermal burn.** This irregular, ulcerated, erythematous area on the palate is due to a burn that was caused by hot soup. Other hot foods such as pizza also cause thermal burns of the palate.

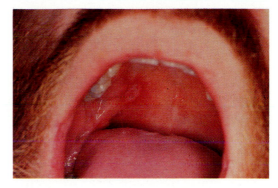

Color Plate 64. **Major aphthous ulcer.** This aphthous ulcer on the right soft palate is larger than a centimeter in diameter.

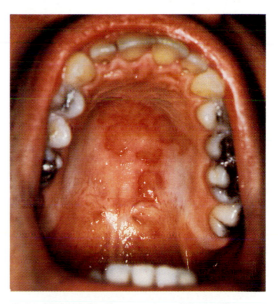

Color Plate 65. **Erythematous candidiasis.** This is an example of the form of candidiasis that is characterized by erythematous mucosa. Diagnosis usually involves the identification of fungal hyphae on a smear taken from the lesion and resolution of the lesion with antifungal medication.

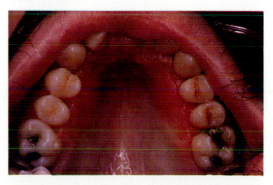

Color Plate 66. **Denture stomatitis.** This erythematous lesion, the most common form of oral candidiasis, is confined to within the borders of an acrylic partial denture ("flipper").

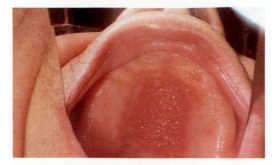

Color Plate 67. **Papillary hyperplasia.** This lesion is associated with an ill-fitting maxillary full denture. Papillary hyperplasia of the palate is characterized by multiple nodular excrescences on the palate. (Courtesy of Dr. Edward V. Zegarelli.)

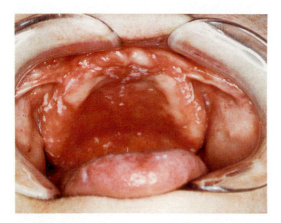

Color Plate 68. **Pseudomembranous candidiasis.** Pseudomembranous candidiasis developed in this patient after she took a systemic corticosteroid because of rheumatoid arthritis. She wore a full denture. Note that the lesions extend beyond the denture borders.

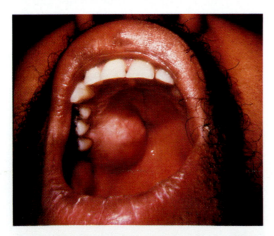

Color Plate 69. **Salivary gland tumor.** The junction of the hard and soft palate is the most common intraoral location for tumors of minor salivary gland origin. The tumor illustrated here was a benign tumor—a pleomorphic adenoma. Biopsy and histologic examination are necessary for diagnosis of this type of lesion.

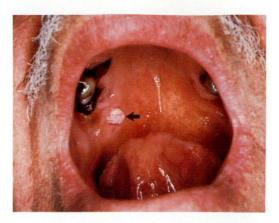

Color Plate 70. **Papilloma.** This benign epithelial lesion is characterized by numerous small finger-like projections of epithelium arranged in a cauliflower-like configuration. Human papillomavirus has been associated with the development of oral mucosal papillomas.

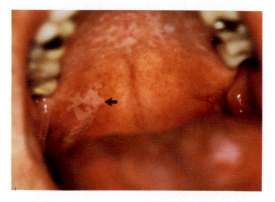

Color Plate 71. **Leukoplakia (epithelial dysplasia).** This white lesion on the soft palate occurred in a patient with lichen planus involving other oral mucosal areas. Biopsy and histologic examination of this lesion revealed epithelial dysplasia, not lichen planus.

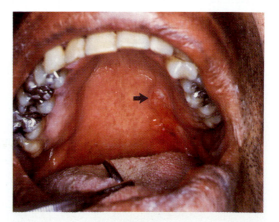

Color Plate 72. **Squamous cell carcinoma.** This somewhat exophytic ulcerated lesion on the left soft palate was diagnosed histologically as squamous cell carcinoma. The patient had a history of both smoking and high alcohol intake for many years.

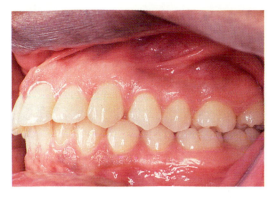

Color Plate 73. **Normal gingiva.** The normal, healthy gingiva in this young patient is characterized by a uniform light-pink color and sharply pointed interdental papillae completely filling the embrasure. The gingival margin is adapted tightly to the tooth surface.

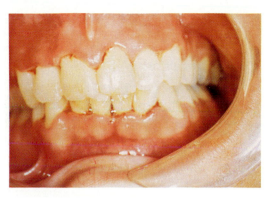

Color Plate 76. **Acute necrotizing ulcerative gingivitis (ANUG).** Ulceration and blunting of the interdental papillae are seen this patient with ANUG. A pseudomembrane resulting from superficial necrosis of the gingiva is present in areas, and bleeding is also seen.

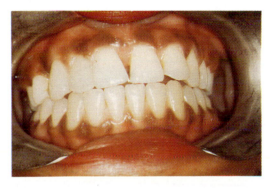

Color Plate 74. **Melanin pigmentation.** Melanin pigmentation of the gingiva is normal in patients with deeply pigmented skin.

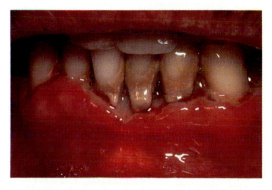

Color Plate 77. **HIV-associated necrotizing ulcerative periodontitis.** Destruction of the bone as well as the gingival tissue is seen in this HIV-infected patient with necrotizing ulcerative periodontitis. (Courtesy of Dr. Stuart R. Epstein.)

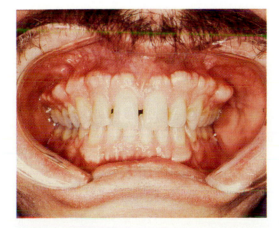

Color Plate 75. **Exostoses.** Exostoses are nodular enlargements of normal bone, which are seen in this patient on the labial and buccal aspect of the maxilla and the labial aspect of the mandible.

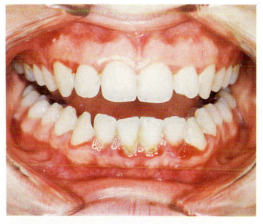

Color Plate 78. **Acute gingivitis.** Gingivitis in this adolescent patient resulted from poor oral hygiene.

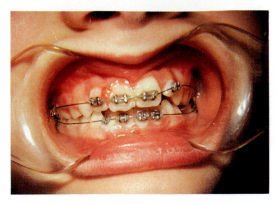

Color Plate 79. **Pyogenic granuloma.** The exophytic lesion located on the gingiva between the maxillary right lateral and central incisors was diagnosed histologically as a pyogenic granuloma. (Courtesy of Dr. Victor M. Sternberg.)

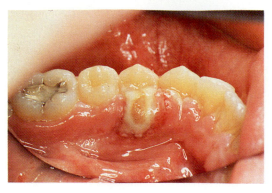

Color Plate 82. **Chickenpox (varicella-zoster infection) of the gingiva.** Lesions of chickenpox occur on the skin and also occasionally involve the oral mucosa. In this patient with chickenpox, many lesions were present on the skin. The lesion illustrated here was seen on the gingiva. (Courtesy of Dr. Roger S. Kitzis.)

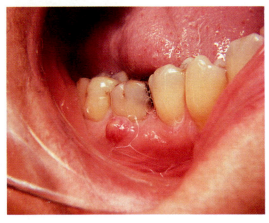

Color Plate 80. **Granulation tissue at external aspect of fistulous tract.** In this patient the fistulous tract was associated with a nonvital tooth and a periapical radiolucency.

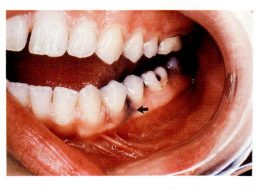

Color Plate 83. **Amalgam tattoo.** The diagnosis of this amalgam tattoo was confirmed by the presence of radiopaque particles on a radiograph of the area.

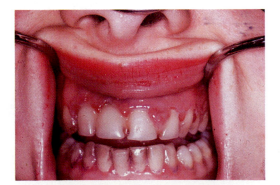

Color Plate 81. **Pregnancy gingivitis (pyogenic granuloma of pregnancy).** Histologically, the gingival enlargement of the papillae seen in this patient between the maxillary left central and lateral incisors is a pyogenic granuloma. (Courtesy of Dr. Edward V. Zegarelli.)

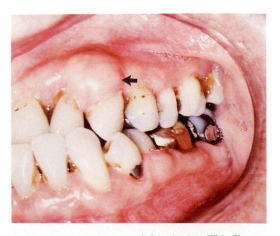

Color Plate 84. **Fibroma of the gingiva.** This fibroma of the gingiva occurred following healing of a periodontal abscess. (Courtesy of Dr. Murray Schwartz.)

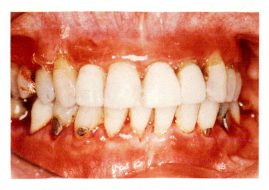

Color Plate 85. Desquamative gingivitis. Desquamative gingivitis may be seen in patients with lichen planus, benign mucous membrane pemphigoid, and occasionally pemphigus vulgaris. The appearance of the oral mucosa in other areas may be helpful in establishing a differential diagnosis. Biopsy is often necessary to establish the diagnosis of desquamative gingivitis. In this patient the histologic diagnosis was benign mucous membrane pemphigoid. (Courtesy of Dr. Victor M. Sternberg.)

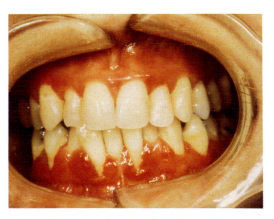

Color Plate 86. Cyclic neutropenia. The gingival lesions in this patient are occurring because of a cyclic (monthly) decrease in circulating neutrophils. At the time of the decrease patients become more susceptible to bacterial infection.

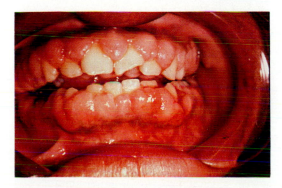

Color Plate 87. Drug-induced gingival hypertrophy. The gingival enlargement in this patient is due to phenytoin (Dilantin). (Courtesy of Dr. Edward V. Zegarelli.)

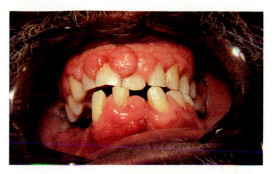

Color Plate 88. Drug-induced gingival hypertrophy. The gingival enlargement in this patient is due to nifedipine (Procardia).

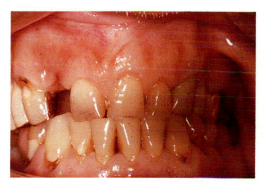

Color Plate 89. Gingival pallor due to anemia. The gingiva of patients with severe anemia of any type may exhibit pallor associated with decreased oxygenation of blood. (Courtesy of Dr. Edward V. Zegarelli.)

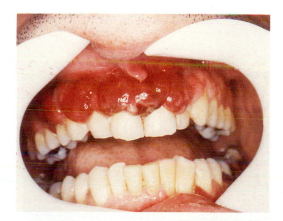

Color Plate 90. Kaposi's sarcoma. This patient with HIV infection has Kaposi's sarcoma of the gingiva. The bluish-red color of this lesion is characteristic of Kaposi's sarcoma, a vascular lesion. The palate and gingiva are the most common intraoral locations for Kaposi's sarcoma. (Courtesy of Dr. Fariba Younai.)

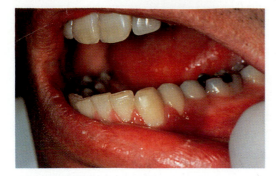

Color Plate 91. **Kaposi's sarcoma.** This small lesion of the gingiva surrounding the mandibular left first bicuspid is Kaposi's sarcoma.

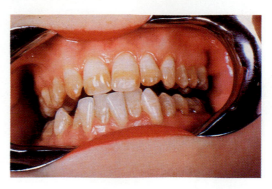

Color Plate 94. **Mottled enamel.** The discoloration of the enamel in this patient occurred as a result of high fluoride intake.

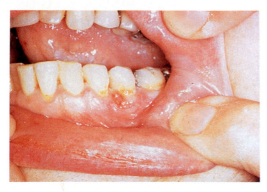

Color Plate 92. **Carcinoma of the gingiva.** Squamous cell carcinoma in this location is rarer than in other intraoral locations. The diagnosis of this lesion was made by biopsy and histologic examination. (Courtesy of Dr. Edward V. Zegarelli.)

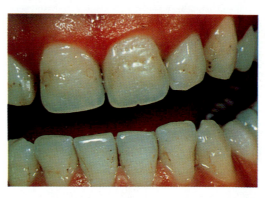

Color Plate 95. **Amelogenesis imperfecta.** The pitting of the enamel illustrated here is due to an inherited disturbance of enamel formation. (From Young WG, Sedano HO: Atlas of Oral Pathology. Minneapolis, MN, University of Minnesota Press, 1981.)

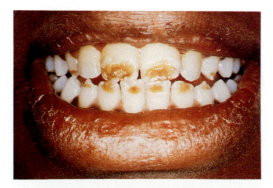

Color Plate 93. **Enamel hypoplasia.** In this patient the enamel hypoplasia follows a pattern that is suggestive of a systemic problem such as a high fever that caused disruption in enamel formation.

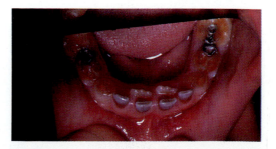

Color Plate 96. **Dentinogenesis imperfecta.** In this patient the discoloration of the teeth was due to an inherited disorder of dentine formation. Note that the primary teeth are more severely involved than the permanent teeth, a common finding in dentinogenesis imperfecta. Radiographs showing short roots and obliteration of pulp chambers would be helpful in diagnosing this disorder.

Oral Pathology
for the
Dental Hygienist

1

Introduction to Preliminary Diagnosis of Oral Lesions

OLGA A. C. IBSEN

Objectives

After studying this chapter, the student should be able to:

1. Define each of the terms in the vocabulary list for this chapter.
2. List and define the eight diagnostic categories that contribute to the diagnostic process.
3. Name a diagnostic category and give an example of a lesion, anomaly, or condition for which this category contributes greatly to the diagnosis.
4. Describe the clinical appearance of Fordyce's granules (spots), torus palatinus, mandibular tori, and lingual varicosities, and identify them on a slide.
5. Describe the radiographic picture and historical data (including the age, sex, and race of the patient) that are relevant to periapical cemental dysplasia (cementoma).
6. Define "variant of normal" and give three examples of such lesions involving the tongue.
7. List and describe the clinical characteristics and identify a clinical picture of fissured tongue, median rhomboid glossitis, geographic tongue, ectopic geographic tongue, and hairy tongue.
8. Describe the clinical and histologic differences between leukoedema and linea alba.

Vocabulary

Clinical Appearance of Lesions Within Soft Tissue

Bulla (adjective, bullous; plural, bullae)   A circumscribed elevated lesion that is more than 5 mm in diameter, usually contains serous fluid, and looks like a blister.

Lobule (adjective, lobulated)   A segment or lobe that is a part of the whole. These lobes sometimes appear fused together (Fig. 1–1).

Macule   An area that is usually distinguished by a color different from that of the surrounding tissue. It is flat and does not protrude above the surface of the normal tissue (e.g., freckles).

Papule   A small circumscribed lesion usually less than 1 cm in diameter that is elevated or protrudes above the surface of normal surrounding tissue.

Pedunculated   Attached by a stem-like or stalk base similar to that of a mushroom (Fig. 1–2).

Pustules   Variously sized circumscribed elevations containing pus.

Sessile   Describing the base of a lesion that is flat or broad instead of stem-like (Fig. 1–3).

Vesicle   A small elevated lesion less than 1 cm in diameter that contains serous fluid.

Soft Tissue Consistency

Nodule   A palpable solid lesion up to 1 cm in diameter found in soft tissue. It can occur above, level with, or beneath the skin surface.

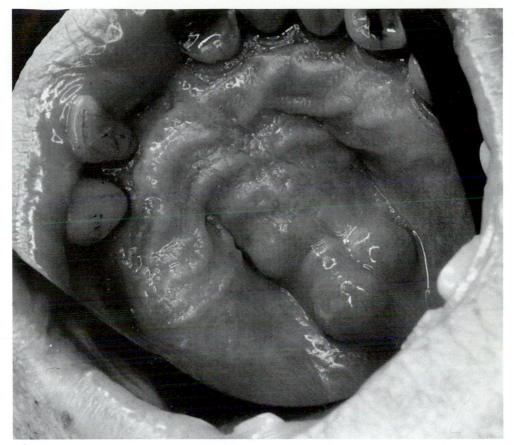

■ *f* i g u r e 1–1   Lobulated torus palatinus.

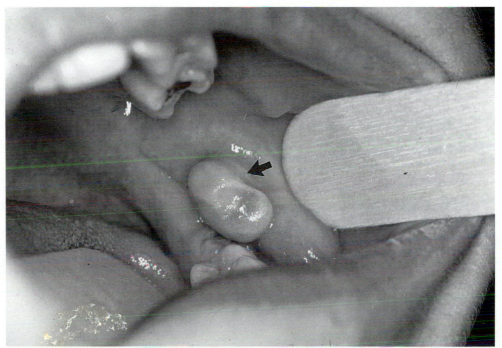

■ *f* i g u r e 1–2   Fibroma with a pedunculated base. Arrow points to the stem-like base.

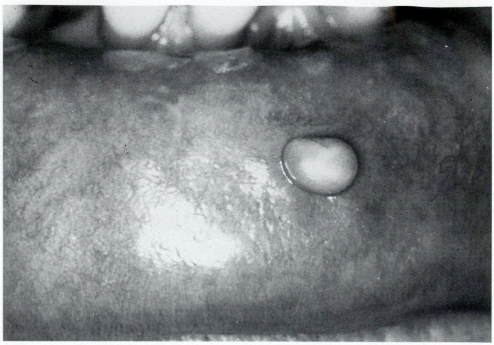

f i g u r e 1–3   Fibroma with a sessile base.

Palpation   The evaluation of a lesion by feeling it with the fingers to determine the texture of the area. The descriptive terms for palpation are soft, firm, semifirm, and fluid filled. These terms also describe the consistency of a lesion.

Color of the Lesion

Colors   Red, pink, salmon, white, blue-black, gray, brown, and black are the colors used most frequently to describe oral lesions. They can be used to identify specific lesions and may also be incorporated into general descriptions.

Erythema   An abnormal redness of the mucosa or gingiva.

Pallor   Paleness of the skin or mucosal tissues. *Sensitive to latex*

White lesion: body trying to build tissue

Size of the Lesion

Centimeter (cm)   One hundredth of a meter. Equivalent to a little less than one-half inch (0.393 of an inch) (Fig. 1–4).

Millimeter (mm)   One thousandth of a meter (a meter is equivalent to 39.3 inches). The periodontal probe is of great assistance in documenting the size or diameter of a lesion that can be measured in millimeters (Fig. 1–5).

General terms such as small, medium, or large are sometimes used, but these terms are not distinct.

Surface Texture

Corrugated   Wrinkled.

Fissure   A cleft or groove, normal or otherwise, showing prominent depth.

Papillary   Resembling small, nipple-shaped projections or elevations found in clusters.

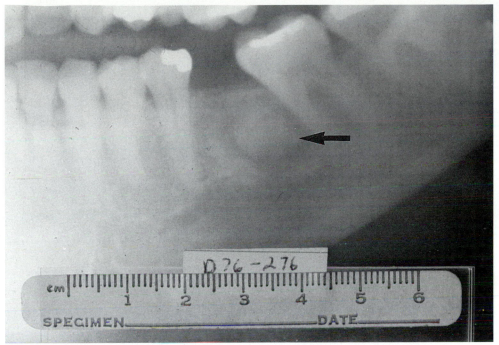

ƒ i g u r e 1-4   A ruler measuring centimeters is used to measure all specimens submitted for microscopic examination. On this radiograph, anterior to the mandibular second molar, the arrow points to a lesion that will be surgically removed and submitted for microscopic evaluation. (Courtesy of Drs. Paul Freedman and Stanley Kerpel.)

Smooth, rough, folded   Terms used to describe the surface texture of a lesion.

Radiographic Terms Used to Describe Lesions in Bone

Coalescence   The process by which parts of a whole join together, or fuse, to make one.

Diffuse   Describes lesion whose borders are not well defined, making it impossible to detect the exact parameters of the lesion. This usually makes treatment much more difficult and, depending on the biopsy results, more radical (Fig. 1–6).

Multilocular   Describes a lesion that extends beyond the confines of one distinct area and is defined as many lobes or parts that are somewhat fused together, making up the entire lesion. A multilocular radiolucency is sometimes described as resembling soap bubbles. An odontogenic keratocyst often presents as a multilocular radiolucent lesion (Fig. 1–7).

Radiolucent   Describes the black or dark areas on a radiograph. Radiant energy can pass through these structures. Less dense tissue, such as the pulp, is seen as a radiolucent structure (Fig. 1–8).

Radiolucent and radiopaque   Terms used to describe a mixture of light and dark areas within a lesion usually denoting a stage in the lesion's development. For example, in a stage I periapical cemental dysplasia (cementoma) (Fig. 1–9A), the lesion is radiolucent; in stage II, it is radiolucent and radiopaque (Fig. 1–9B).

Radiopaque   Describes the light or white area on a radiograph that results from the inability of radiant energy to pass through the structure. The more dense the structure, the more light or white it appears on the radiograph. This is illustrated in Figure 1–10.

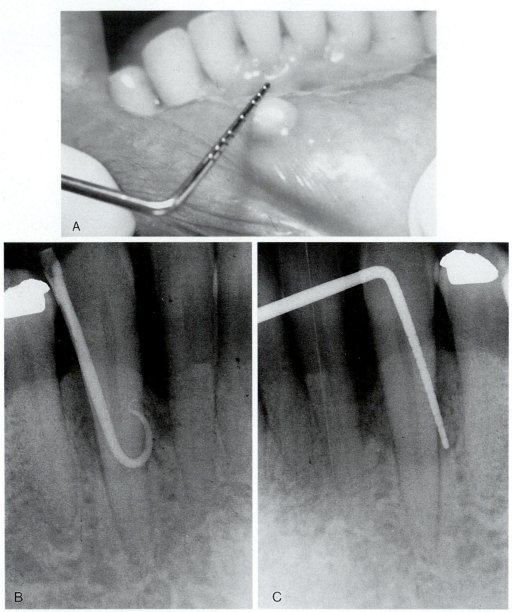

f i g u r e 1-5　*A*, Probe measuring the diameter of a fibroma with a sessile base. *B*, Gutta-percha point used to explore a radiographic defect. *C*, Periodontal probe placed prior to a radiograph.

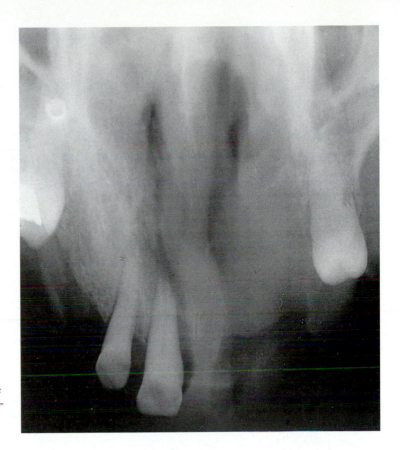

ƒ i g u r e 1–6
Squamous cell carcinoma of the hard palate showing diffuse borders. (Courtesy of Drs. Paul Freedman and Stanley Kerpel.)

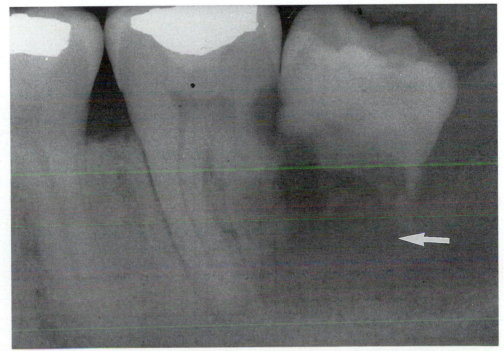

ƒ i g u r e 1–7 Odontogenic keratocyst *(arrow)*, illustrating a multilocular lesion. (Courtesy of Dr. Victor M. Sternberg.)

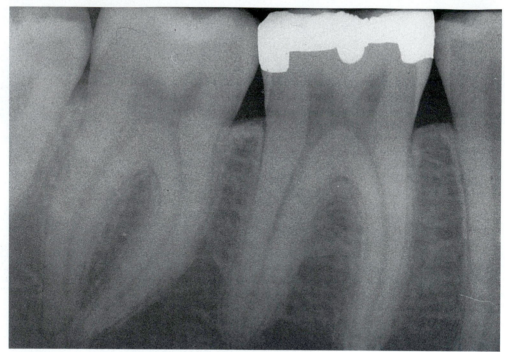

■ *f* i g u r e 1-8   Prominent pulp chambers, horns, and canals in mandibular molars.

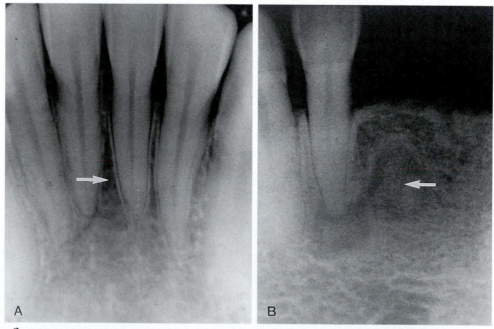

■ *f* i g u r e 1-9   *A*, Stage I periapical cemental dysplasia (cementoma). *B*, Stage II periapical cemental dysplasia (cementoma).

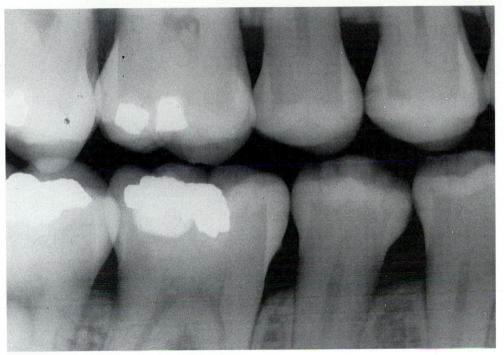

f i g u r e **1–10**   Amalgam restorations on the occlusal surfaces of the maxillary and mandibular molars.

Root resorption   Observed radiographically when the apex of the tooth appears shortened or blunted and irregularly shaped. It occurs as a response to stimuli, which can include a cyst, tumor, or trauma. Figure 1–11 illustrates resorption of the roots as a result of a rapid orthodontic procedure (see also Fig. 1–27). External resorption arises from tissues outside the tooth, such as the periodontal ligament, whereas internal resorption is triggered by pulpal tissue reaction from within the tooth. In the latter, the pulpal area can be seen as a diffuse radiolucency beyond the confines of the normal pulp area.

Scalloping around the root   A radiolucent lesion that extends between the roots, as seen in a traumatic bone cyst. This lesion appears to extend up the periodontal ligament (Fig. 1–12).

Unilocular   Having one compartment or unit that is well defined or outlined as in a simple radicular cyst (Fig. 1–13).

Well circumscribed   Term used to describe a lesion whose borders are specifically defined, and in which one can clearly see the exact margins and extent (Fig. 1–14).

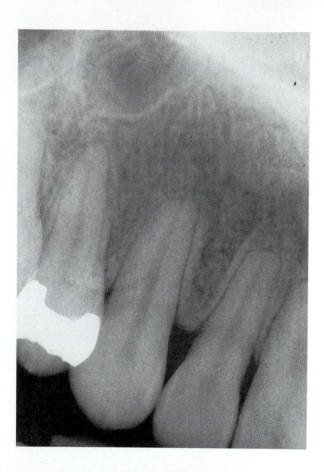

ƒ i g u r e 1–11
Resorption of the roots on maxillary anteriors as a result of rapid orthodontic movement.

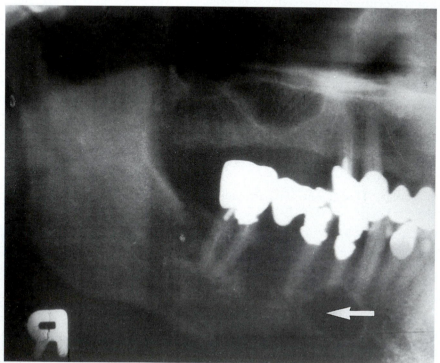

ƒ i g u r e 1–12   Traumatic bone cyst around the roots. (Courtesy of Drs. Paul Freedman and Stanley Kerpel.)

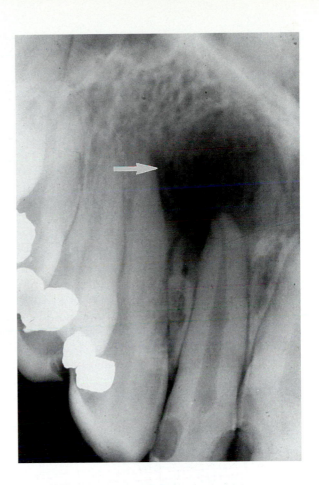

ƒigure 1-13
Radicular cyst at the apex of the maxillary lateral incisor illustrating a unilocular lesion.

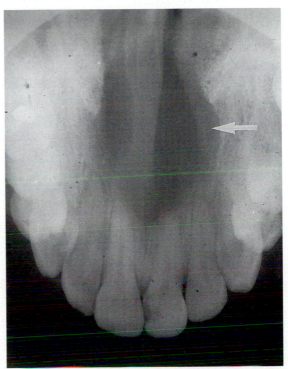

ƒigure 1-14
Well-circumscribed median palatal cyst.

To understand the material in this text, it is imperative that you approach the material in a systematic manner. Significant time is spent in the dental hygiene curriculum identifying and describing normal structures. Before one can identify the abnormal condition, it is necessary to have a solid understanding of the basic and dental sciences, such as human anatomy and physiology, histology, and dental anatomy. Once you have a solid understanding of normal structures and those that are variants of normal, findings that deviate from normal and pathologic conditions are more easily recognized. The preliminary evaluation and description of these lesions are within the scope of dental hygiene practice and are truly among the most challenging experiences in clinical practice.

In the first part of this chapter, the definitions of commonly used terms that describe the clinical and radiographic features of a lesion, including terms used for normal, variants of normal, and pathologic conditions discussed throughout this text, are presented. You are encouraged to use these terms in the clinical setting so that they become part of your everyday professional vocabulary and thereby facilitate communication between you and other dental practitioners in the clinical setting.

The second part of this chapter focuses on the eight diagnostic categories that provide a systematic approach to the preliminary evaluation of oral lesions. Each area is described and the strength of that area in the diagnostic process illustrated through specific examples of lesions.

The final part of the chapter includes conditions that are considered variants of normal and those that are benign conditions of unknown cause. Most are diagnosed from their distinct clinical appearance and history.

THE DIAGNOSTIC PROCESS

Making a Diagnosis

How is a diagnosis made? What are the essential components? The answers to these questions begin with **data collection.** The process of diagnosis requires gathering information that is relevant to the patient and the lesion being evaluated, this information coming from various sources. There are eight distinct diagnostic categories that should be thought of as pieces in a puzzle, each piece playing a significant role in the final diagnosis.

The eight categories that contribute segments of information leading to the definitive or final diagnosis are composed of clinical, radiographic, historical, laboratory, microscopic, surgical, therapeutic, and differential findings. It is important to note that usually one area alone does not provide sufficient information to make a diagnosis; the strength of the diagnosis is often derived from one or two areas. As you become more aware of the diseases and conditions discussed in this text, it will be most helpful to use the diagnostic categories as a guide to the evaluation of a lesion.

Clinical Diagnosis

Clinical diagnosis suggests that the strength of the diagnosis comes from the clinical appearance of the lesion. By observing the area in a well-illuminated clinical setting and **palpating** the area if necessary, the clinician can establish a diagnosis for some lesions on the basis of color, shape, location, and history of the lesion. Because a diagnosis can be made based on these unique clinical features, there is no need for biopsy or surgical intervention. Examples of lesions that can be clinically diagnosed are Fordyce's granules (Fig. 1–15; Color Plate 25), torus palatinus (Fig. 1–16; Color Plate

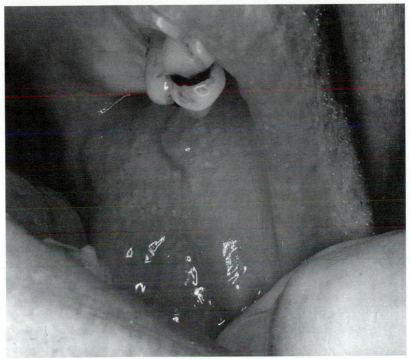

▪ *f* **i g u r e** **1–15**   Fordyce's granules.

61), mandibular tori (Fig. 1–17; Color Plate 53), melanin pigmentation (Fig. 1–18; Color Plate 74), retrocuspid papillae (Fig. 1–19), and lingual varicosities (Color Plate 40). These lesions are described later in this chapter. Other benign conditions of unknown cause that are recognized by their distinct clinical appearance include fissured tongue (Fig. 1–20*A,B*), median rhomboid glossitis (Fig. 1–21; Color Plate 39), geographic tongue (Fig. 1–22; Color Plate 35), and hairy tongue (Fig. 1–23*A–C*; Color Plates 36 and 37). These conditions are also discussed later in this chapter.

Sometimes the diagnostic process requires historical information in addition to the clinical findings. For example, an amalgam tattoo can be observed as a blue to gray patch on the gingiva or mucosa at the point at which there is or has been an amalgam restoration (Fig. 1–24; Color Plate 83). Although this condition is usually easily

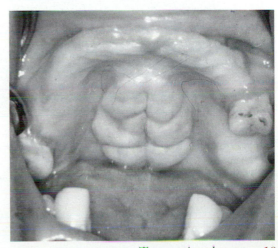

▪ *f* **i g u r e** **1–16**
Lobulated torus palatinus. (Courtesy of Dr. Edward V. Zegarelli.)

Text continued on page 18

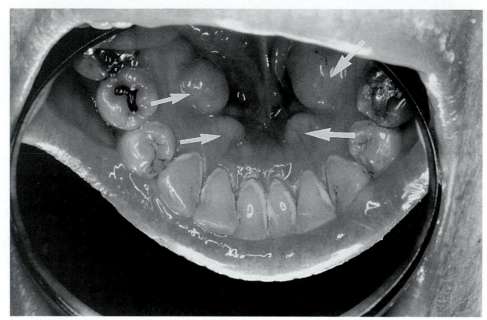

▪ *f* **i g u r e 1–17**   Arrows point to mandibular tori.

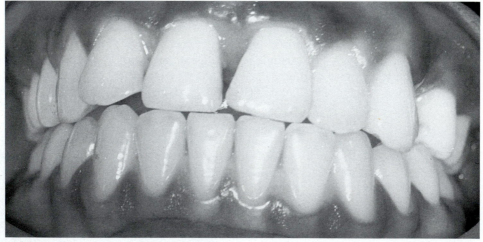

▪ *f* **i g u r e 1–18**   Melanin pigmentation.

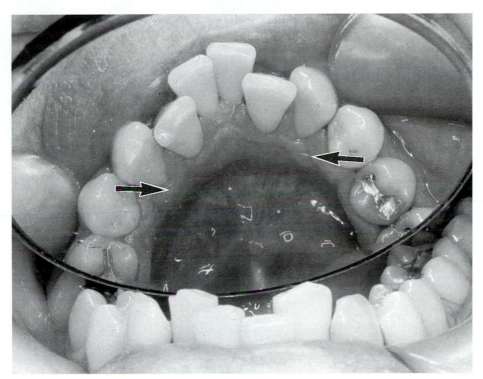

◾ *f* i g u r e **1–19**   Arrows point to the retrocuspid papillae on the gingival margin of the lingual aspect of the mandibular cuspids.

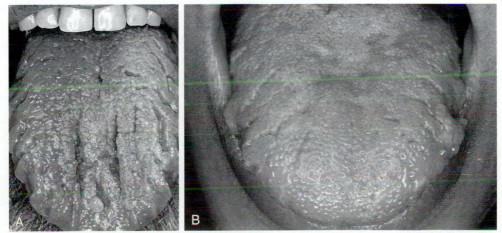

◾ *f* i g u r e **1–20**   *A* and *B*, Fissured tongue.

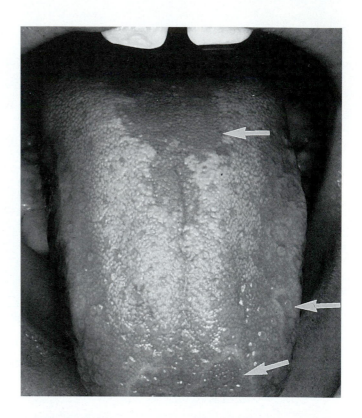

■ *f* i g u r e 1–21
Median rhomboid glossitis *(top arrow)*
and geographic tongue *(bottom arrows)*.

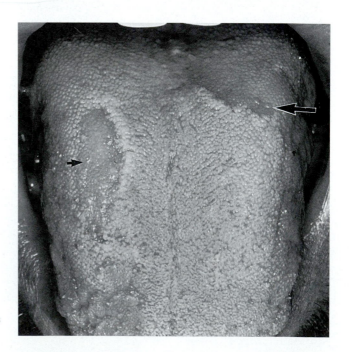

■ *f* i g u r e 1–22
Geographic tongue. Arrows point to areas
of depapillation.

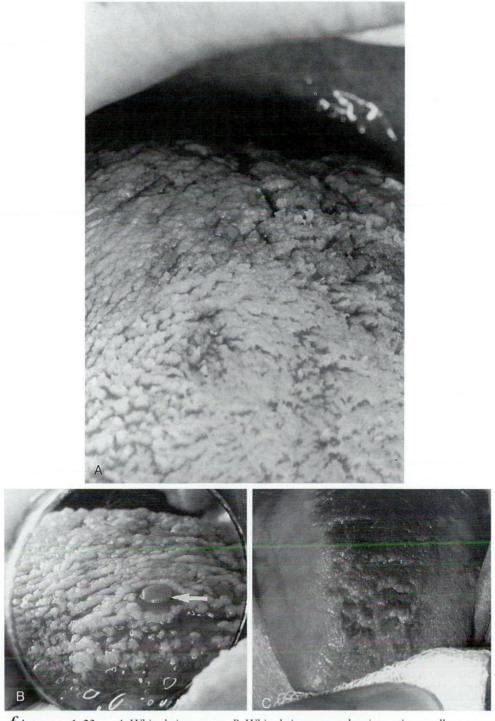

■ *f* i g u r e 1–23   *A*, White hairy tongue. *B*, White hairy tongue showing a circumvallate papilla *(arrow)*. *C*, Black hairy tongue.

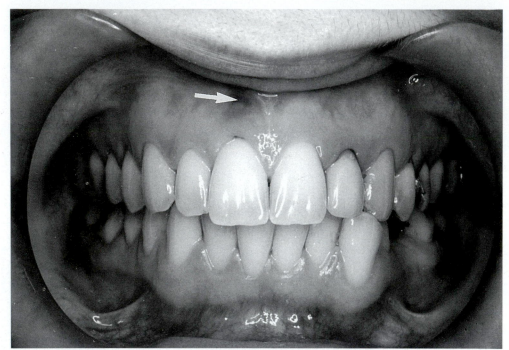

▪ *f* i g u r e **1–24**   Arrow points to an amalgam tattoo at the apical area of the patient's maxillary right central incisor. This patient had a root canal procedure on a deciduous tooth. There is no other amalgam restoration in the area; therefore, it was helpful to know the patient's past dental history to confirm this diagnosis.

observed and a clinical diagnosis made, there are times when the history involving the area can be very helpful, confirming the clinical impression. The patient in Figure 1–24 had root canal therapy and a retrograde amalgam on a deciduous tooth. The amalgam tattoo is observed in the apical area of the permanent central incisor. There is no evidence of an amalgam restoration in the entire anterior area.

Radiographic Diagnosis

In a radiographic diagnosis, the radiograph provides sufficient information to establish the diagnosis. Although additional clinical and historical information may contribute, the diagnosis is obtained from the radiograph. Conditions for which the radiograph provides the most significant information include periapical pathosis (PAP) (Fig. 1–25A,B), internal resorption (Fig. 1–26), external resorption (Fig. 1–27), heavy interproximal calculus (Fig. 1–28), dental caries (Fig. 1–29A–C), compound odontoma (Fig. 1–30), complex odontoma (Fig. 1–31A,B), supernumerary teeth (Fig. 1–32A,B), impacted or unerupted teeth (Fig. 1–33A,B), and calcified pulp (Fig. 1–34).

Normal anatomic landmarks are also easily observed radiographically. In some cases the radiograph may show very distinct and well-defined structures—for example, the nutrient canals that are seen in Figure 1–35A,B and the mixed dentition that is seen in Figure 1–35C. Unusual radiographic findings are illustrated in Figure 1–36A–I.

Historical Diagnosis

Historical data constitute an important component in every diagnosis. However, there are times when, combined with the clinical appearance of a lesion, they are the most important contribution. Personal history, family history, past and present medical

Text continued on page 25

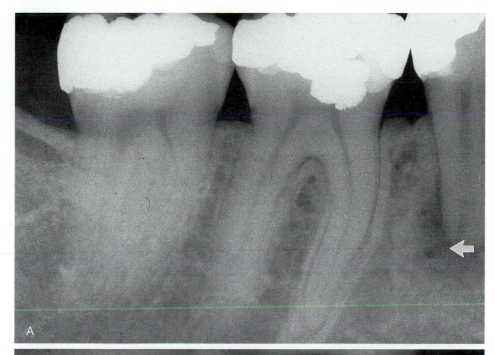

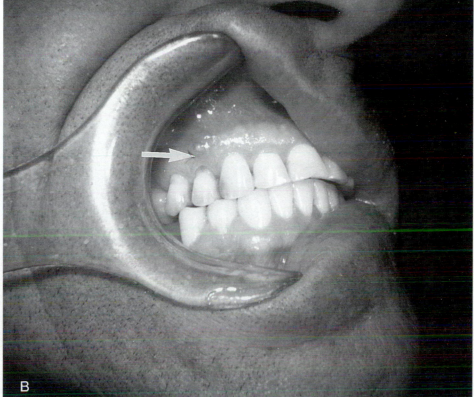

▪ *f* **i g u r e** **1–25**   *A*, Periapical pathosis (PAP); there is a radiolucency at the apex of the mandibular second premolar. *B*, In another patient the arrow points to a fistula that is seen clinically. A fistula is usually an indication of PAP. When a fistula is observed clinically, a radiograph is necessary for diagnostic and treatment purposes.

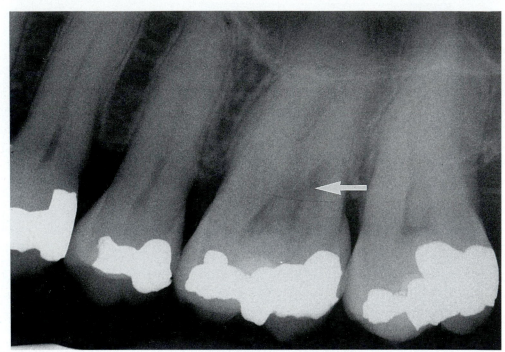

▪ *f* i g u r e 1–26   Arrow points to the area of internal resorption on the maxillary first molar.

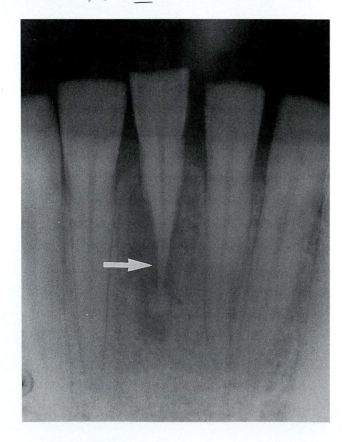

▪ *f* i g u r e 1–27
External resorption on a mandibular central incisor. (Courtesy of Dr. Gerald P. Curatola.)

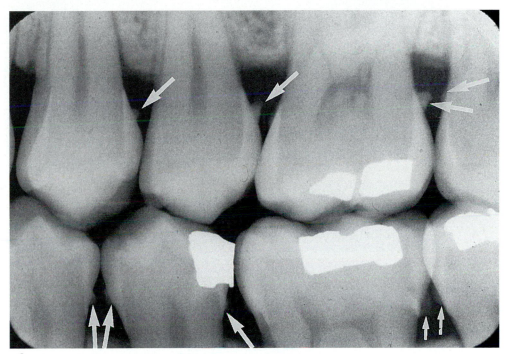

▪ *f* i g u r e 1–28   Heavy interproximal calculus.

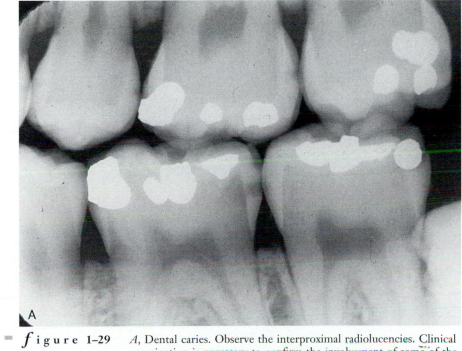

▪ *f* i g u r e 1–29   *A,* Dental caries. Observe the interproximal radiolucencies. Clinical examination is necessary to confirm the involvement of some of the areas.

Illustration continued on following page

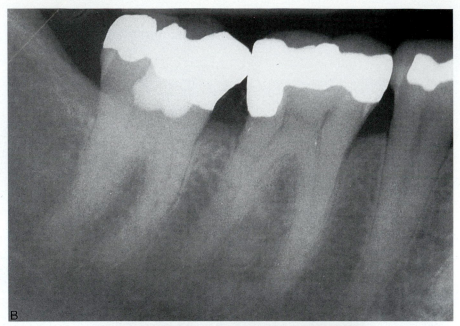

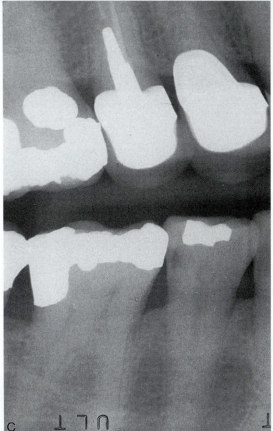

■ *f* i g u r e 1–29 *Continued B*, Periapical radiograph taken September 1989. Observe the subtle carious area on the distal aspect of the mandibular second premolar. *C*, The patient in *B* was seen in June 1990. During the scaling procedure a defect on the distal aspect of the mandibular second premolar was detected. This vertical bite-wing radiograph was taken. Note the definite radiolucent, carious area on the distal aspect of the mandibular second premolar. This example emphasizes the need for careful clinical as well as radiographic evaluation. (*B* and *C*, Courtesy of Dr. Victor M. Sternberg.)

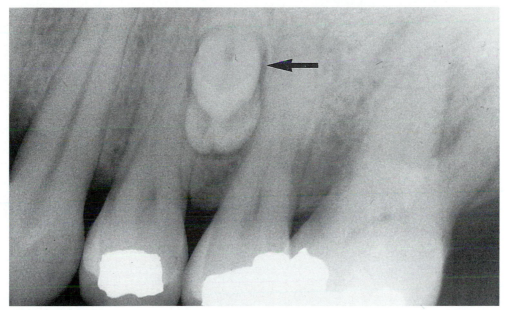

■ *f i g u r e* 1–30   Arrow points to compound odontoma.

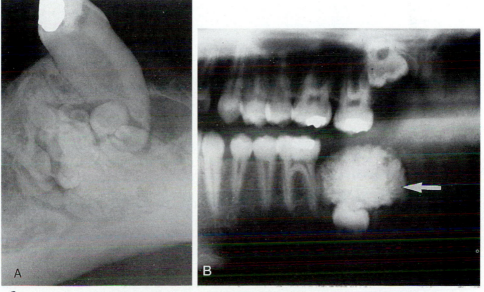

■ *f i g u r e* 1–31   *A,* Complex odontoma rather easily diagnosed from the radiograph alone. *B,* Complex odontoma not diagnosed from the radiograph alone. (*B,* Courtesy of Drs. Paul Freedman and Stanley Kerpel.)

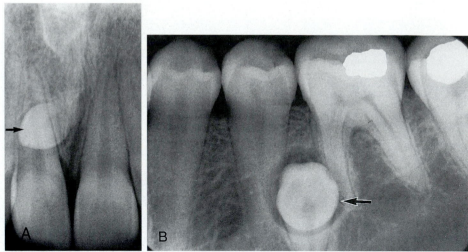

▪ *f* **i g u r e** **1–32**   *A*, Mesiodens. A supernumerary tooth between the maxillary central incisors. *B*, A radiograph showing a supernumerary mandibular premolar *(arrow)*. Clinically, this area was thought to be a mandibular torus (until the radiograph was taken).

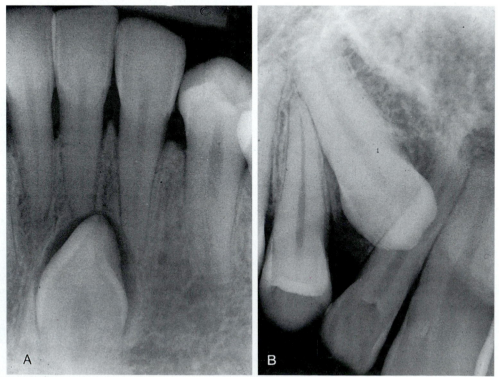

▪ *f* **i g u r e** **1–33**   *A*, Impacted mandibular cuspid. *B*, Impacted maxillary cuspid.

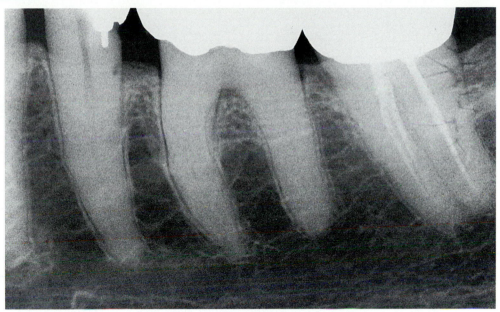

▪ **f i g u r e 1–34**   Calcified pulp in the mandibular first molar.

and dental histories, history of drug ingestion, and history of the presenting disease or lesion can provide information necessary for the final diagnosis. Thorough medical and dental histories must be a part of every patient's permanent record. The clinician should carefully review these documents and update them with the patient at each visit. Pathologic conditions in which the family history contributes a significant role in the diagnosis include amelogenesis imperfecta (Fig. 1–37*A,B*; Color Plate 95) and dentinogenesis imperfecta (Fig. 1–38; Color Plate 96) as well as many other genetic disorders.

A patient's medical or dental status can also contribute significant information to a diagnosis. A history of ulcerative colitis may contribute to the diagnosis of oral ulcers (Fig. 1–39*A*), which could be related to this medical condition. Another patient (Fig. 1–39*B*; Color Plate 18) experienced a chemical burn during an endodontic procedure.

A history of a skin graft from the hip to the ridge and mucobuccal fold area in the anterior mandible in a black patient can provide significant information relevant to the diagnosis of a brown pigmented area on the mandibular anterior ridge and vestibule (Fig. 1–40; Color Plate 54).

Periapical cemental dysplasia (cementoma) is another lesion in which the patient's personal history contributes significantly. It is found most frequently in black women in the third decade of life. Other characteristics of the lesion reveal that it is asymptomatic and that the teeth involved are vital (see Fig. 1–9).

Laboratory Diagnosis

Laboratory tests, including blood chemistries and urinalysis, can provide information that contributes to a diagnosis. An elevated serum alkaline phosphatase level is significant in the diagnosis of Paget's disease. This feature, in addition to a distinctive radiographic appearance (Fig. 1–41), provides conclusive information for a definitive diagnosis. Laboratory cultures are also helpful in determining the diagnosis of oral infections.

Text continued on page 31

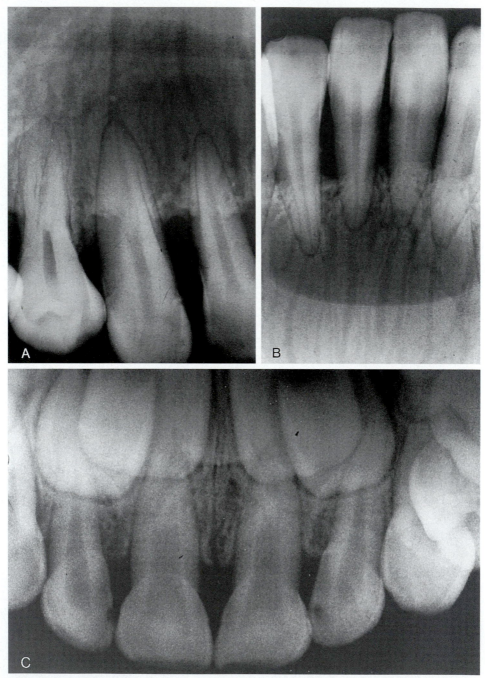

■ *f i g u r e* 1-35   *A*, Nutrient canals in the anterior maxillary arch. *B*, Nutrient canals in the mandibular anterior area. *C*, The mixed dentition of a 5-year-old child is observed in this radiograph.

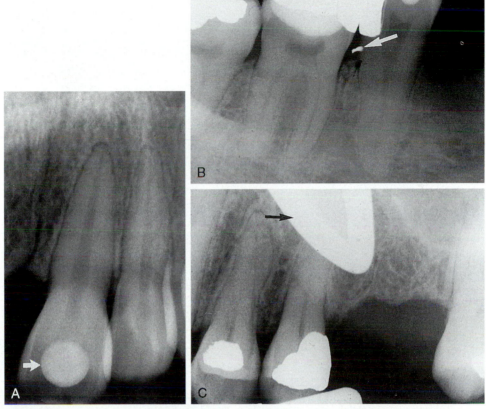

■ ƒ i g u r e 1–36   *A*, Arrow points to a 7-carat cubic zirconia (a round stone) that was glued to this patient's maxillary left central incisor. *B*, The radiopaque area on the distal aspect of the mandibular second premolar *(arrow)* is an amalgam fragment. There was a subtle clinical amalgam tattoo in the interproximal papilla that was not detected or charted on initial examination, which included a full-mouth series of radiographs and some scaling that was incomplete. When the radiographs were viewed after the patient was dismissed, the radiopaque area was thought to be the tip of a broken instrument. Further evaluation of the instruments used at that appointment ruled out the possibility of a broken instrument. When the patient returned for an additional appointment 2 weeks later, another radiograph, using the same long cone and precision Rinn instruments, was taken of the area. The radiopaque fragment remained in the exact same place. Clinically, a very close look at the interproximal papilla in the area then revealed a subtle bluish-black area. The dentist surgically slit the papilla on the buccal aspect and revealed the amalgam particle. *C*, This patient kept on her wide-framed eyeglasses during the radiographic procedure. The arrow points to a U-shaped radiopacity from the eyeglass frame.

Illustration continued on following page

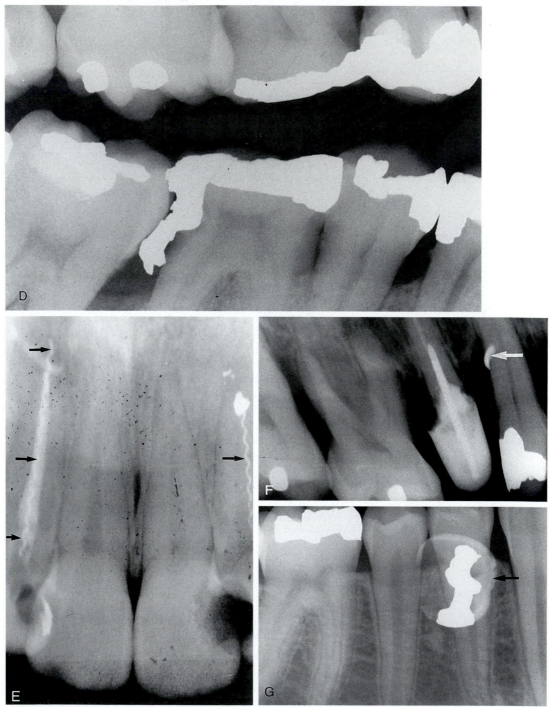

▬ *f* i g u r e 1-36   *Continued D,* This radiograph reveals an obvious radiopaque overhang from the amalgam restoration on the distal aspect of the mandibular first molar. *E,* Instruments from a root canal procedure were broken in these two maxillary lateral incisors *(arrows). F,* The broken tip of a curet *(arrow)* is observed as a radiopaque area on the distal aspect of the maxillary first premolar. *G,* The arrow points to a retained deciduous tooth with an amalgam restoration.

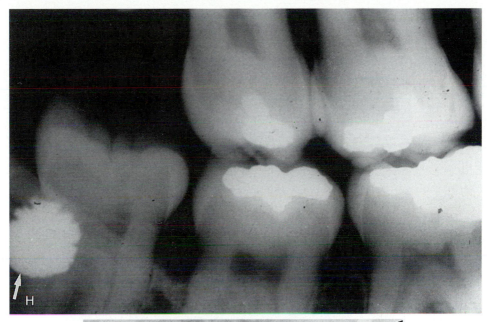

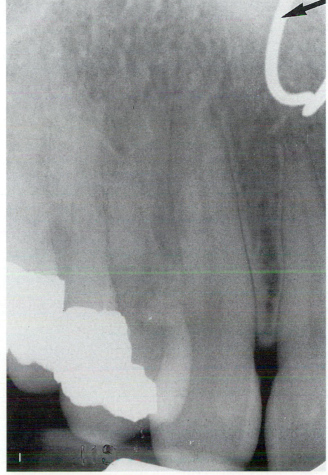

▪ *f* i g u r e 1–36 *Continued H,* The arrow points to a radiopaque area that identifies a retained shotgun pellet on the distal aspect of the mandibular third molar. *I,* The arrow points to a radiopaque circular area that is a nose ring.

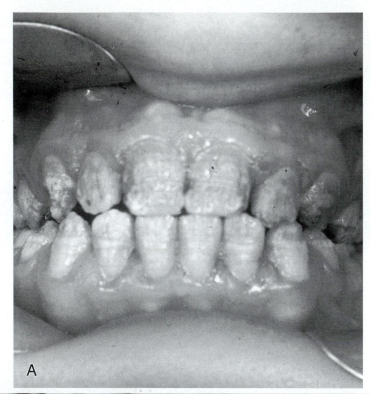

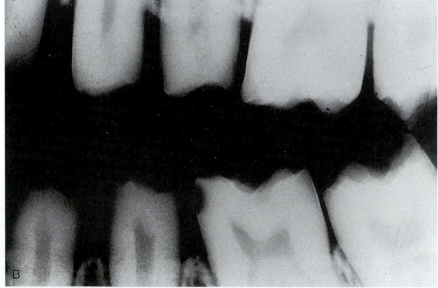

▪ *f i g u r e* **1-37**   *A*, One of the clinical appearances of amelogenesis imperfecta. *B*, The radiographic aspect of amelogenesis imperfecta. (Courtesy of Dr. Edward V. Zegarelli.)

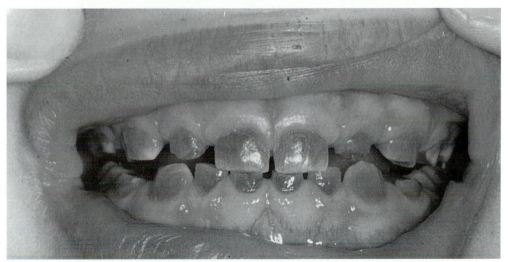

■ *f* i g u r e 1–38   The clinical aspect of dentinogenesis imperfecta. (Courtesy of Dr. Edward V. Zegarelli.)

Microscopic Diagnosis

Microscopy is of particular importance in the diagnostic process and therefore is discussed separately from laboratory diagnosis. The microscopic evaluation of the biopsy specimen taken from the lesion in question contributes significant information. This procedure is often the main component of the definitive diagnosis. However, the skill of the practitioner performing the biopsy is of equal importance. It is most important that an adequate tissue sample be removed for microscopic evaluation. If other diagnostic information, for example, clinical features and history of the lesion, indicates the strong possibility of malignancy and the biopsy report does not concur, a second biopsy should be performed.

A white lesion (Fig. 1–42) cannot be diagnosed on the basis of its clinical appearance alone. The microscopic appearance of this type of white lesion can vary from a thickening of the epithelium or surface keratin layer to epithelial dysplasia, which can be premalignant (Color Plate 49).

Surgical Diagnosis

The strength of a surgical diagnosis comes from surgical intervention. Diagnosis is made using the information gained during the surgical procedure—for example, **traumatic bone cyst** (Fig. 1–43) and **lingual mandibular bone concavity,** static or Stafne's bone cyst (Fig. 1–44). A traumatic or simple bone cyst may appear as a radiolucency that scallops around the roots. Surgical intervention provides conclusive evidence when the lesion is opened and an empty void within the bone is found. The void usually fills with bone and heals after the surgical procedure. Lingual mandibular bone concavity is a developmental anomaly and is often bilateral. Surgical examination of the well-circumscribed radiolucent area reveals salivary gland tissue entrapped during development; no treatment is indicated.

Therapeutic Diagnosis

Nutritional deficiencies are common conditions to be diagnosed by therapeutic means. Although angular cheilitis (Fig. 1–45) may be associated with a deficiency of

Text continued on page 36

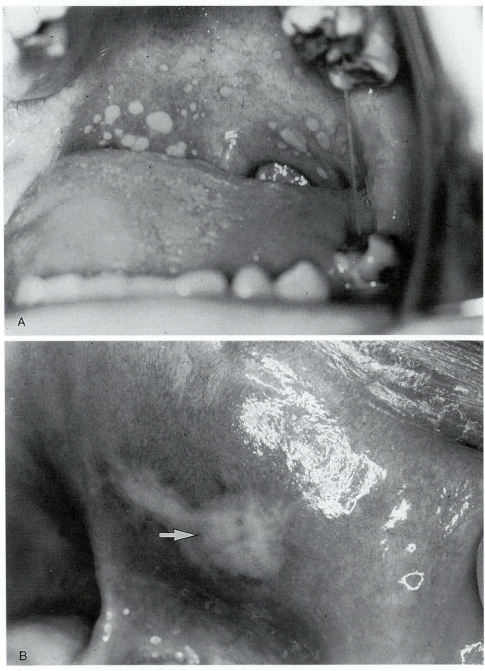

▪ *ƒ* i g u r e **1–39**   *A,* Oral ulcers on the soft palate associated with ulcerative colitis. (Courtesy of Dr. Edward V. Zegarelli.) *B,* Chemical burn of the mucosa *(arrow)* caused by irrigation during root canal procedure.

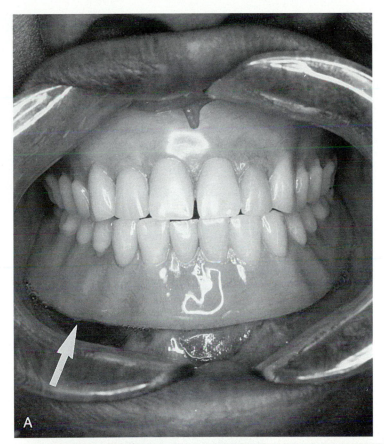

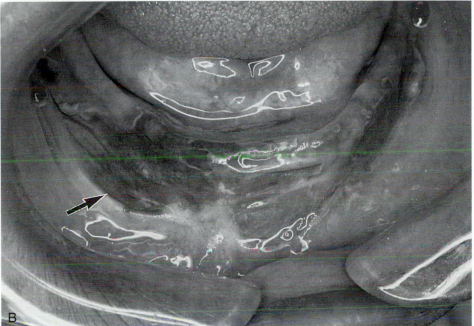

▪ *f* i g u r e **1–40**   *A,* Arrow points to skin graft area of the patient with denture in place. Note the unusually dark area on the mandibular right ridge. *B,* Same patient with the denture removed. There is an obvious darkened area *(arrow)* on the right mandibular alveolar ridge. Without the patient's past medical and dental histories, it would be difficult to diagnose this anomaly of melanosis accurately.

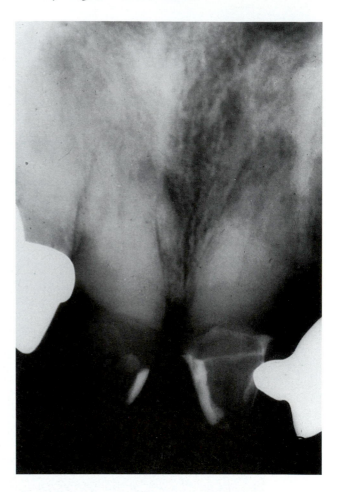

▪ *ƒ* i g u r e **1–41**
The radiographic appearance of Paget's disease showing the traditional "cotton-wool" radiopaque appearance of bone.

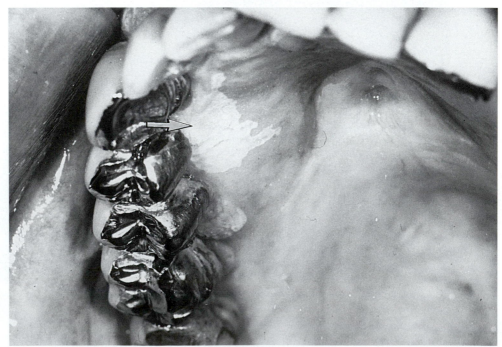

▪ *ƒ* i g u r e **1–42**   Arrow points to a white lesion on the palate.

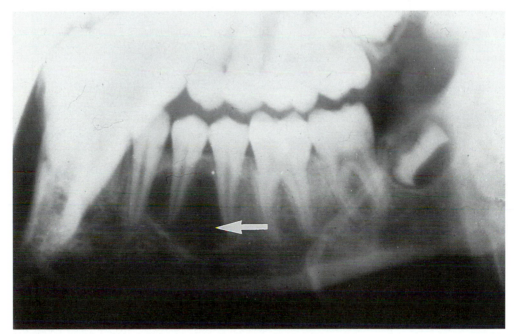

▪ *f* i g u r e 1–43   Traumatic bone cyst *(arrow)*. (Courtesy of Dr. Edward V. Zegarelli.)

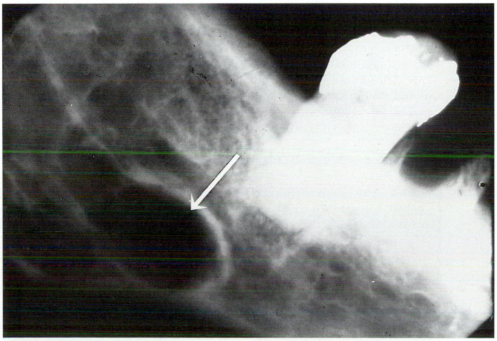

▪ *f* i g u r e 1–44   Arrow points to static bone cyst. (Courtesy of Dr. Edward V. Zegarelli.)

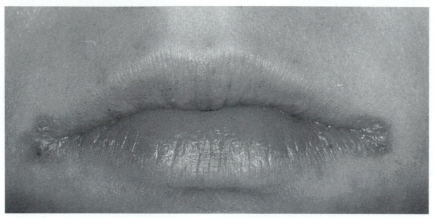

▪ *f* i g u r e 1–45   Angular cheilitis.

the B-complex vitamins, it is most commonly a fungal condition and responds to topical application of an antifungal cream such as nystatin (Color Plate 3). A thorough patient history should be obtained to rule out contributory nutritional deficiency.

Acute necrotizing ulcerative gingivitis (ANUG) has distinct clinical features (Fig. 1–46*A–D*; Color Plate 76) and constitutional signs. It responds to hydrogen peroxide rinses because the anaerobic bacteria that cause ANUG cannot survive in an oxygenated environment. Prescribing hydrogen peroxide rinses without culturing the bacteria applies the principle of therapeutic diagnosis because it is based solely on clinical and historical information.

Differential Diagnosis

The differential diagnosis is that point in the diagnostic process when the practitioner decides which test or procedure is required to rule out the conditions originally suspected and establish the definitive or final diagnosis. All the previously discussed components are applied to the differential diagnosis. The final diagnosis emerges from a thorough evaluation of the suspected lesions.

The following case study illustrates how the diagnostic processes work together and how the differential diagnosis is used.

CASE STUDY

An 11-year-old white girl comes to the dental office with her mother. The mother is concerned about the interdental papilla on the child's labial aspect between the maxillary right central and lateral incisors (Fig. 1–47; Color Plate 79). There is nothing in the child's medical history to explain the condition. She has been wearing orthodontic appliances for about a year. Clinically, the interdental papilla is enlarged and has a papillary surface that bleeds easily when probed. The sessile lesion measures 5 mm cervicoincisally by 3 mm mesiodistally. There is no pain in the area. Information pertinent to the history of the lesion is secured from the mother. The lesion has been there for about a year and was first noticed around the time the child began wearing braces. At times, tags of the lesion or pieces of it "fell off" during brushing. The orthodontist "pulled most of it off" at one point, but it was never surgically removed or submitted for microscopic examination, and it seemed to grow back. Additional questioning reveals that the child has had a wart on her foot within the last year. A biopsy is performed, and

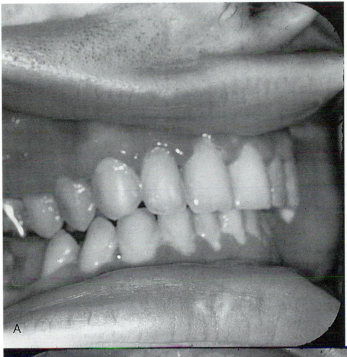

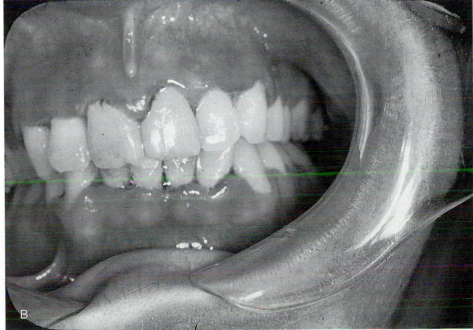

▪ *f* i g u r e **1–46**   *A*, Acute necrotizing ulcerative gingivitis (ANUG). *B*, ANUG. Note the gingival contours and punched-out papillae.

Illustration continued on following page

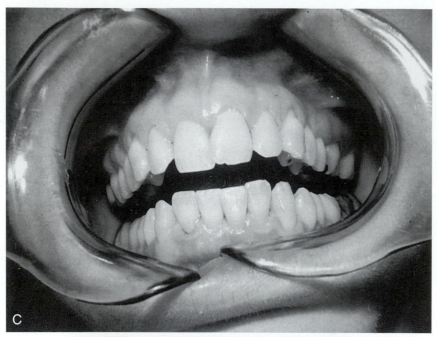

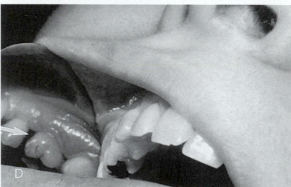

■ *f i g u r e* **1–46**   *Continued C,* Anterior view of a rather healthy mouth. *D,* Patient in *C* with a localized area of ANUG *(arrow)* on the mesial aspect of the maxillary second premolar and molar. (*C* and *D,* Courtesy of Dr. Victor M. Sternberg.)

the tissue sample is placed in formalin and sent to an oral pathology laboratory with the following diagnostic impressions:

■ Papilloma: Based on the papillary surface texture of the lesion, it was thought to be a papilloma.
■ Verruca vulgaris: Since the child had a wart and could have spread the virus, verruca vulgaris was suggested. Also, histologically a wart has lateral lipping, and it was thought that this could explain why pieces of the lesion fell off periodically during brushing. However, the surface of a verruca vulgaris is usually keratinized and therefore whiter than the lesion illustrated in Figure 1–47 and Color Plate 79.
■ Pyogenic granuloma: The spongy inflammatory tissue was possibly caused by the mechanical irritation from the orthodontic bands, thereby causing pyogenic granuloma.

The microscopy report revealed stratified squamous epithelium covering a core

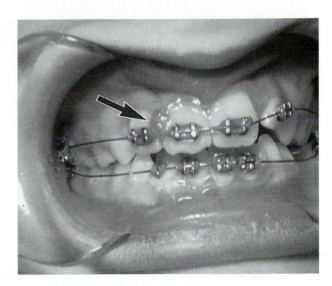

figure 1–47
Arrow points to a pyogenic granuloma between the patient's right maxillary central and lateral incisors. (Courtesy of Dr. Victor M. Sternberg.)

of loose and edematous fibrous connective tissue. The stroma contained numerous endothelium-lined, blood-filled capillaries and a dense infiltrate of lymphocytes, plasma cells, and neutrophils.

The definitive or final diagnosis was pyogenic granuloma.

In order to arrive at a diagnosis, the data collection included the patient's medical and dental health histories, the history of the lesion in question, a clinical description and evaluation, and biopsy and microscopy reports. This case illustrates the fact that arriving at a diagnosis involves a process. As stated previously, it can be thought of as a puzzle, since the information from each diagnostic category becomes part of the entire diagnostic process. In this case, the microscopy report contributed most significantly to the definitive or final diagnosis. Having arrived at three diagnostic impressions, the biopsy and microscopic examinations provided conclusive information in the diagnostic process.

The hygienist can be effective in the preliminary evaluation of the lesion by calling it to the attention of the dentist and then gathering and preparing all the data for the clinician who will perform the biopsy. Additionally, it is both challenging and stimulating to discuss diagnostic impressions with other professionals based on the data available at the time.

VARIANTS OF NORMAL

Fordyce's Granules

Clusters of ectopic sebaceous glands are called **Fordyce's granules.** They are most commonly observed on the lips and buccal mucosa. Clinically, they appear as yellow lobules in clusters and are usually distributed over the buccal mucosa or vermilion border of the involved lips. Surrounding tissue is normal, and since more than 75% of adults over 20 years of age have Fordyce's granules, they are considered a variant of normal. Microscopically, Fordyce's granules appear as normal sebaceous glands. They are asymptomatic and require no treatment (Fig. 1–48; Color Plate 25).

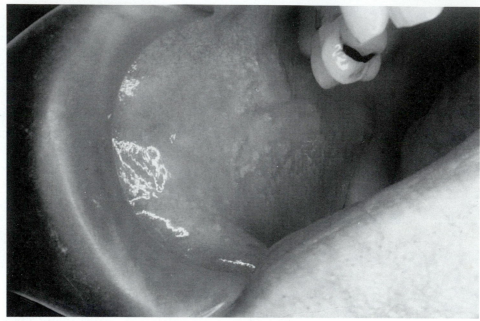

■ *f i g u r e* **1–48**   Fordyce's granules on the buccal mucosa.

Torus Palatinus

Torus palatinus or palatal tori are exophytic growths of normal compact bone. They are inherited and occur more frequently in women. They are asymptomatic and develop gradually. **Torus palatinus** is observed clinically in the midline of the hard palate. These palatal tori may take on various shapes and sizes, may be lobulated, and are covered by normal soft tissue. It is not unusual for the torus to be traumatized, which can cause discomfort and possible ulceration on the surface of the torus. When the lesion is large, it may be seen as a radiopaque mass on the radiograph. There is no treatment indicated unless the torus interferes with speech, swallowing, or a prosthetic appliance (Fig. 1–49*A,B*; Color Plate 61).

Mandibular Tori

Outgrowths of dense bone found on the lingual aspect of the mandible in the area of the premolars above the mylohyoid ridge are **mandibular tori.** They are usually bilateral, often lobulated or nodular, and can appear fused together. There is no predilection for either sex. Mandibular tori do not usually require treatment unless the patient needs a prosthodontic appliance (denture) and the tori interfere with proper fabrication and placement (Fig. 1–50*A,B*; Color Plate 53).

Melanin Pigmentation

Melanin is the pigment that gives color to the skin, eyes, hair, mucosa, and gingiva. **Melanin pigmentation** of the oral mucosa or gingiva is most commonly observed in dark-skinned individuals (Fig. 1–51; see also Fig. 1–18 and Color Plate 74).

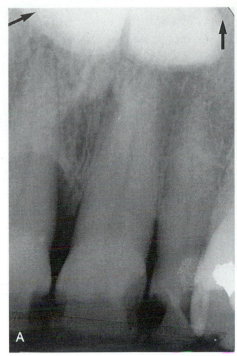
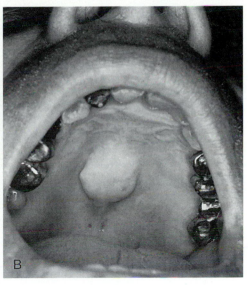

■ *f* i g u r e 1–49   *A*, The radiopaque appearance of torus palatinus. *B*, The clinical appearance of a torus palatinus.

Retrocuspid Papilla

A **retrocuspid papilla** is a sessile nodule on the gingival margin of the lingual aspect of the mandibular cuspids (see Fig. 1–19).

Lingual Varicosities

Prominent lingual veins, called **lingual varicosities,** are usually observed on the ventral and lateral surfaces of the tongue. Clinically, red to purple enlarged vessels or clusters are seen. There is no association with other systemic diseases; however, a relationship between varicosities in the legs and prominent lingual veins has been reported. Lingual varices are most commonly observed in individuals older than 60 years of age and are therefore believed to be related to the aging process (Fig. 1–52; Color Plate 40).

Linea Alba

Linea alba is a "white line" that extends anteroposteriorly on the buccal mucosa along the occlusal plane. It may be bilateral and can be more prominent in patients who have a clenching or bruxing habit (Fig. 1–53; Color Plate 24).

Leukoedema

A generalized opalescence is imparted to the buccal mucosa by **leukoedema.** It is most commonly observed in black individuals but can also be seen in whites. Clinically,

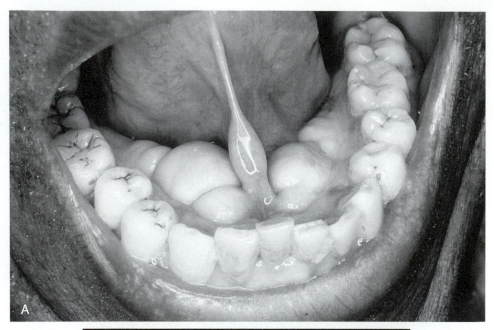

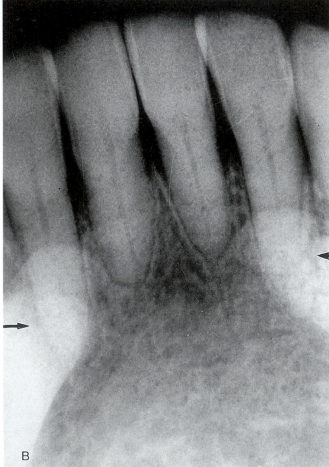

▪ *f i g u r e* **1–50**   *A,* The clinical appearance of lobulated mandibular tori. *B,* The radiopaque appearance of mandibular tori *(arrows).*

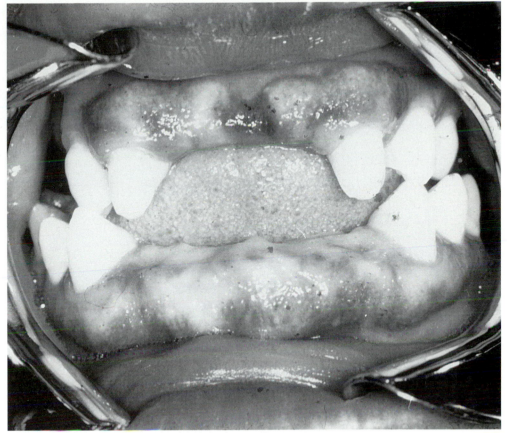

■ *f* i **g u r e** 1–51   Melanin pigmentation of the gingiva.

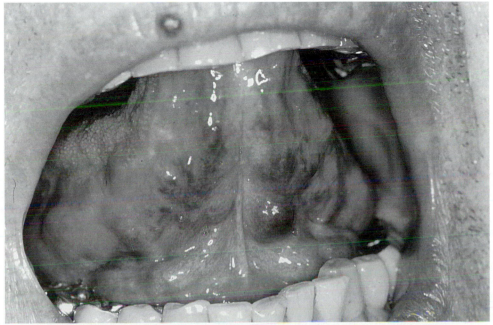

■ *f* i **g u r e** 1–52   Lingual varices. (Courtesy of Dr. David Zegarelli.)

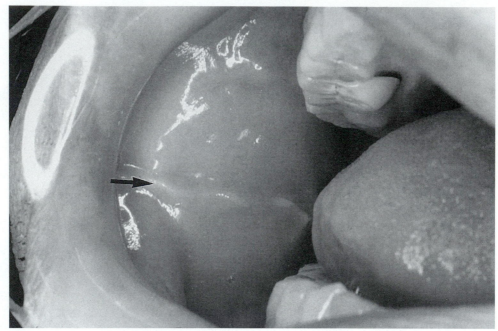

■ *f* i g u r e 1–53   Arrow points to linea alba on the buccal mucosa.

a gray-white film is diffused equally throughout the buccal mucosa, which gives the mucosa an opaque quality. If the mucosa is stretched, the opalescence becomes less prominent. The film is an integral part of the buccal tissue and cannot be removed. Histologically, there is significant intracellular edema in the spinous cells and acanthosis of the epithelium. It is a benign anomaly that requires no treatment. (Fig. 1–54; Color Plate 12).

BENIGN CONDITIONS OF UNKNOWN CAUSE

Lingual Thyroid Nodule

When thyroid tissue becomes entrapped in the tissue that makes up the tongue, **lingual thyroid nodule** results. The thyroid tissue is thought to be a remnant associated with a developmental anomaly. Research has indicated a high predilection in females and has linked the condition with hormonal changes, since its onset appears to be associated with puberty, pregnancy, and menopause. Clinically, lingual thyroid nodule is observed as a mass in the midline of the dorsal surface of the tongue posterior to the circumvallate papillae in the area of the foramen caecum. The lesion usually has a sessile base and is 2 to 3 cm in width. On histologic examination, normal thyroid tissue is found. Treatment requires careful evaluation of the lesion to determine whether the thyroid gland is normal. Surgical intervention is not always required.

Fissured Tongue

The cause of **fissured tongue** is unknown, but it is considered a variant of normal. There are theories that it may be associated with a vitamin deficiency or chronic

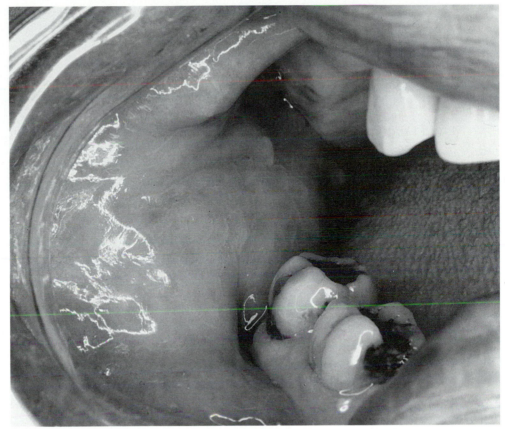

▪ *f* i g u r e 1-54   Leukoedema of the buccal mucosa showing an opalescent, velvety texture.

trauma over a long period. Clinically, the dorsal surface of the tongue appears to have deep fissures or grooves that may become irritated if food debris collects in them. There is no treatment indicated for the condition. However, a patient who presents with a fissured tongue may be advised to brush the tongue gently with a soft toothbrush to keep the fissures clean of debris and irritants (Fig. 1-55; see also Fig. 1-20).

Median Rhomboid Glossitis

In the past, **median rhomboid glossitis** has been described as a developmental anomaly that occurs as a result of entrapment of the tuberculum impar during fusion of the lateral portions of the tongue. However, today there is a great deal of doubt associated with this theory, since the condition has not been observed in young children. More recent evidence and research have suggested that it may be associated with a chronic fungal infection from *Candida albicans*. Clinically, median rhomboid glossitis appears as a flat or slightly raised oval or rectangular erythematous area in the midline of the dorsal surface of the tongue, beginning at the junction of the anterior and middle thirds and extending posterior to the circumvallate papillae. It is devoid of filiform papillae, and therefore its texture is smooth. If the remaining surface of the tongue is coated, the rectangular area appears more prominent. There is no specific treatment. Sometimes an antifungal agent is applied and the lesion resolves. However, this is not always the case. Sometimes the condition resolves with no specific treatment at all (Fig. 1-56; Color Plate 39).

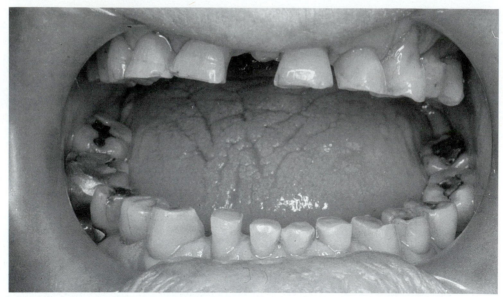

▪ *figure* **1-55**   Fissured tongue and attrition.

Geographic Tongue

The cause of **geographic tongue** is unknown. Some investigators suggest that it is induced by stress, and there are studies that associate the histologic findings with those found in psoriasis. The clinical appearance involves the dorsal and lateral borders of the tongue. Diffuse areas of desquamation of the filiform papillae can be observed. Erythematous patches are surrounded by a white or yellow perimeter, and the fungiform papillae appear distinct within the erythematous patch. The condition does not remain static; there appears to be remission and changes in the depapillated areas.

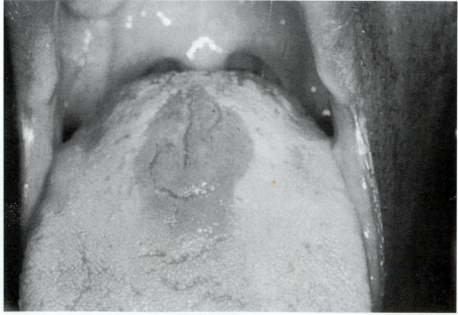

▪ *figure* **1-56**   Median rhomboid glossitis; Color Plate 39. (Courtesy of Dr. Edward V. Zegarelli.)

Occasionally, a patient complains of a burning discomfort associated with geographic tongue. Usually, no treatment is indicated (Fig. 1–57*A*; Color Plate 35).

Ectopic geographic tongue is the term used to describe the condition when it is found on mucosal surfaces other than the tongue. In Figure 1–57*B*, it is seen in the mandibular anterior mucobuccal fold.

Hairy Tongue

In **hairy tongue,** the filiform papillae become elongated and can appear white, yellow, brown, or black. The color of black hairy tongue is due to chromogenic bacteria

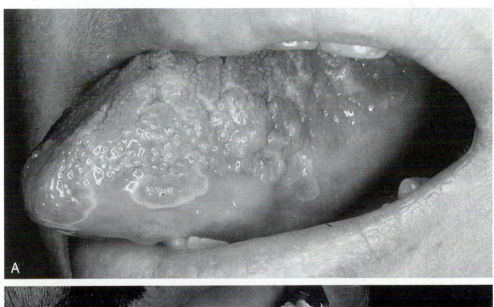

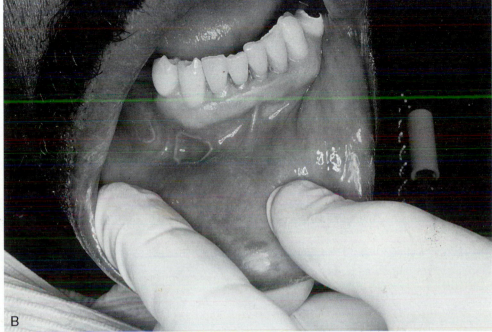

■ *figure 1-57*   *A,* Geographic tongue. *B,* Ectopic geographic tongue observed in the mandibular anterior mucobuccal fold.

(Fig. 1–58*A*; Color Plates 36 and 37). White hairy tongue describes the dorsal surface when the filiform papillae are elongated, resulting in a white appearance (Fig. 1–58*B*). Although the cause is unknown, tobacco, chemical rinses (e.g., hydrogen peroxide), alcohol, and certain foods have been associated with hairy tongue. Additionally, hairy tongue may result from systemic antibiotic therapy, corticosteroid therapy, or radiation therapy to the head and neck areas. *Candida albicans* has also been found in histologic

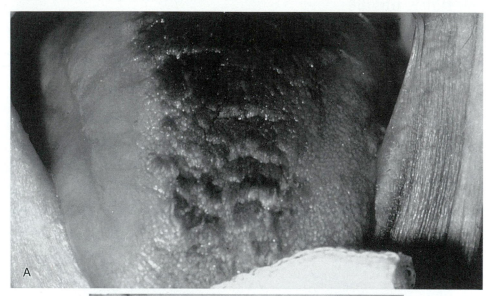

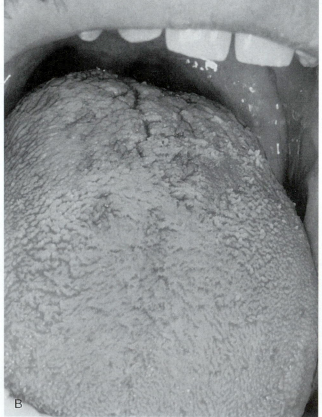

■ *f* i g u r e 1–58   *A*, Black hairy tongue. *B*, White hairy tongue.

examination, but this does not constitute a cause-and-effect condition. However, there is an alteration in the general microbial flora of the tongue (see also Fig. 1–23A–C).

Treatment involves directing the patient to brush the tongue gently with a toothbrush (wet with water only) to remove debris. The condition usually clears completely but may recur.

SELECTED REFERENCES

BOOKS

Darby ML: Mosby's Comprehensive Review of Dental Hygiene, 3rd ed. St. Louis, CV Mosby, 1994.

Neville BW, Damm DD, Allen CM, Bouquot JE: Oral and Maxillofacial Pathology. Philadelphia, WB Saunders, 1995.

Neville BW, Damm DD, White DK, Waldron CA: Color Atlas of Clinical Oral Pathology. Philadelphia, Lea & Febiger, 1991.

Regezi JA, Sciubba JJ: Oral Pathology: Clinical Pathologic Correlations. Philadelphia, WB Saunders, 1989.

Ritchie AC: Boyd's Textbook of Pathology, 9th ed, Vols I and II. Philadelphia, Lea & Febiger, 1990.

Shafer WG, Hine MK, Levy BM: A Textbook of Oral Pathology, 4th ed. Philadelphia, WB Saunders, 1983.

Sonis ST, Fazio RC, Fang L: Principles and practice of oral medicine, 2nd ed. Philadelphia, WB Saunders, 1995.

JOURNAL ARTICLES

Chapnick L: External root resorption: An experimental radiographic evaluation. Oral Surg Oral Med Oral Pathol 67:578–582, 1989.

Comfort M, Wu PC: The reliability of personal and family medical histories in the identification of hepatitis B carriers. Oral Surg Oral Med Oral Pathol 67:531–534, 1989.

Kaugars GE, Miller ME, Abbey LM: Odontomas. Oral Surg Oral Med Oral Pathol 67:2172–2176, 1989.

Lydiatt DD, Hollins RR, Peterson GP: Multiple idiopathic root resorption: Diagnostic considerations. Oral Surg Oral Med Oral Pathol 67:208–210, 1989.

Neupert EA, Wright JM: Regional odontodysplasia presenting as a soft tissue swelling. Oral Surg Oral Med Oral Pathol 67:193–196, 1989.

Pogrel MA, Cram D: Intraoral findings in patients with psoriasis with a special reference to ectopic geographic tongue (erythema circinata). Oral Surg Oral Med Oral Pathol 66:184–189, 1988.

REVIEW QUESTIONS

1. After arriving at a differential diagnosis, information from which one of the following categories will best establish a final or definitive diagnosis?
   - (A) Clinical
   - (B) Historical
   - (C) Microscopic
   - (D) Radiographic

2. A freckle is an example of which one of the following terms?
   - (A) Bulla
   - (B) Vesicle
   - (C) Lobule
   - (D) Macule

3. Which one of the following terms describes the base of a lesion that is stalk-like?
   - (A) Sessile
   - (B) Lobulated
   - (C) Bullous
   - (D) Pedunculated

4. Clinical diagnosis can be used to determine the final or definitive diagnosis of all of the following *except*
   (A) Fordyce's granules
   (B) Unerupted supernumerary teeth
   (C) Mandibular tori
   (D) Geographic tongue

5. Radiographic diagnosis would most likely be sufficient to determine the final or definitive diagnosis of
   (A) Internal resorption
   (B) Periapical cemental dysplasia
   (C) Odontomas
   (D) All of the above

6. To determine the presence of blood dyscrasias, which one of the following would provide the most definitive information?
   (A) Laboratory blood tests
   (B) Bleeding during probing
   (C) Pallor of the gingiva and mucosa
   (D) Patient complaint of weakness

7. When an antifungal ointment or cream is applied (before any culture) to areas of angular cheilitis, which one of the following diagnostic categories is being used?
   (A) Clinical
   (B) Historical
   (C) Therapeutic
   (D) Differential

8. Yellow clusters of ectopic sebaceous glands commonly observed on the buccal mucosa and evaluated through clinical diagnosis are most likely
   (A) Lipomas
   (B) Fordyce's granules
   (C) Cheek bites
   (D) Linea alba

9. A slow-growing, bony, hard exophytic growth in the midline of the hard palate is developmental and hereditary in origin. The diagnosis is determined through clinical evaluation. You suspect
   (A) Torus palatinus
   (B) Mixed tumor
   (C) Palatal cyst
   (D) Nasopalatine cyst

10. The "white line" observed clinically on the buccal mucosa that extends from anterior to posterior along the occlusal plane is
    (A) Leukoedema
    (B) Leukoplakia
    (C) Linea alba
    (D) Lichen planus

11. Which one of the following is a variant of normal that at one time was thought to be a developmental anomaly but is now suggested to be associated with *Candida albicans*? Clinically, there is a rectangular area on the midline of the dorsal surface of the tongue devoid of filiform papillae.
    (A) Median rhomboid glossitis
    (B) Geographic tongue

(C) Fissured tongue
(D) Lingual thyroid

12. Which one of the following diagnostic categories would the hygienist most easily apply to the preliminary evaluation of oral lesions?
(A) Microscopic
(B) Clinical
(C) Therapeutic
(D) Differential

13. These examples of exostoses are found on the lingual aspect of the mandible in the area of the premolars. They are benign, bony, and hard and require no treatment. Radiographically, they appear as radiopaque areas and are often bilateral. You suspect
(A) Mandibular tori
(B) Lingual mandibular bone concavity
(C) Genial tubercles
(D) Mandibular fossa

14. Which one of the following terms is most often used when describing mandibular tori?
(A) Bullous
(B) Lobulated
(C) Sessile
(D) Pedunculated

15. Leukoedema is considered a variant of normal and is observed clinically as a diffuse gray to white film on the buccal mucosa that gives an opalescent character to the tissue. It is most commonly found in
(A) Whites
(B) Asians
(C) Native Americans
(D) Blacks

16. A patient presents with the clinical signs of acute necrotizing ulcerative gingivitis. Other constitutional signs are also evident. You have the patient begin hydrogen peroxide rinses without culturing the bacterial flora. This action applies which one of the following diagnostic categories?
(A) Therapeutic
(B) Microscopic
(C) Clinical
(D) Final or definitive

17. A small circumscribed lesion usually less than 1 cm in diameter that is elevated and protrudes above the surface of normal surrounding tissue is called a
(A) Bulla
(B) Macule
(C) Vesicle
(D) Papule

18. A sessile-based lesion is
(A) Broad and flat
(B) Stem-like
(C) Corrugated
(D) Lobulated

19. The identification of which one of the following is not determined by clinical diagnosis?
    (A) Fordyce's granules
    (B) Tori
    (C) Compound odontoma
    (D) Retrocuspid papilla

20. Another term for geographic tongue is
    (A) Migratory glossitis
    (B) Median rhomboid glossitis
    (C) Scalloped tongue
    (D) White hairy tongue

21. The cause of supernumerary teeth is most likely
    (A) Genetic
    (B) Traumatic
    (C) Cystic
    (D) Developmental

22. Historical diagnosis can include the patient's
    (A) Age and sex
    (B) Sex and family history
    (C) Race and medical history
    (D) All of the above

23. Which condition is most often seen on the buccal mucosal?
    (A) Melanin pigmentation
    (B) Fordyce's granules
    (C) Nicotine stomatitis
    (D) Retrocuspid papilla

2

Inflammation and Repair

MARGARET J. FEHRENBACH
·

ULLA E. LEMBORN
·

JOAN A. PHELAN
·

Objectives

After studying this chapter, the student should be able to:

1. Define each of the words in the vocabulary list for this chapter.
2. List the five "cardinal signs" of inflammation that are visible at the site of inflammation.
3. List three systemic signs of inflammation.
4. Describe the microscopic events that are associated with each of the cardinal signs of inflammation.
5. List and describe the microscopic events of the inflammatory process, beginning with injury and ending with phagocytosis of foreign and necrotic substances.
6. Define the terms "flare" and "wheal."
7. List the types of white blood cells that participate in inflammation and describe the function of neutrophils and monocytes.
8. Describe the differences between acute and chronic inflammation.
9. Define and contrast hyperplasia and hypertrophy.
10. Describe the microscopic events that occur during the repair of a mucosal wound.
11. Describe and contrast healing by primary intention, healing by secondary intention, and healing by tertiary intention.
12. Describe and contrast attrition, abrasion, and erosion.
13. Describe the pattern of erosion seen in bulimia.
14. Describe the relationship between bruxism and abrasion.
15. Describe the cause, clinical features, and treatment of each of the following:
    Aspirin and phenol burns
    Electric burn
    Traumatic ulcer
    Frictional keratosis
    Linea alba
    Nicotine stomatitis
16. Describe the clinical features, cause (when known), treatment, and histologic appearance of each of the following:
    Traumatic neuroma
    Postinflammatory melanosis
    Solar cheilitis
    Mucocele
    Ranula
    Necrotizing sialometaplasia
    Pyogenic granuloma
    Giant cell granuloma
    Chronic hyperplastic pulpitis
    Irritation fibroma
17. Describe the difference between a mucocele and a ranula.
18. Define sialolithiasis.
19. Describe the difference between acute and chronic sialadenitis.
20. Describe the clinical features, radiographic appearance, and histologic appearance of a periapical abscess, a periapical granuloma, and a periapical (radicular) cyst.
21. Describe and contrast internal and external tooth resorption.

Vocabulary

Acute (ah-kūt)   Of short duration or of short and relatively severe course

Central (sen′tral)   Within bone

Chemotaxis (ke″mo-tak′sis)   The directed movement of white blood cells to the area of injury along a chemical concentration gradient

Chronic (kron′ik)   Persisting over a long time

Emigration (em″ĭ-gra′shun)   The passage of white blood cells through the endothelium and wall of small blood vessels

Erythema (er″ĭ-the′mah)   Redness of the skin or mucosa

Exudate (eks′u-dāt)   Inflammatory exudate; fluid with a relatively high content of serum proteins and leukocytes formed as a reaction to injury of tissues and blood vessels

Fever (fe′ver)   An elevation of body temperature to greater than the normal of 98.6° F (37° C)

Flare (flār)   Redness of the skin or mucosa around an area of an irritant

Hyperemia (hi″per-e′me-ah)   An excess of blood in a part of the body

Hyperplasia (hi″per-pla′ze-ah)   The abnormal multiplication or increase in the number of normal cells in normal arrangement in a tissue

Know difference

Hypertrophy (hi-per′tro-fe)   An enlargement of a tissue or organ resulting from an increase in size but not in number of cells

Leukocytosis (loo″ko-sī-to′sis)   A temporary increase in the number of white blood cells circulating in blood

Local (lo′kal)   Confined to a limited part, not general or systemic

Lymphadenopathy (lim-fad″ĕ-nop′-ah-thē)   Any disease process that affects lymph nodes such that they become enlarged and palpable.

Margination (mar″jĭ-nā′shun)   A phenomenon that occurs during the relatively early phases of inflammation in which white blood cells tend to occupy the periphery of the blood vessels and adhere to endothelial cells that line the vessels

Necrosis (nĕ-kro′sis)   The pathologic death of one or more cells or a portion of tissue or organ resulting from irreversible damage

Pavementing (pāv′ment-ing)   Adherence of white blood cells to the endothelial cells lining an injured blood vessel

Peripheral (pĕ-rif′er-al)   Located away from the center—indicates that the location of a lesion is in the soft tissue surrounding a bone

Phagocytosis (fag″o-sī-to′sis)   A process of ingestion and digestion by cells

Purulent (pu′roo-lent)   Containing or forming pus

Repair (re-pār′)   The restoration of damaged or diseased tissues

Serous (se′rus)   Having a watery consistency—relating to serum

Systemic (sis-tem′ik)   Pertaining to or affecting the body as a whole

Wheal (hwēl) A localized swelling of tissue due to edema during inflammation, often accompanied by severe itching

Inflammation and **repair** are the body's responses to injury. Inflammation allows the human body to eliminate injurious agents, contain injuries, and heal defects. The specific lesions included in this chapter occur in response to injury. Many of these lesions are quite common and are likely to be encountered when the dental hygienist examines the hard and soft tissues of the oral cavity. Lesions that occur as a result of infection or as a result of destruction through activity of the immune system are included in Chapter 3.

INJURY

Injury is an alteration in the environment that causes tissue damage. Injury to oral tissues can be caused by many different factors. Physical injury can affect teeth, soft tissue, and bone. Chemical injury can occur from the application of caustic materials to oral tissues. Microorganisms can cause injury by invading oral tissues. Nutritional deficiencies can render oral tissues more susceptible to injury from other sources.

most

INFLAMMATION

Inflammation is a nonspecific response to injury and occurs in the same manner regardless of the nature of the injury. The extent and duration of the injury determine the extent and duration of the inflammatory response. The inflammatory response may be local and limited to the area of injury, or it may become systemic if the injury is extensive. The inflammatory response may be acute or chronic. If the injury is minimal and brief and its source is removed from the tissue, only acute inflammation occurs. The tissue may return to its original state, or repair of the tissue may begin immediately. Chronic inflammation occurs if injury to the tissue continues. Sometimes acute and chronic inflammatory responses are superimposed on each other. Repair of the tissue occurs only if the persistent source of injury is removed. Inflammation of a specific tissue is denoted by the suffix **"itis"** following the name of the tissue (e.g., pulpitis, gingivitis).

Acute Inflammation

Microscopic Events and Clinical Signs of Inflammation

Microscopic events occur within the injured tissues during both acute and chronic inflammation. These events cause changes that can be seen clinically. Local clinical changes visible at the site of injury are called the **cardinal signs of inflammation**—redness, heat, swelling, pain, and loss of normal tissue function (Table 2–1). Systemic signs of inflammation may be present when the response is more extensive and include an increase in body temperature (fever), an increase in the number of white blood cells (leukocytosis), and enlargement of lymph nodes (lymphade-

Know

Pyrogens

56

TABLE 2–1 Local and Systemic Clinical Signs of Inflammation and Their Associated Microscopic Events

Clinical Feature	Associated Microscopic Events
Local Signs of Inflammation	
Redness (erythema) and heat	Dilation of microcirculation leads to hyperemia in the tissues
Swelling	Permeability of microcirculation leads to exudate formation in the tissues
Pain	Pressure on nerves by exudate formation
	Release of chemical mediators
Loss of normal tissue function	Events associated with swelling and pain
Systemic Signs of Inflammation	
Fever	Pyrogens affect hypothalamus, which influences body temperature
Leukocytosis	Increased circulating white blood cells from increased formation and release from bone marrow
Lymphadenopathy	Hyperplasia and hypertrophy of lymphocytes

nopathy) (Fig. 2–1). The microscopic events involve the small blood vessels in the area of injury, certain white blood cells, and chemicals called chemical mediators. The underlying microscopic events proceed faster than the clinical changes. A summary of the sequence of microscopic events that occur during the inflammatory response follows:

1. Injury
2. Constriction of the microcirculation   *Stops bleeding, promotes clot*
3. Dilation of small blood vessels

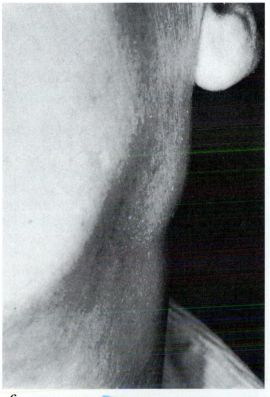

f i g u r e 2–1   Enlarged cervical lymph node.

4. Increase in permeability of small blood vessels
5. Exudate leaves small blood vessels
6. Increased blood viscosity
7. Decreased blood flow through the microcirculation
8. Margination and pavementing of white blood cells
9. White blood cells leave small blood vessels and enter tissue
10. White blood cells ingest foreign material
11. Cellular and tissue debris is removed

diabetics have lazy leukocytes

The first microscopic event of the inflammatory response is a brief, immediate reflex **constriction** of the microcirculation (arterioles, capillaries, and venules) in the area of the injury. This occurs immediately following tissue injury and is followed by a dilation of the same small blood vessels. **Dilation** is an increase in the diameter of the vessels and is caused by chemical mediators that are released at the time of the injury. Dilation of the microcirculation results in increased blood flow through the vessels. The increased blood flow that floods the capillary beds in the injured tissue is called **active hyperemia.** Hyperemia is responsible for two clinical signs of inflammation: redness (erythema) and heat. **Erythema** is easily visible in most oral tissues. A red **flare** is seen surrounding the injury. Local temperature changes may be difficult to recognize.

While hyperemia is occurring, there is also an increase in the permeability of the microcirculation, which is caused by blood vessel injury, chemical mediators, or an opening of the junctions of the endothelial cells that line the vessels. This increased permeability allows blood plasma and proteins to flow into the injured tissues. The plasma fluids and proteins that leave the blood vessels and enter the surrounding tissue are called **exudate.** The presence of exudate in the injured tissue helps to dilute injurious bacterial agents that may be present. There are two main types of exudate—serous and purulent. **Serous exudate** is composed mainly of plasma fluids and proteins with a few white blood cells. **Purulent exudate** contains tissue debris and many white blood cells in addition to plasma fluids and proteins.

Swelling of the injured area occurs as the exudate escapes into the tissue (Fig. 2–2). This is called **edema.** Clinically, this swelling is called a **wheal.** If the swollen tissue area is injured further, the exudate flows out of the tissue as either a thin clear fluid (serous exudate) or a thick white to yellow pus (purulent exudate).

The formation of exudate may be so excessive that it interferes with repair of the tissue. The injured tissue may allow the excess exudate to drain by formation of a natural drainage passage that bores through the tissue, allowing drainage to the outside. This channel through the tissue is called a **fistula** (Fig. 2–3; Color Plate 80); it is formed at the expense of healthy, functioning tissue in the area, which is lost as the tissue becomes necrotic. Sometimes excessive exudate in damaged tissue has to be mechanically drained by making an incision in the surface of the swollen area, often placing a drainage tube in the site of the incision. This procedure is called **incision and drainage** and is usually accompanied by the administration of medication to reduce inflammation (Fig. 2–4). Exudate formation also results in pain as the exudate presses on sensory nerves in the area. In addition, some chemical mediators in inflamed tissue can cause pain. The swelling and pain in tissue resulting from the inflammatory process may cause a loss of normal tissue function—another clinical sign of inflammation.

In addition to exudate formation, blood vessel permeability also leads to increased blood viscosity because of the loss of plasma fluids. The blood becomes thicker and cannot flow as easily. This eventually results in decreased flow through the microcirculation. As the blood flow slows down, the red blood cells begin to pile up in the center of the blood vessels and the white blood cells are displaced to the vessel walls. The movement of the white blood cells to the periphery of the vessel walls is called **margination.** The white blood cells are now in position to attach themselves to

Red Bld cells - Center

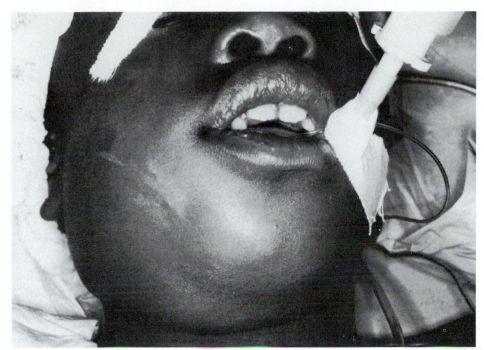

■ *f i g u r e* 2–2   Swelling resulting from a dental infection. The patient was hospitalized for treatment of the swelling. (Courtesy of Dr. Sidney Eisig.)

the injured, "sticky" walls of the blood vessel. This lining of the walls by white blood cells is called **pavementing** (Fig. 2–5).

After pavementing the peripheral walls, the white blood cells begin to escape from the blood vessels along with the plasma fluids and enter the injured tissue. This process is called **emigration**. Emigration occurs from a combination of events: increased blood flow in the microcirculation causing increased pressure, opening of the junctions of the endothelial cells that line the blood vessels, increased mobility of the white blood cells involved, and chemical mediators in the injured tissue that cause directed movement of the white blood cells in the injured tissue.

This directed movement is called **chemotaxis**, and substances that enhance this directed movement are called **chemotactic factors**. Emigration of the white blood cells to the area of injury allows these cells to participate in the body's defense against the injury. At first these cells try to wall off the site of the injury from the surrounding healthy tissue. After emigration the white blood cells remove foreign substances from the site by ingesting them. This is called **phagocytosis** (Fig. 2–6). The ingested substances may be foreign substances such as pathogenic microorganisms or tissue debris. Their presence interferes with the repair process; therefore they must be removed for the inflammation to resolve and any necessary tissue repair to proceed.

Cells Involved in the Acute Inflammatory Response

Emigration of white blood cells, also called **leukocytes**, from the blood vessels into the site of injury is an important part of the process of inflammation. There are six different kinds of white blood cells: neutrophils, monocytes, lymphocytes, plasma cells, eosinophils, and mast cells. The **neutrophil**, also called the **polymorphonuclear leukocyte**, is the first cell to emigrate to the site of injury and is the primary cell involved in acute inflammation. The **monocyte** or **macrophage** is the second cell to

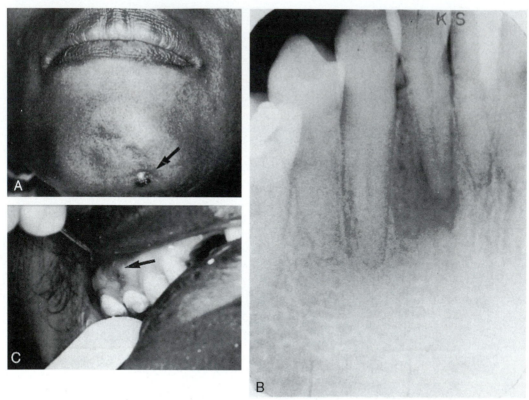

▪ *f* i g u r e 2–3   Fistula formed from a periapical abscess to the skin. *A,* The opening of the fistulous tract is seen on the skin. *B,* A radiolucency is seen in the mandibular anterior area. *C,* In another patient a fistula formed from the periapical area to the buccal attached gingiva. (See Color Plate 80.)

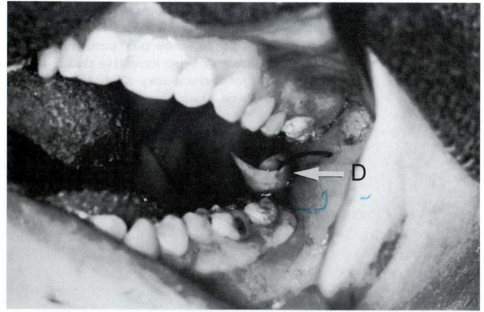

▪ *f* i g u r e 2–4   The abscess has been incised and a drain (D) placed to allow the escape of purulent exudate from the tissue. (Courtesy of Dr. Sidney Eisig.)

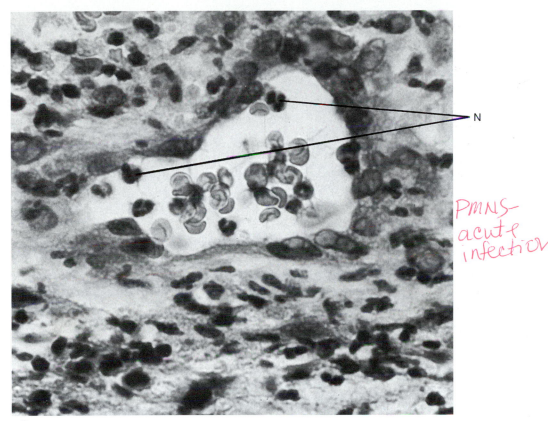

N

*PMNS—
acute
infection*

■ *f* i g u r e 2–5   Margination and pavementing during inflammation. Neutrophils (N) are seen at the periphery of a blood vessel (high magnification).

participate in the inflammatory response. The **lymphocyte** and **plasma cell** are involved in both chronic inflammation and the immune response, and the **eosinophil** and **mast cell** participate in both inflammatory and immune responses. *Starts to turn into chronic infect.*

As inflammation begins and as it continues, there are changes in the types of white blood cells present in the tissue (Fig. 2–7). At first the neutrophil is the primary inflammatory cell present (Fig. 2–8). The monocyte, which circulates in blood, becomes the macrophage as it enters the tissue, becoming the second white blood cell at the site of injury. As inflammation continues, the number of neutrophils dwindles. If the injury persists and chronic inflammation occurs, macrophages, lymphocytes, and plasma cells become the predominant cells in the tissue instead of neutrophils (Fig. 2–9).

Neutrophils. Neutrophils constitute 60% to 70% of the entire white blood cell population. Like all white blood cells, the neutrophil is derived from a precursor cell called a **stem cell**, which is located in the bone marrow (Fig. 2–10). Neutrophils possess a multilobed nucleus, which is the reason they are also called polymorphonuclear leukocytes, and a granular cytoplasm, which contains enzymes called lysosomal enzymes (Fig. 2–11). Neutrophils are produced throughout life and have the ability to move by ameboid actions, which involve extending portions of their cytoplasm.

The main function of the neutrophil is phagocytosis of substances such as pathogenic microorganisms and tissue debris. The cells move into the area of injury in response to chemotactic factors. Lysosomal enzymes contained within vacuoles in the cytoplasm destroy substances after they have been engulfed by the cell. The removal of these substances from the site of injury is necessary to allow the process of healing to occur.

The neutrophil dies shortly after phagocytosis, during which lysosomal enzymes

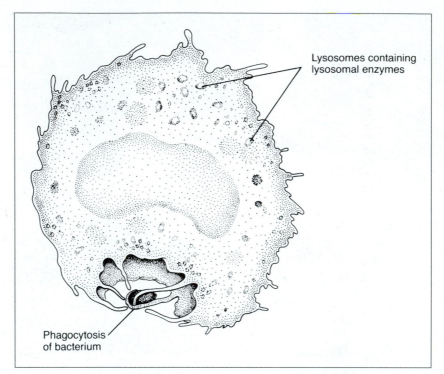

▪ *f* i g u r e **2–6**   Phagocytosis of a foreign substance (bacterium) by a white blood cell. The foreign substance will later be destroyed within the cell by lysosomal enzymes that are contained within lysosomes.

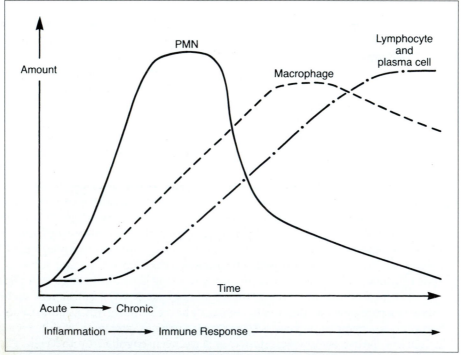

▪ *f* i g u r e **2–7**   Changes in the injured tissue's white blood cell population over time, starting with acute inflammation and continuing to chronic inflammation. PMN = polymorphonuclear neutrophils.

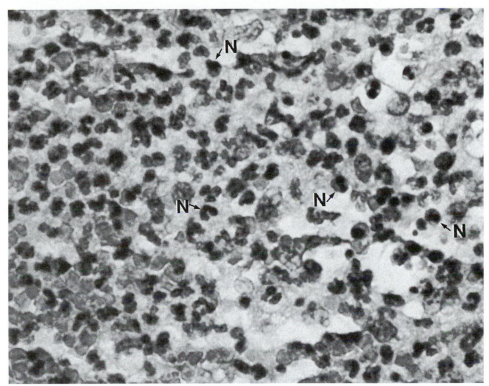

■ *f i g u r e* 2–8   Microscopic view of acute inflammation showing a predominance of neutrophils (N) (medium magnification).

and other damaging cellular substances, which were meant only for intracellular destruction of foreign substances, leak from the cells. These substances are also released into the tissue when the cells die. This leakage can cause further tissue damage, leading to the spread of infection or tissue death (necrosis).

Monocytes. The monocyte is the second white blood cell to emigrate from the blood vessels into the injured tissue, where it becomes a **macrophage.** Like the neutrophil, the monocyte is derived from the stem cell in the bone marrow (see Fig. 2–10), responds to chemotactic factors, is capable of phagocytosis, and has lysosomal enzymes in its cytoplasm that assist in the destruction of foreign substances. The macrophage has a single round nucleus and a nongranular cytoplasm (Fig. 2–12). It constitutes 3% to 8% of the entire white blood cell population. The macrophage has a somewhat longer life span than the polymorphonuclear leukocyte. In addition to its role in phagocytosis, it acts as a helper during the immune response.

Chemical Mediators of Inflammation

Many of the events involved in the inflammatory response are caused by chemical agents called **chemical mediators.** These agents start or enhance the inflammatory response. Some are derived from blood, some come from white blood cells, and others are produced by certain pathogenic microorganisms as they injure the tissue.

Three systems in the blood may be activated during inflammation: the kinin system, the clotting mechanism, and the complement system. These systems are interrelated, and there is much interaction among their activation, their products, and their actions.

Kinin System. The kinin system mediates inflammation by causing increased

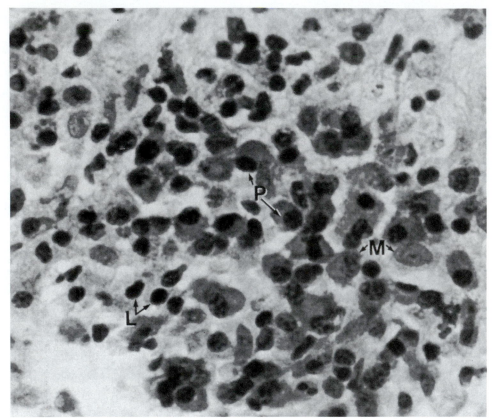

▪ *f* i g u r e 2–9   Microscopic view of chronic inflammation showing mainly macrophages (M), lymphocytes (L), and plasma cells (P) (high magnification).

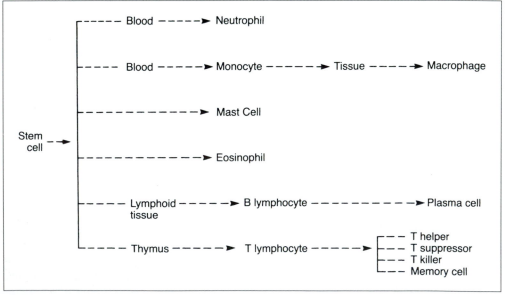

▪ *f* i g u r e 2–10   The derivation of white blood cells from a stem cell in the bone marrow.

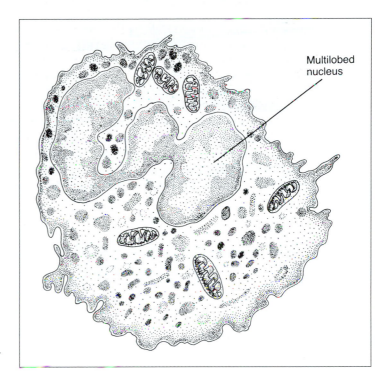

Multilobed
nucleus

▪ *f* i g u r e **2-11**
A neutrophil has a multilobed nucleus and granular cytoplasm.

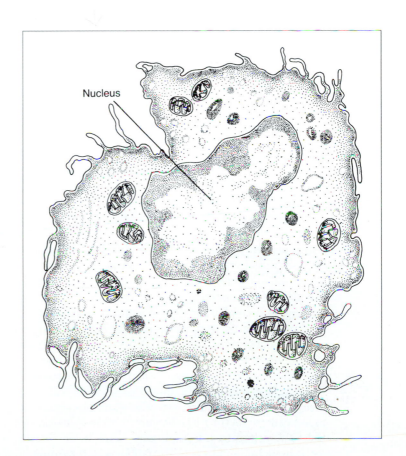

Nucleus

▪ *f* i g u r e **2-12**
Macrophage.

dilation of the blood vessels at the site of injury and increasing the permeability of local blood vessels by widening the gaps between endothelial cells. This system is rapidly activated both by substances present in plasma and by substances present in injured tissues. Its role is limited to the early phases of inflammation. Components of the kinin system also induce pain.

Clotting Mechanism. The clotting mechanism functions primarily in the clotting of blood. It also mediates inflammation since certain of its products that are activated when tissue is injured cause local vascular dilation and permeability by activating the kinin system. The clotting mechanism is also important in the repair process.

Complement System. This system involves the production of a sequential cascade of plasma proteins that are present in blood in an inactivated form. Many of these plasma proteins function in both inflammation and immunity. Components of the complement system cause the white blood cells called mast cells to release the granules in their cytoplasm that contain the chemical histamine. Histamine causes an increase in vascular permeability and vasodilation. Other components of the complement system cause cell death (cytolysis) by creating holes in the cell's membrane. They also form chemotactic factors for white blood cells and enhance phagocytosis.

Other Chemical Mediators of Inflammation. In addition to the chemical mediators already mentioned, others are formed in the body during inflammation. Prostaglandins are involved in the inflammatory response by causing increased vascular dilation and permeability, tissue pain and redness, and changes in connective tissues. Lysosomal enzymes are released from the granules in white blood cells. They act as chemotactic factors and can cause damage to connective tissues and to the clot.

Endotoxin and lysosomal enzymes that are released by pathogenic microorganisms may also serve as chemical mediators. Endotoxin is produced from gram-negative bacteria and can serve as a chemotactic factor, can activate complement, and can function as an antigen and damage bone tissue. During infection the lysosomal enzymes released from pathogenic microorganisms have a similar chemical composition and action to those released by the white blood cells.

Systemic Manifestations of Inflammation

In addition to the local features of inflammation, systemic signs may also occur. These include fever, an increase in the number of white blood cells (leukocytosis), and involvement of lymph nodes (lymphadenopathy) (see Table 2–1).

Fever. Body temperature is controlled by a regulatory center in the brain called the **hypothalamic thermoregulatory center.** Fever is an elevated body temperature (higher than 100° F or 37.7° C) and is associated with a systemic inflammatory response. Fever-producing substances, called **pyrogens**, are produced by white blood cells and pathogenic microorganisms. Pyrogens exert their effects by action on the regulatory center in the brain that increases the temperature of the body, producing fever. The function of this increased body temperature is not clear. A moderately high fever may be helpful in combating some infections, since many pathogenic microorganisms cannot tolerate increased temperatures. The body cannot tolerate excessively high fever for very long, however, and such fever could prove fatal. Medications can be given to reduce high fever. Measuring body temperature with a thermometer is helpful in assessing whether a systemic inflammatory response is present.

Leukocytosis. The number of white blood cells circulating in the blood can be measured by a laboratory test—the white blood cell count. The normal number of white blood cells is 4000 to 10,000/mm³ of blood. A systemic inflammatory response, particularly a response to infection, may result in an increase in the number of white blood cells circulating in blood from 10,000 to 30,000/mm³. This increase is called **leukocytosis** and usually primarily involves the neutrophil. The body increases the number of circulating white blood cells by increasing their formation and releasing immature forms from the bone marrow into the blood. This increase in the number of circulating white blood cells is an attempt by the body to provide more cells for phagocytosis.

Lymphadenopathy. Involvement of lymph nodes is clinically identified by enlarged and palpable lymph nodes **(lymphadenopathy)** and may also be present clinically in persons with systemic inflammatory disease. The enlarged lymph node or nodes can be felt (palpated) as a mass or masses in the area of inflammation and possibly along the associated lymphatic drainage route (Fig. 2–13). When palpated, the involved node feels firm and larger than normal and is tender.

An enlarged lymph node results from changes in its lymphocytes. Lymphocytes are white blood cells that mature in lymphoid tissue and also travel from the node to the tissue, in which they are involved in the immune response. The changes in the lymphocytes cause the change in size of the lymph nodes. These changes include an increase in the number of cells **(hyperplasia)**, resulting from increased cell division, and an enlargement of individual cells **(hypertrophy)**, resulting from cellular maturation. These changes in the lymphocyte population occur during prolonged or chronic inflammation. Lymphocytes are also the primary cells of the immune response.

Chronic Inflammation

Chronic inflammation results from injuries that persist, often for weeks or months. In addition to neutrophils and monocytes, other white blood cells are involved, as is

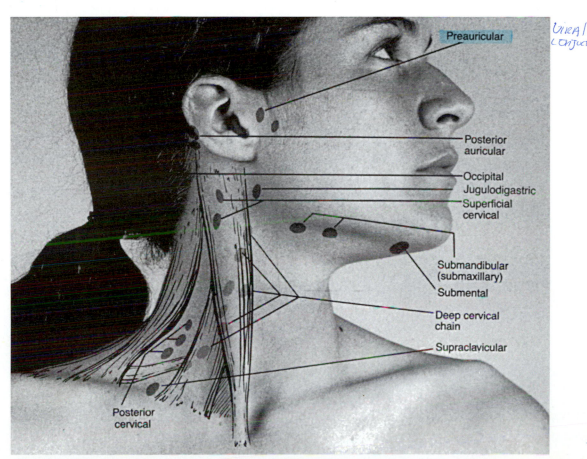

Preauricular

Viral Conjuctivitis

Posterior auricular

Occipital
Jugulodigastric
Superficial cervical

Submandibular (submaxillary)

Submental

Deep cervical chain

Supraclavicular

Posterior cervical

▪ *figure* 2-13   Location of lymph nodes in the neck. (From Jarvis C: Physical Examination and Health Assessment. Philadelphia, WB Saunders, 1992, p 281.)

the proliferation of fibroblasts. Repair takes place at the same time that the chronic inflammation proceeds, but it cannot be completed until the source of the injury is removed. The cells involved in chronic inflammation include macrophages, lymphocytes, and plasma cells.

A distinctive form of chronic inflammation is called **granulomatous inflammation**. It is characterized by the formation of granulomas, which are microscopic groupings of macrophages surrounded by lymphocytes and occasional plasma cells. They usually contain large macrophages that have multiple nuclei called **multinucleated giant cells**. Certain infections—for example, tuberculosis—tend to stimulate the formation of granulomas.

Hyperplasia and Hypertrophy

Hyperplasia is defined as an increase in the number of cells in a tissue or organ. Pathologic hyperplasia frequently occurs in oral tissues. The increase in the number of epithelial cells and the increased thickness of the epithelium occur in response to chronic irritation or abrasion. As surface epithelial cells are lost, there is increased division of basal epithelial cells to replace the lost cells. The production of new cells is in excess of the original number of cells, so the epithelium becomes thickened and the tissue appears paler or whiter (Fig. 2–14). When the irritation subsides, the proliferation ceases, the epithelium returns to its normal size, and the color of the tissue appears normal. Hyperplasia of fibrous connective tissue may also occur in response to chronic injury and is common in the oral cavity. Oral lesions caused by epithelial and fibrous hyperplasia are described later in this chapter.

Hypertrophy is different from hyperplasia. **Hypertrophy** is defined as an increase in the size of a tissue or organ due to an increase in the size, not the number, of cells. However, hypertrophy and hyperplasia are often seen together.

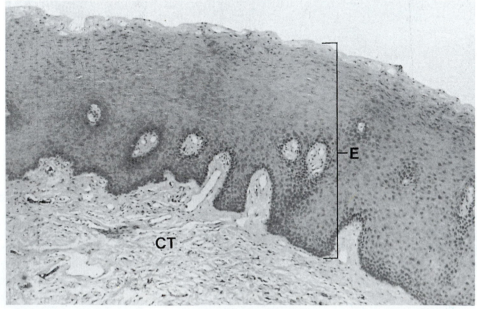

■ *f i g u r e* **2–14**   Microscopic appearance of epithelial hyperplasia (low power). The epithelium (E) is thickened, and the underlying connective tissue is identified as CT.

REGENERATION AND REPAIR *healing phase*

When tissue damage has been slight, the inflamed area may return completely to its normal structure and function. This is the most favorable end to acute inflammation and involves complete removal of all cells, breakdown products, and inflammatory exudate that enter the tissue during inflammation and return of the small blood vessels to their preinflammatory state. Thus, the injured area returns to normal.

The process of repair takes place when complete return of the tissue to normal is not possible because the damage has been too great. Some tissues, such as epithelium, fibrous connective tissue, and bone, have the ability to undergo repair. Other tissues, such as teeth, do not.

Repair

Repair is the body's final defense mechanism in its attempt to restore injured tissue to its original state. During the repair process, destroyed cells and tissue are replaced with live cells and new tissue components, but the repair process cannot be completed until the source of injury is removed or the injurious agents are destroyed. Repair is not always a perfect process. Functioning cells and tissue components may be replaced by nonfunctioning scar tissue.

Microscopic Events That Occur During Repair

After an injury microscopic events occur in both the epithelium and connective tissue (Fig. 2–15). These events are different for each of these tissues but occur almost simultaneously and are dependent on each other for optimal healing. If the source of the injury is removed, the repair process for both tissues is usually completed in 2 weeks. The repair process is slightly different in mucosa than in skin because mucosal tissues are wet and a scab does not form.

Day of Injury.   A clot forms as the blood flows into the injured tissue. The clot consists of locally produced fibrin, clumped (aggregated) red blood cells, and platelets. The clot or meshwork of fibrin is produced in the area of injury as a result of activation of the clotting mechanism. **Platelets,** also called **thrombocytes,** are found in blood and are extremely important in the formation of a clot. Hereditary factors, drugs, extensive injury, or certain diseases may affect the formation of the clot and prevent or delay tissue repair.

One Day After Injury.   Acute inflammation is taking place in the area of repair. The neutrophils emigrate from the microcirculation into the injured tissue, and phagocytosis of foreign substances and necrotic tissue occurs as part of the inflammatory response.

Two Days After Injury.   The monocytes emigrate from the microcirculation into the injured area as macrophages. Macrophages continue phagocytosis in a manner similar to that of the neutrophils, which are now dwindling in number as the inflammatory process proceeds. Fibroblasts increase in number within the injured connective tissue. They begin to produce new collagen fibers, using the fibrin meshwork as a scaffold.

The initial tissue formed in the connective tissue portion of the injury is called **granulation tissue.** It is an immature tissue, with many more capillaries and fibroblasts than mature connective tissue. Sometimes the growth of this tissue is excessive (exuberant). Lesions resulting from **exuberant granulation tissue** are described later in this

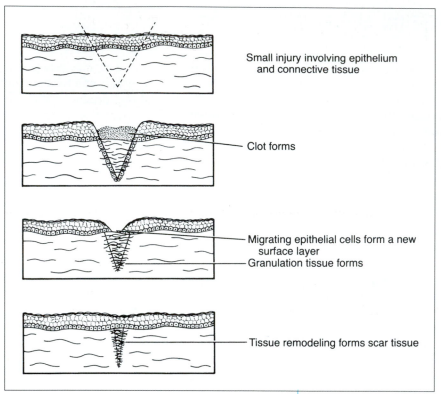

Small injury involving epithelium
and connective tissue

Clot forms

Migrating epithelial cells form a new
surface layer
Granulation tissue forms

Tissue remodeling forms scar tissue

▪ *f i g u r e* **2–15**   The underlying microscopic events of the repair process from the
day of injury to 2 weeks later.

section. Exuberant granulation tissue is a vivid red. It may interfere with the repair
process until it is removed surgically.

If the surface epithelium has been destroyed by the injury, the epithelial cells
create a new surface tissue at the same time that granulation tissue forms in the injured
connective tissue. The epithelial cells from the borders of the healing injured area lose
their cell junctions and become mobile. They then divide and migrate across the
injured tissue, using the fibrin meshwork as a guide to form a new surface layer.

In addition to serving as a guide for migrating epithelial cells and as a scaffold for
forming connective tissue, the fibrin meshwork serves to protect the two newly formed
tissues from further injury. Thus, it is important for the clot to remain in place during
this time to allow optimal repair in both tissues. Dressings placed over the clot may
prove beneficial to the healing process in some injuries.

At the end of 2 days, lymphocytes and plasma cells begin to emigrate from the
surrounding blood vessels into the injured area as chronic inflammation and an immune
response begin. The macrophages already present in the area now assist the lymphocytes in the immune response occurring at the site of injury.

Seven Days After Injury.   The fibrin is digested by tissue enzymes and sloughs
off, and the initial repair of the tissues is completed. Clinically, the surface of the
repaired injury remains redder because of the thinness of the new epithelium and the
increased vascularity of the new connective tissue. If the source of the injury has been
completely removed, the inflammatory and immune responses in the tissue are nearly
complete.

Two Weeks After Injury.   The initial granulation tissue and its fibers have been
remodeled, giving the tissue its full strength. The new tissue is now called **scar tissue**
and appears whiter or paler at the surface of the repaired injury because of the
increased number of collagen fibers and decreased vascularity. The amount of scar

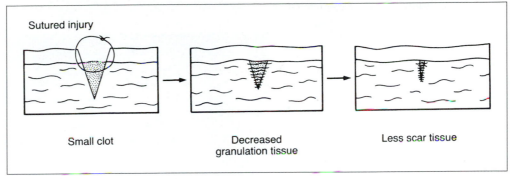

Sutured injury

Small clot   Decreased granulation tissue   Less scar tissue

f i g u r e 2–16   The use of sutures in an unintentional injury to encourage healing by primary intention.

tissue remaining after an injury depends on many factors, such as heredity, the strength and flexibility needed in the tissue, and the type of repair that has occurred.

Types of Repair

Healing by Primary Intention.   This refers to the healing of an injury in which there is little loss of tissue, such as in a surgical incision. In this type of healing, the clean edges of the incision are joined with sutures to form only a small clot, and very little granulation tissue forms (Fig. 2–16). Thus, there is less scar tissue and a higher retention of normal tissue. The use of sutures in an accidental injury is an attempt to try to join the edges of the injury surgically so that healing by primary intention occurs and scarring is minimized.

Healing by Secondary Intention.   This involves injury in which there is loss of tissue, so the edges of the injury cannot be joined during healing. A large clot slowly forms, resulting in increased formation of granulation tissue (e.g., extraction site) (Fig. 2–17). After healing there is increased scar tissue and greater loss of normal tissue function. Scar tissue formation can be so excessive in the epithelium and connective tissue that surgical correction is sometimes needed. Excessive scarring in skin is called **keloid formation** (Fig. 2–18).

Healing by Tertiary Intention.   If infection occurs at the site of a surgical incision that is healing by primary intention, healing by secondary intention may ensue. This transformation occurs because of an enlargement of the injured area and an increase in the magnitude and duration of the inflammatory and immune responses triggered by the presence of pathogenic microorganisms. In some cases an infected injury is left open and the edges are not surgically joined until the infection is controlled. Waiting to perform surgical tissue repair until the infection is resolved is called healing by tertiary intention.

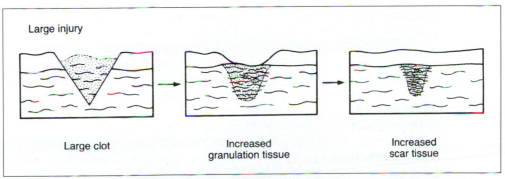

Large injury

Large clot   Increased granulation tissue   Increased scar tissue

f i g u r e 2–17   Healing by secondary intention in a large injury.

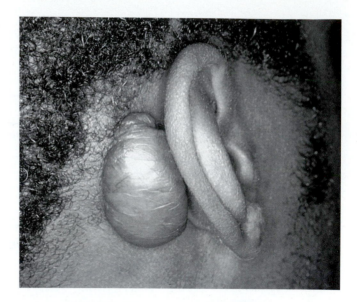

▪ *figure* 2–18

An example of keloid formation following an injury. (Courtesy of Dr. Harold Baurmash.)

Bone Tissue Repair

Repair of a bone injury is similar to the process that takes place in fibrous connective tissue except that it involves the creation of bone tissue. This tissue is produced by bone-forming cells called **osteoblasts,** which are found on the inner and outer surfaces of bone. Healing of a bone injury can be interrupted by removal of osteoblast-producing tissues or increased movement of the bone and can be delayed by the presence of hemorrhage or infection in the tissue.

PHYSICAL AND CHEMICAL INJURIES OF THE ORAL TISSUES

Injuries to Teeth

Attrition

Attrition is the wearing away of tooth structure during mastication. It is a normal occurrence and happens as an individual ages. It occurs on the incisal, occlusal, and proximal surfaces of the teeth and is rarely seen on any other tooth surfaces unless teeth are abnormally placed in the arch (Fig. 2–19). It occurs in both deciduous and permanent dentitions and is usually a slow process that starts as soon as the teeth are in contact and continues for the duration of the contact.

The first sign of attrition is the disappearance of the mamelons (Fig. 2–20) on incisal teeth and the flattening of the occlusal cusps. The rate of attrition is influenced by diet. A diet of more fibrous food causes greater attrition. Attrition is accelerated by bruxism, the use of chewing tobacco, and certain occupations and environments in which abrasive dust particles enter the mouth. The rate of attrition has been reported to be greater in men than in women.

Bruxism. Grinding and clenching the teeth together for nonfunctional purposes is called **bruxism.** The signs and symptoms resulting from bruxism and their extent are related to the intensity of the grinding and clenching. They are varied and include "wear facets" visible on enamel surfaces, an abnormal rate of attrition (Fig. 2–21),

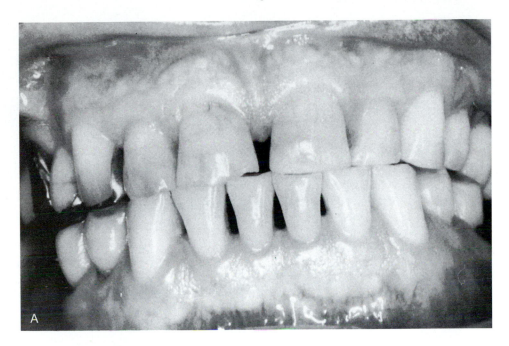

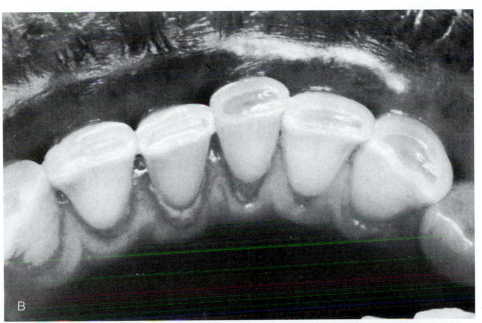

▪ *figure* **2–19**   *A,* Attrition of adult dentition (full view). *B,* Attrition of adult dentition (incisal view).

hypertrophy of masticatory muscles (especially the masseter muscle), increased muscle tone, muscle tenderness, muscle fatigue, cheek biting, pain in the temporomandibular joint area (see Chapter 8), tooth mobility, and pulpal sensitivity to cold.

The incidence of bruxism varies greatly according to the population studied. In a university student population, 5% of individuals showed signs and symptoms of bruxism. In studies of patients with periodontal disease, 60% to 90% had evidence of bruxism. In children aged 2 to 5, the average incidence reported was 20% to 30%, but the highest incidence reported was 78%.

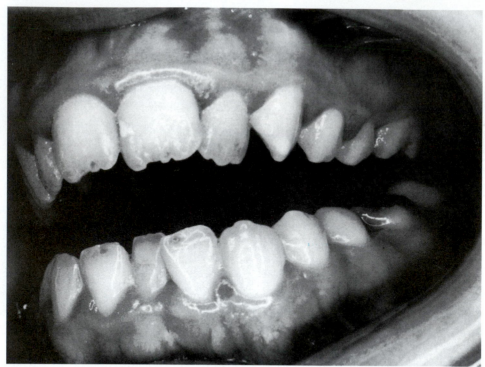

▪ *f i g u r e* **2–20**   Mamelons are present on the anterior teeth.

The cause of bruxism is unclear. Local factors such as occlusal interferences in combination with stress and tension are considered to be triggering factors. A relationship has been reported between bruxism and anxiety, hostility, and hyperactivity. Other studies have characterized the individual who engages in bruxism as emotionally fragile with meticulous character traits, more headaches and muscle pains, and more success

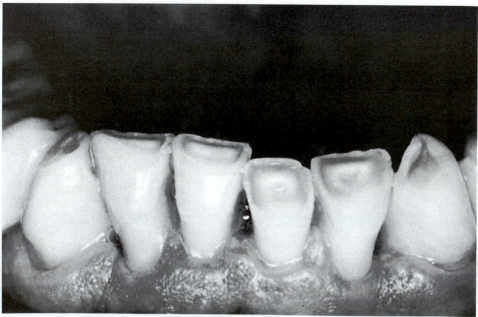

▪ *f i g u r e* **2–21**   Attrition resulting from bruxism.

in school. Certain conditions such as seizure disorders have been related to bruxism. The higher prevalence of bruxism reported in certain occupations is possibly related to the amount of stress associated with those occupations.

Management of the individual with bruxism includes eliminating the occlusal interferences through occlusal adjustments and protecting the teeth and supporting tissues from further destruction by fabricating an acrylic splint that can be worn as a protective device.

The dental hygienist may identify signs of bruxism while taking the patient's history and during the oral examination. Active wear facets, muscle tenderness, and excessive attrition are clues to the presence of bruxism.

Abrasion

Abrasion is the pathologic wearing away of tooth structure that results from a repetitive mechanical habit. It is most commonly seen in exposed root surfaces because the cementum and dentin are not as hard as enamel; however, abrasion occurs on enamel surfaces as well. The process of abrasion is usually slow, and the dentin responds by laying down a protective layer of secondary dentin. Therefore, pulpal exposure does not usually result.

Abrasion most frequently presents as a notching of the root surface in areas of gingival recession and may occur from an improper tooth-brushing technique, most commonly a back-and-forth scrubbing motion using excessive pressure. The use of an abrasive dentifrice or a hard toothbrush may also cause abrasion (Fig. 2–22). Today most dentifrices manufactured in the United States have a very low abrasive index and

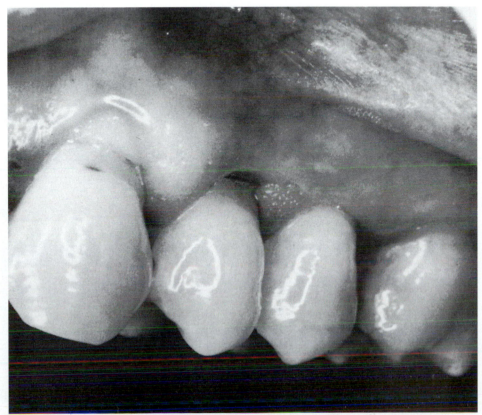

f i g u r e 2–22   Abrasion caused by brushing of teeth.

toothbrushes with soft bristles are recommended. Other causes of abrasion include opening bobby pins with the teeth or holding needles or pins in the teeth. These practices result in a notching of the maxillary incisors. Musicians who play wind instruments may also exhibit forms of abrasion of the teeth in the area of the mouth where the instrument is placed, and pipe smokers may show evidence of abrasion in the area of pipe placement.

The diagnosis of abrasion can often be made by correlating the clinical appearance of the lesions with information gained from questioning the patient about possible factors that may be causing the lesions. The patient should be informed of the cause of the abrasion, and corrective measures should be taken to prevent further destruction of tooth structure. Restorative dental treatment to repair the defect may be appropriate.

Erosion

Erosion is the loss of tooth structure resulting from chemical action. The loss may occur on the smooth facial or lingual surfaces of the teeth as well as on the proximal and occlusal surfaces (Fig. 2–23). The area of erosion appears smooth and polished and is usually large, involving several teeth. If erosion occurs in an area where there are restorations, the tooth structure is lost around the restoration, making it appear as if the restoration is standing on its own. This phenomenon is not seen in abrasion or attrition, since the restoration would be worn down along with the tooth surface.

Erosion may be seen in individuals who work in industries in which acid is used, such as battery manufacturing, plating companies, and soft-drink manufacturing. The

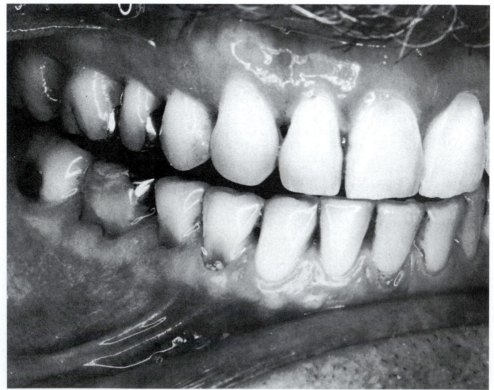

▪ *f i g u r e 2-23*   Erosion of buccal and labial surfaces of teeth that occurred as a result of accidental exposure to sulfuric acid.

erosion occurs because the workers breathe the acid in the air. Proteolytic enzymes in the workplace have also caused abrasion and erosion. Erosion of teeth associated with intraorally applied cocaine hydrochloride has been reported. Erosion of the facial surfaces of the teeth may also occur as a result of frequently sucking on lemons; erosion of the lingual surfaces of the teeth may occur as a result of chronic vomiting. The location of erosion and abrasion cannot reliably identify the cause. The patient's history must be correlated with the location and cause.

Bulimia is an eating disorder characterized by food binges, usually of very high caloric intake (sweets), followed by self-induced vomiting. Because of the pattern of erosion of the lingual surfaces of the teeth caused by frequent vomiting (Fig. 2–24), the dental hygienist may be the first health care professional to identify a patient with bulimia and may assist in encouraging the patient to seek treatment. Bulimia differs from anorexia nervosa, another eating disorder, which is characterized by a distorted perception of body image, along with depression, intense fear of gaining weight, and self-imposed starvation. The patient with bulimia maintains a normal body weight but is secretive about eating habits. Vomiting after eating is a component of bulimia and not of anorexia nervosa. Electrolyte imbalance and signs of malnutrition may be present. Irritation of the oral mucosa and lips may occur, and there may be lesions on the back of the fingers caused by their continual use to induce vomiting. Generalized erosion of the lingual surfaces of teeth is common and results from frequent vomiting.

Dental management of patients who vomit frequently includes an effort to minimize the effects of acid on tooth enamel by encouraging the daily use of fluoride rinse and toothpaste containing fluoride. Rinsing the mouth with water and thoroughly cleaning the teeth immediately after vomiting episodes also lessens the effects of acid.

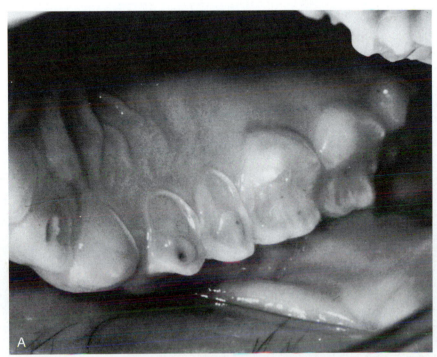

f i g u r e **2–24**   Erosion caused by bulimia. *A,* Erosion of maxillary lingual surfaces of teeth.

Illustration continued on following page

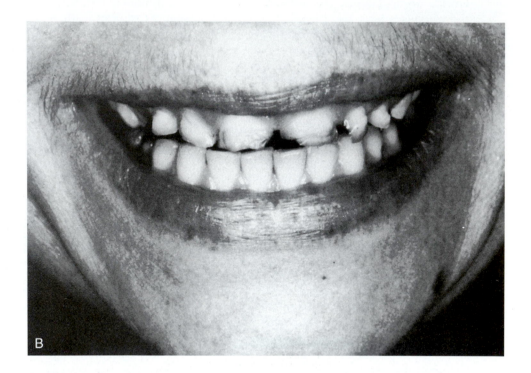

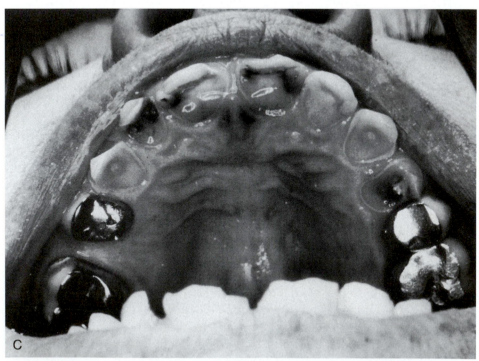

▪ *f i g u r e* **2–24**   *Continued B*, Decreased tooth size. *C*, Erosion of maxillary lingual surfaces.

Injuries to Oral Soft Tissues

Aspirin Burn

leukoplakia in Buccal vestibul next to tooth.

An aspirin burn generally occurs when a patient with a toothache places an aspirin tablet directly on the painful tooth instead of swallowing it. Aspirin (acetylsalicylic acid) is an analgesic (pain reliever) and anti-inflammatory agent that must be ingested to be effective. Topical application is a common misuse of aspirin. As a result of placing the aspirin on the soft tissue, the tissue becomes necrotic and white. The lesion is painful, and the necrotic tissue may separate from the underlying connective tissue and slough off, resulting in a large ulcer (Fig. 2–25; Color Plate 29). Questioning the patient should reveal the cause of the lesion, and the diagnosis is generally made without the need for biopsy of the tissue. An aspirin burn is painful and heals slowly because of the extent of destruction. However, the ulcer usually heals spontaneously in 7 to 21 days. The patient requires appropriate treatment of the painful tooth and medication for symptomatic relief of pain until the ulcer heals.

Phenol Burn

Phenol is used in dentistry as a cavity-sterilizing agent and a cauterizing agent. When phenol comes into contact with the soft tissues, a whitening of the exposed area occurs as a result of destruction of the epithelium. The surface tissue may slough off, exposing the underlying connective tissue. The resulting ulcer is painful, and the duration of healing depends on the extent of the destruction. The phenol should be removed immediately to minimize the destruction. If phenol is ingested, the patient should drink large amounts of water.

Phenol is also a component of some over-the-counter products that are advertised for relief of oral pain. Patients frequently use these preparations for oral ulcers, and the resulting destruction, in addition to being quite painful, may mask the diagnostic characteristics of the original ulcer.

Electric Burn

Electric burns in the oral area are usually seen in young children who have bitten or chewed a live electric cord or have inserted something into an electric socket. The electric current can cause a great deal of destruction of the oral tissues. Any tissue in the area may be damaged, including the permanent tooth buds. Permanent disfigurement and scarring may result from this type of injury.

Treatment. The treatment of electric burns may require a multidisciplinary approach that includes plastic surgery, oral surgery, and orthodontics.

Other Burns

Mucosal burns from hot food are common. They occur most often on the palate and tongue (Fig. 2–26).

Lesions from Self-Induced Injuries

Habits of which the patient may or may not be aware can cause injury. Chronic lip, cheek, or tongue biting and trauma to the gingiva by a fingernail are examples of habits that may cause oral lesions. These lesions range from ulceration to epithelial hyperplasia and hyperkeratosis. Ulcers caused by continual self-induced injuries may

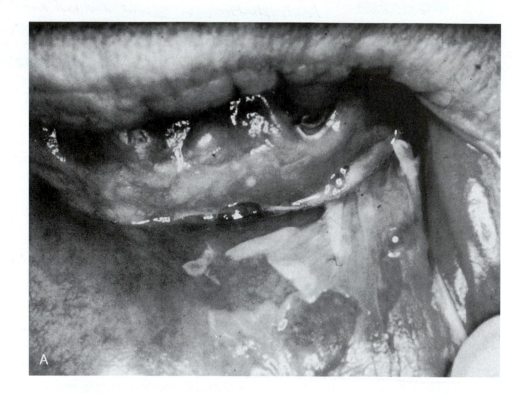

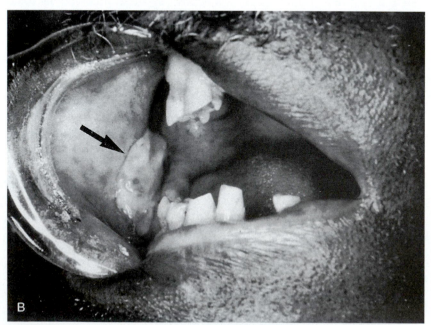

▪ *f i g u r e* 2–25   Aspirin burns. *A*, Lower labial mucosa. *B*, Posterior buccal mucosa.

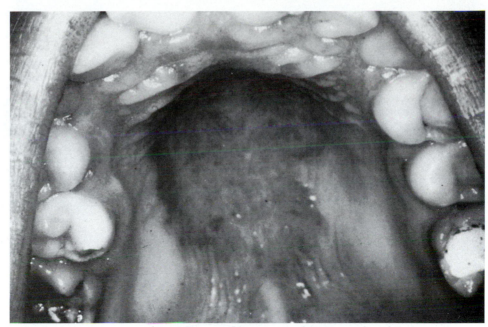

▪ *f* i g u r e 2–26   Burn of palatal mucosa from hot food.

be of long duration and may require biopsy and histologic examination to confirm the diagnosis.

   Treatment.   Treatment of self-induced lesions depends on the amount and type of destruction and may involve psychotherapy.

Lesions Associated with Cocaine Use

   Lesions located at the midline of the hard palate that vary from ulcers to keratotic lesions to exophytic reactive lesions have been reported to result from the smoking of crack cocaine. When crack cocaine is smoked, the crack pipe directs extremely hot smoke to the mid–hard palate. Identification of these lesions is based on their location and the history of recent smoking of crack cocaine. Necrotic ulcers of the tongue and epiglottis related to smoking free-base cocaine have also been reported.

Traumatic Ulcer

   A traumatic ulcer occurs as a result of some form of trauma (Fig. 2–27). Sources of trauma vary. Biting the cheek, lip, or tongue may result in a traumatic ulcer, as can irritation from a complete or partial denture or mucosal injury from sharp edges of food. The removal of a dry cotton roll from the oral tissue following a dental procedure can cause a traumatic ulcer, and it is not uncommon to see a patient present for a dental hygiene appointment with a traumatic injury to the gingival tissues or vestibular mucosa that results from overzealous brushing prior to the appointment. Persistent trauma may result in a hard (indurated), raised lesion called a **traumatic granuloma** (Color Plate 23).

   Traumatic ulcers are usually diagnosed on the basis of the relationship of the history to the lesion. Healing is usually uneventful and occurs in 7 to 14 days unless the trauma persists. If trauma persists, ulcers may last for weeks to months. The patient is followed until healing is ensured. If an ulcer does not heal in 7 to 14 days, a biopsy is usually indicated. Microscopically, the inflammatory infiltrate associated with a

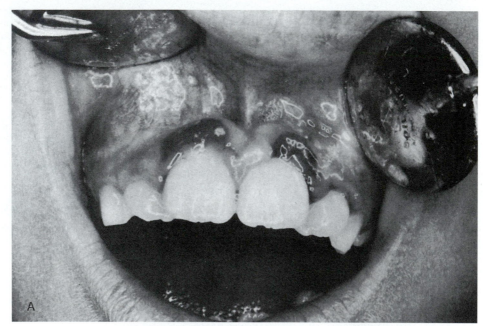

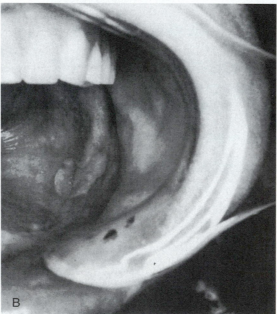

■ *f* i g u r e 2–27   *A*, Traumatic ulceration caused by irritation of gingiva by fingernails. *B*, Traumatic ulcer caused by denture.

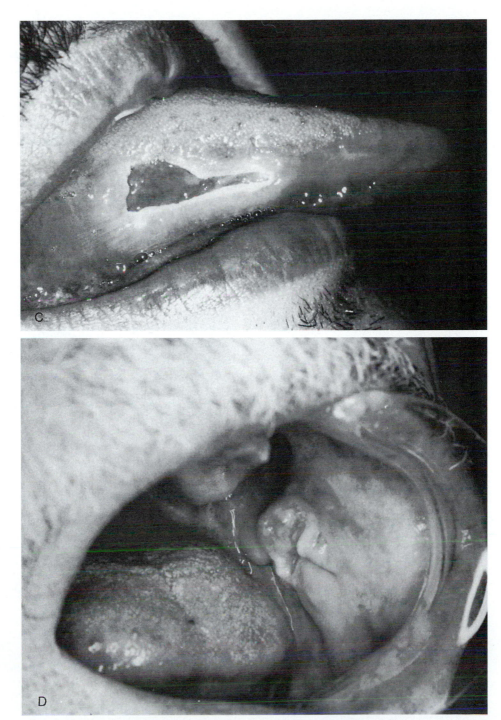

▪ *f* i g u r e **2–27**   *Continued C,* Traumatic ulcer on lateral tongue caused by chronic trauma to tongue by teeth. *D,* Traumatic ulcer (traumatic granuloma) of buccal mucosa.

traumatic ulcer includes many eosinophils in addition to neutrophils, lymphocytes, and plasma cells.

Frictional Keratosis

Chronic rubbing or friction against an oral mucosal surface may result in a thickening of the keratin on the surface, which is called **hyperkeratosis.** This results in an opaque, white appearance of the tissue and represents a protective response. It is analogous to a callus on the skin. An example of frictional keratosis is an increase in surface keratin that results from chronic cheek and tongue chewing and chewing on edentulous alveolar ridges (Fig. 2–28). Frictional keratosis is not associated with malignancy.

The diagnosis of frictional keratosis is made by identification of the trauma causing

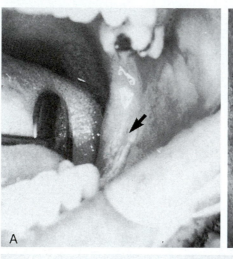
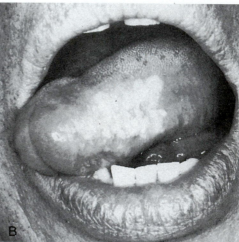
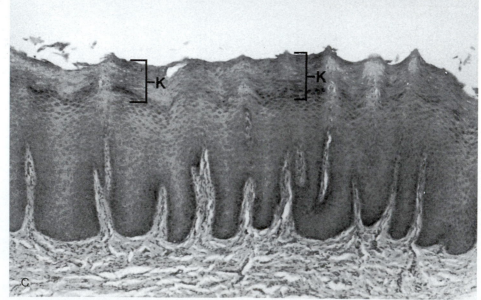

f i g u r e **2–28**   Frictional keratosis caused by an opposing third molar, as indicated by arrow *(A)*, and chronic tongue chewing *(B)*. *C*, Microscopic appearance of hyperkeratosis (low power) showing an increase in the amount of surface keratin (K).

the lesion, elimination of the cause, and observing the resolution of the lesion. The keratosis may take a while to disappear on keratinized surfaces such as the gingiva. Frictional keratosis must be distinguished from other white lesions that arise spontaneously and are not caused by trauma because idiopathic leukoplakia may be a premalignant lesion. Biopsy is indicated for any questionable lesion.

Linea Alba

Linea alba is a white, raised line that forms most commonly on the buccal mucosa at the occlusal plane (Fig. 2–29; Color Plate 24). In some patients the line becomes prominent as a result of a teeth-clenching habit. The line follows the pattern of the teeth at the occlusal plane. Although it is most commonly seen on the buccal mucosa, linea alba may form on the labial mucosa as well. Histologically, the white raised line is due to epithelial hyperplasia and hyperkeratosis.

Treatment. No treatment is indicated. However, the prominence of linea alba may be helpful in evaluating the severity of the clenching or bruxing.

Nicotine Stomatitis

Nicotine stomatitis is a benign lesion on the hard palate associated with smoking—most typically pipe and cigar smoking, but it occurs with cigarette smoking as well. The development of the lesion indicates that the patient is smoking heavily. The intensity of smoking required to produce this lesion increases the patient's risk for development of malignancy elsewhere in the oral cavity and respiratory tract.

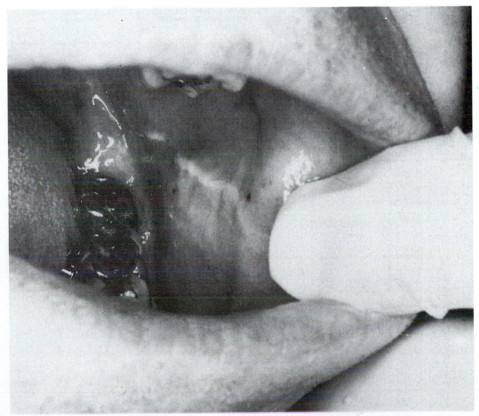

▪ *f i g u r e* **2–29**   Linea alba.

The palatal mucosa's initial response to the heat from these substances is an erythematous appearance. Over time keratinization occurs, resulting in increasing opacification. Following the increase in keratinization, raised red dots are seen at the openings of the ducts of the minor salivary glands on the palatal surface (Fig. 2–30; Color Plate 62). The minor salivary glands become inflamed as a result of obstruction by keratin at the mucosal opening of the ducts. The palate may develop a very similar clinical appearance as a result of the chronic intake of very hot liquids.

Tobacco Chewer's White Lesion

Individuals who chew tobacco may experience a white lesion in the area where the tobacco is habitually placed. The mucobuccal fold is the most common location. The epithelium usually has a granular or wrinkled appearance in early lesions. Long-standing lesions may be more opaquely white and have a corrugated surface (Fig. 2–31; Color Plate 20). The lesion often disappears when the tobacco is no longer placed in the area. There is a risk of malignancy with long-term exposure to smokeless tobacco. Lesions that do not resolve require biopsy and may show atypical epithelium. In addition there is an increased risk of caries, periodontal disease, attrition, and staining with this habit.

ulcerated area be suspicious of.

Traumatic Neuroma

A **traumatic neuroma** is a lesion caused by injury to a peripheral nerve. Nerve tissue is encased in a sheath composed of Schwann cells and their fibers. When this

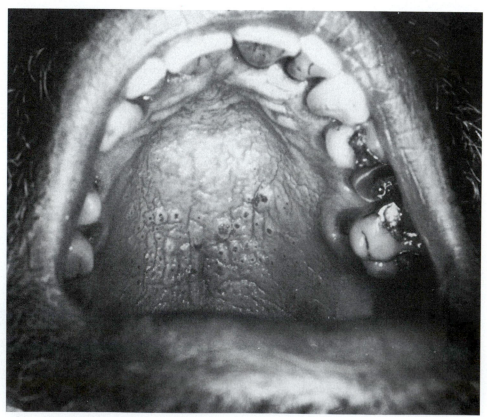

▪ *f i g u r e 2–30*   Nicotine stomatitis.

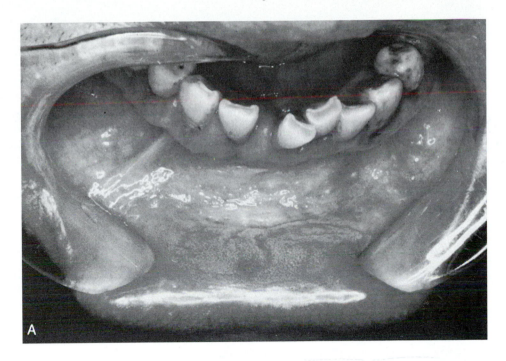

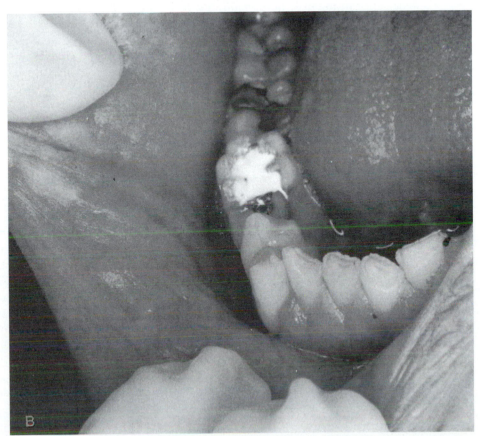

■ f i g u r e 2–31   Tobacco chewer's white lesion. Note the rough texture of the surface.
A, Labial mucosa. B, Anterior buccal mucosa.

sheath is disrupted, the nerve loses its framework. When a nerve and its sheath are damaged, the proximal end of the damaged nerve proliferates into a mass of nerve and Schwann cells mixed with dense fibrous scar tissue. In the oral cavity, injury to a nerve may occur from injection of local anesthesia, surgery, or other sources of trauma.

Traumatic neuromas are often painful. The pain may range from pain on palpation to severe and constant pain. Most traumatic neuromas occur in adults, and the mental foramen is the most common location. However, a traumatic neuroma may occur in other locations as well. Although the clinical features, particularly the pain that is characteristic, may suggest that a lesion is a traumatic neuroma, the diagnosis is made on the basis of a biopsy and microscopic examination.

a lot in nerves

Treatment. Traumatic neuromas are treated by surgical excision. Recurrence is rare.

Amalgam Tattoo

An **amalgam tattoo** is a flat, bluish-gray lesion of the oral mucosa that results from the introduction of amalgam particles into the tissues (Fig. 2–32; Color Plate 83). This may occur at the time of placement or removal of an amalgam restoration or at the time of tooth extraction if a piece of amalgam fractures off a restoration and remains in the tissue. The metallic particles disperse in the tissue and result in a permanent area of pigmentation. Over time the mercury-silver-tin amalgam changes, and it is mainly silver that remains in the tissue.

Amalgam tattoos may be seen in any location in the oral cavity but are most commonly found on the gingiva or edentulous ridge. The posterior region of the mandible is the most common location.

An amalgam tattoo is usually diagnosed on the basis of the clinical appearance of the pigmented area. Often the particles of amalgam can be seen on a periapical radiograph (see Fig. 2–32). As amalgam particles diffuse in the tissue over time, the size of the amalgam tattoo may increase. Biopsy may be necessary to distinguish an amalgam tattoo from a melanocytic lesion, particularly if it is located in an area other than the gingiva or alveolar ridge. Once the diagnosis of amalgam tattoo has been established, treatment is generally not indicated.

Melanosis

Normal, physiologic pigmentation of the oral mucosa is common, particularly in dark-skinned individuals (Color Plate 74). Melanin pigmentation may also occur following inflammation (Fig. 2–33). The **oral melanotic macule** is a flat, well-circumscribed brown lesion of unknown etiology. These are usually small (<1 cm in diameter) and may require biopsy and histologic examination for diagnosis. A similar lesion may occur on the vermilion of the lips. When occurring on the lips, the lesion may darken with exposure to sunlight. Another type of melanosis is called **smoker's melanosis** or **smoking-associated melanosis**. In this type of melanosis, the melanin pigmentation is associated with smoking, and the intensity is related to the amount and duration of smoking. The pigmentation fades when smoking is discontinued. However, this may take months to years. The anterior labial gingiva is the most commonly affected site. Women are affected more frequently than men. A relationship to female hormones and birth control pills has been suggested.

Solar Cheilitis

Sun exposure, particularly in fair-skinned individuals, can result in degeneration of the tissue of the lips, called **solar cheilitis** (Fig. 2–34). The development of this

white on lower lip

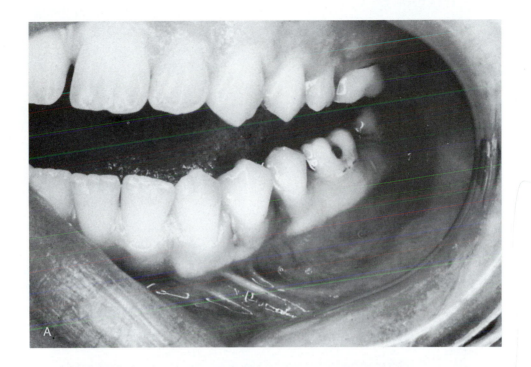

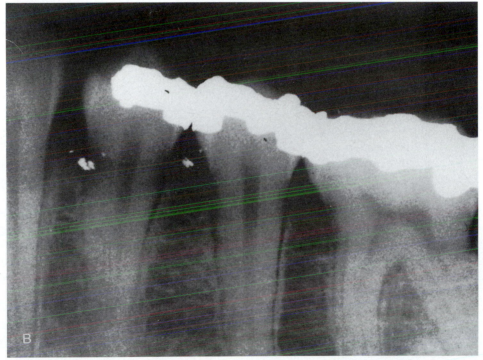

▪ *f i g u r e* 2–32   *A,* This blue-gray pigmentation of the gingiva is an amalgam tattoo. *B,* Periapical radiograph showing amalgam particles in the gingival tissue.

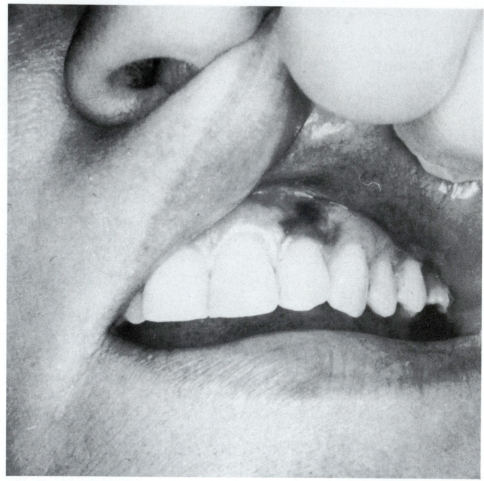

ƒ i g u r e 2–33   Post-traumatic melanin pigmentation. This area of melanin pigmentation
followed the healing of a traumatic injury.

condition is related to the total cumulative exposure to sunlight and the amount of
skin pigmentation and therefore may be seen in young as well as in older individuals.
The lower lip is usually more severely involved than the upper lip. The epithelium is
thinner than normal, and degenerative changes can be seen microscopically in the
connective tissue.

The vermilion border of the lips is affected. The color appears pale pinkish and
mottled. The interface between the lips and the skin is indistinct, with fissures appearing
at right angles to the skin–vermilion border junction. The lips are dry and cracked.

Treatment.   No specific treatment is indicated. However, there is a strong relationship between these degenerative changes and the development of basal cell carcinoma of the skin or squamous cell carcinoma of the lips and skin. Smoking may
increase this risk. Biopsy is indicated for persistent scaling or ulceration. Identification
of patients at high risk and with early indications of sun damage can be helpful in
preventing future lesions. Patients at risk should be advised to avoid sun exposure and
use sun block for protection.

Mucocele

A **mucocele** is a lesion that forms when a salivary gland duct is severed and the
mucous salivary gland secretion spills into the adjacent connective tissue. Granulation

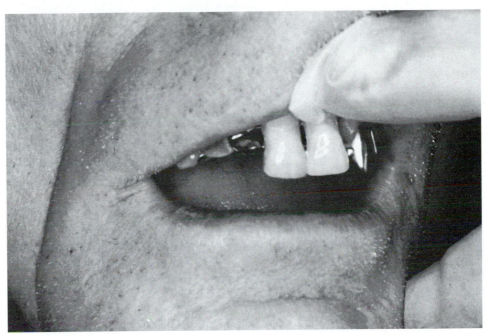

■ *f* i g u r e 2–34   Solar cheilitis.

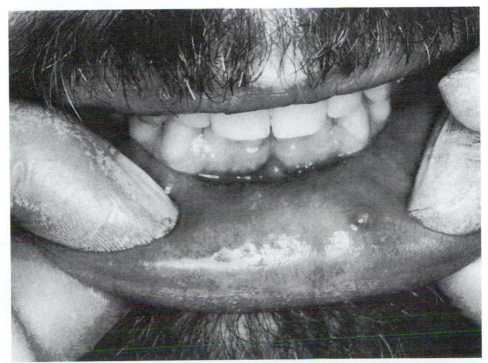

■ *f* i g u r e 2–35   Mucocele of the lower lip.

tissue forms in response to the mucus and forms the lining of a cyst-like structure. This is not a true cyst because the cystic space is not lined by epithelium.

A mucocele presents as a swelling in the tissue that often increases and decreases in size over time. The lower lip is the most common site of occurrence (Fig. 2–35; Color Plate 13). However, mucoceles may form in any area of the oral mucosa in which minor salivary glands are found. On the lower lip they are usually lateral to the midline. If a mucocele is near the surface, it may appear bluish. The color of the mucosa is normal if the mucocele is deeper in the tissue. A mucoepidermoid carcinoma may clinically resemble a mucocele and should be considered in the differential diagnosis. Most mucoceles occur in children and adolescents. However, they may occur in adults as well. If they are chronic or persistent, treatment is by surgical excision and removal of the adjacent minor salivary glands.

Occasionally, an epithelium-lined cystic structure occurs in association with a salivary gland duct. This is also called a mucocele, **mucous cyst**, or **mucous retention cyst** (Fig. 2–36) and occurs much less frequently than the type described above. It is not a true cyst but a dilated salivary gland duct and is thought to develop as a result of obstruction of a salivary gland duct. A ballooning of the duct occurs, which appears microscopically as an epithelium-lined cyst. Mucous cysts usually occur in adults who are older than 50 years of age. They may occur anywhere in the oral cavity where minor salivary glands are found and are treated by removal of the affected minor salivary glands.

Ranula is a term used for a mucocele-like lesion that forms unilaterally on the

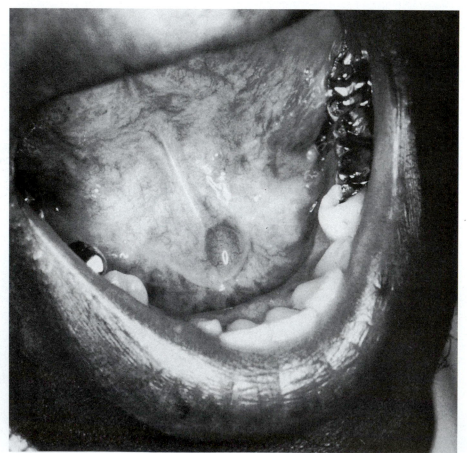

■ *figure 2–36*   Mucocele (mucous cyst) of the floor of the mouth.

floor of the mouth (Fig. 2–37). It is associated with the ducts of the sublingual and submandibular glands. "Ranula" refers to its clinical resemblance to a frog's belly. Although obstruction of the duct is considered to be the most likely cause for its development, histologically a ranula may resemble either a mucocele or a mucous cyst. Ranulas are treated by surgery, and the cause of obstruction, often a salivary gland stone, must be removed.

Necrotizing Sialometaplasia

Necrotizing sialometaplasia is a benign condition of the salivary glands characterized by moderately painful swelling and ulceration in the affected area (Fig. 2–38). Histologically, there is necrosis of the salivary glands. The salivary gland duct epithelium is replaced by squamous epithelium (metaplasia) and appears microscopically as islands of squamous epithelium deep in the connective tissue. If the duration of the ulcer is prolonged, a biopsy is needed to establish the diagnosis. However, the ulcer heals spontaneously, usually within 2 weeks. The junction of the hard and soft palates is most often affected. Necrotizing sialometaplasia is thought to result from blockage of the blood supply to the area of the lesion.

Sialolith

A **sialolith** is a salivary gland stone. Sialoliths occur in both major and minor salivary glands and form by precipitation of calcium salts around a central core. They may cause obstruction of the involved salivary gland; when they occur in the floor of the mouth, they can often be seen as a radiopaque structure on an occlusal radiograph (Fig. 2–39).

Acute and Chronic Sialadenitis

Both acute and chronic **sialadenitis** may occur as a result of obstruction of a salivary gland duct. They may also occur as a result of infection. In some cases the

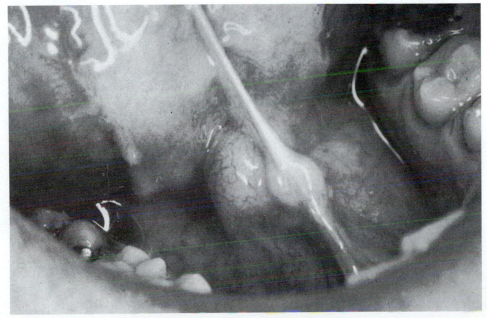

■ *figure* 2–37   Ranula.

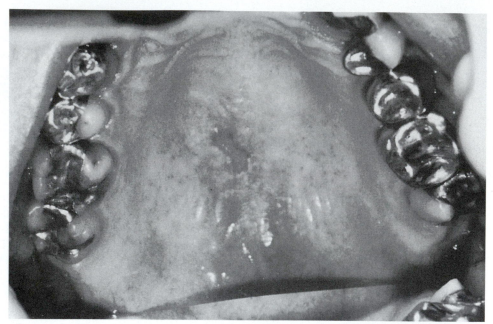

▪ *f* i g u r e 2–38   Necrotizing sialometaplasia.

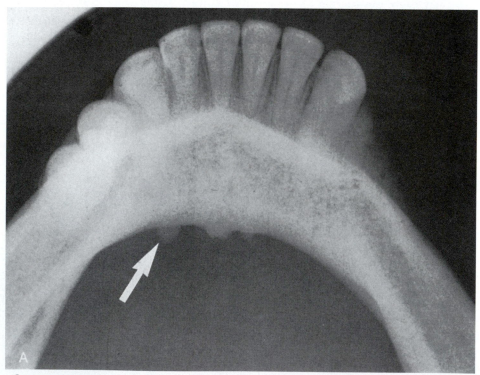

▪ *f* i g u r e 2–39   Sialoliths. *A,* Occlusal radiograph showing a sialolith *(arrow)* in Wharton's duct.

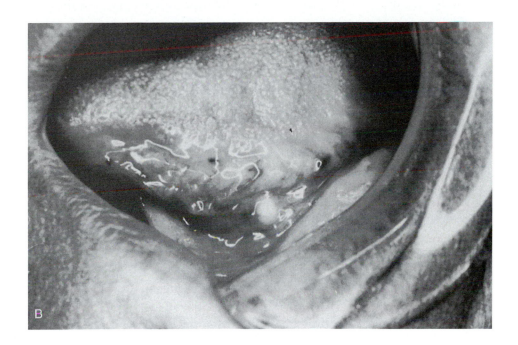

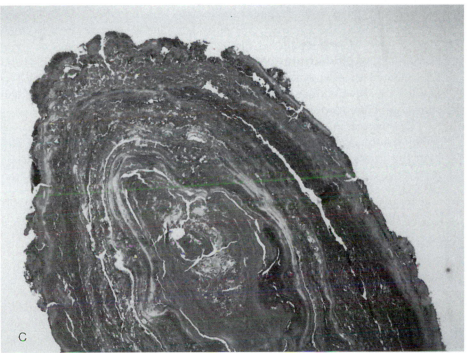

▪ *f* i g u r e 2-39   *Continued B*, Sialolith in a minor salivary gland on the floor of the mouth. *C*, Microscopic appearance of a sialolith showing concentric rings.

cause cannot be identified. Sialadenitis presents as a painful swelling of the involved salivary gland, usually one of the major glands. Diagnosis may require injection of a radiopaque dye into the gland, followed by taking a radiograph of the gland (sialography).

Treatment.   Antibiotics may be necessary in cases of infection.

Reactive Connective Tissue Hyperplasia

Reactive connective tissue hyperplasia consists of proliferating, exuberant granulation tissue and dense fibrous connective tissue. These lesions result from overzealous repair. They may occur as a response to a single event or as a chronic low-grade injury. The reason for the exuberant overgrowth of reparative tissue is not known.

Periapical inflammation, radicular cyst, and internal and external **tooth resorption** are included in this classification because they are also examples of lesions associated with proliferating inflamed tissue.

Pyogenic Granuloma

A **pyogenic granuloma** is a commonly occurring intraoral lesion that is characterized by a proliferation of connective tissue containing numerous blood vessels and inflammatory cells. It occurs as a response to injury. The term "pyogenic granuloma" is a misnomer. The lesion does not produce pus (pyogenic) and is not a true granuloma.

The pyogenic granuloma (Fig. 2–40; Color Plate 79) is usually ulcerated and soft to palpation, and bleeds easily. It is deep red to purple because of the vascularity of the proliferating tissue. It is generally elevated and may be either sessile or pedunculated. When ulcerated, the fibrin membrane on the surface appears yellowish white. The gingiva is the most common location of occurrence, but the lesion also occurs in other areas, such as the lips, tongue, and buccal mucosa. Pyogenic granulomas may vary considerably in size, from a few millimeters to several centimeters. They usually develop rapidly and then remain static. They may occur at any age, and some studies show a predominance in females.

Pyogenic granulomas often occur in pregnant women and have been called **pregnancy tumors** (Fig. 2–41; Color Plate 81). The lesions are identical to those seen in men and in nonpregnant women and may be caused by changing hormonal levels and increased response to plaque. However, they often regress after delivery. Similar gingival lesions also occur during puberty.

Treatment.   The pyogenic granuloma is treated by surgical excision if it does not resolve spontaneously. Occasionally, the lesion may recur if the injurious agent (e.g., calculus) remains.

Giant Cell Granuloma

A **giant cell granuloma** is a lesion that contains many multinucleated giant cells and well-vascularized connective tissue. Red blood cells and chronic inflammatory cells are also seen in this lesion. The cause of the giant cell granuloma is not clear. It occurs only in the jaws and seems to originate from the periodontal ligament or the periosteum and is thought to be a response to injury. The giant cell granuloma occurs both on the gingiva (peripheral giant cell granuloma) and within bone (central giant cell granuloma). The term **peripheral** pertains to those lesions occurring outside the bone, generally on the gingiva or alveolar mucosa, and the term **central** refers to a lesion occurring within the maxilla and mandible.

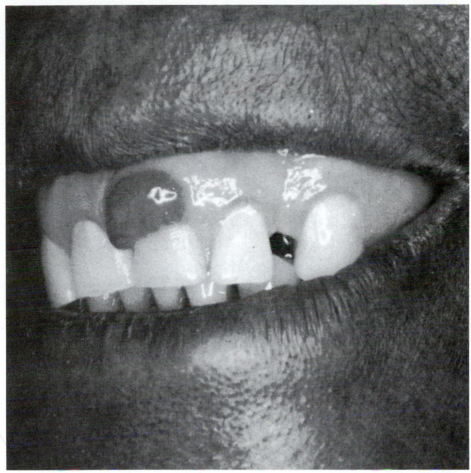

■ *f i g u r e* **2–40**   Pyogenic granuloma.

Peripheral Giant Cell Granuloma

The **peripheral giant cell granuloma** always occurs on the gingiva or alveolar process, usually anterior to the molars. It may resemble the pyogenic granuloma in clinical appearance (Fig. 2–42). Peripheral giant cell granulomas may vary in size from 0.5 to 1.5 cm in diameter and are usually dark red because of the numerous blood vessels present. The lesion may occur at any age but has been reported to be more frequent in people younger than 30 years of age and more common in women than in men. The peripheral giant cell granuloma may cause superficial destruction of the alveolar bone.

Treatment. Peripheral giant cell granulomas are treated by surgical excision of the lesion. They generally do not recur.

Central Giant Cell Granuloma

The **central giant cell granuloma** occurs within the bone of the maxilla or mandible, primarily in children and young adults. Studies have reported its occurrence more commonly in females than in males. These granulomas are common in the anterior segments of the maxilla and mandible and are uncommon in the ramus of the mandible. Patients with central giant cell granulomas may complain of discomfort from the lesions, but pain is not a common feature. The lesion is destructive and produces

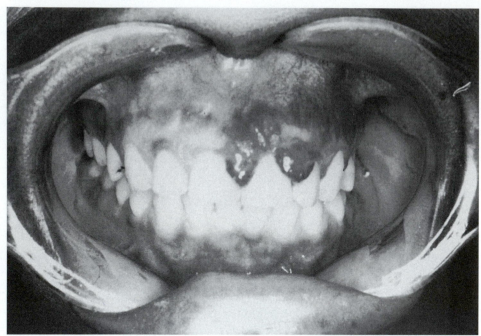

f i g u r e 2-41   Pyogenic granuloma of pregnancy (pregnancy tumor).

a radiolucency in the bone. The borders can be either ragged or sclerotic, and definite locules are often present (Fig. 2–43). Displacement of teeth is often seen.

Treatment.   Central giant cell granulomas are treated by surgical removal. Lesions occasionally recur.

A lesion of bone identical to the central giant cell granuloma (often called **brown tumor**) occurs in patients with hyperparathyroidism (discussed in Chapter 7). They are not surgically removed because they resolve when the underlying disease is successfully treated.

Irritation Fibroma

The **irritation fibroma** (also known as **fibroma** or **traumatic fibroma**) is a broad-based, persistent exophytic lesion that is composed of dense, scar-like connective tissue containing few blood vessels. It occurs as a result of chronic trauma or an episode of trauma such as habitual cheek chewing or cheek biting (Fig. 2–44; Color Plates 21 and 84). The irritation fibroma is usually a small lesion. Most are less than a centimeter in diameter, and fibromas greater than 2 cm in diameter are rare. It is the most common mass on the gingiva. It also occurs on the buccal mucosa, tongue, lips, and palate. The color of the irritation fibroma is usually lighter than that of the surrounding mucosa. The surface is covered by stratified squamous epithelium and may appear opaque and white if it has a thick keratin surface, or it may be ulcerated because of local secondary trauma.

Treatment.   An irritation fibroma is surgically removed. Many benign soft tissue tumors resemble the irritation fibroma in clinical appearance. Excision and microscopic examination of the tissue are important for diagnosis if there is any question about the nature of the lesion. Irritation fibromas usually do not recur at the same site, but additional lesions may occur as a response to additional trauma. Since the fibroma is the most commonly occurring mass on the gingiva, it is frequently encountered by the dental hygienist.

Text continued on page 103

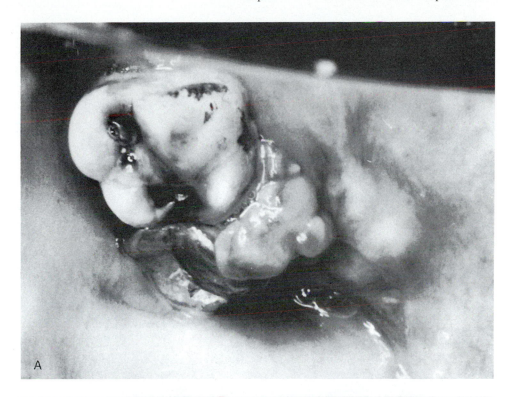

A

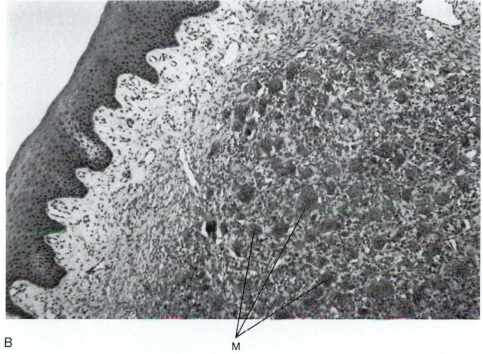

B   M

■ **f i g u r e 2–42**   *A,* Peripheral giant cell granuloma. *B,* Microscopic appearance of a peripheral giant cell granuloma showing multinucleated giant cells (M), capillar-
ies, and fibroblasts.

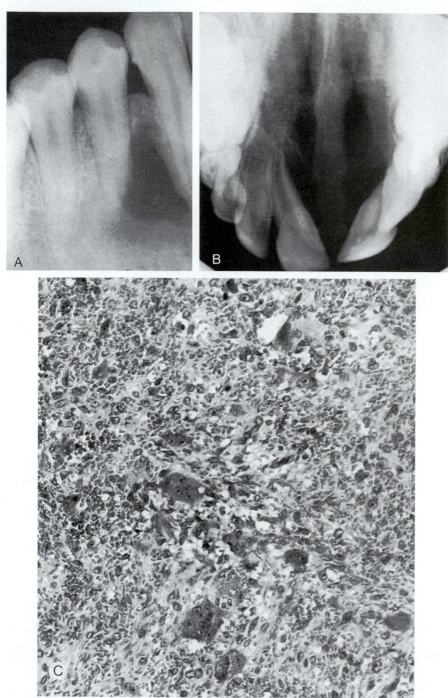

▪ *f* i g u r e 2–43   Radiographs of central giant cell granulomas showing multilocular radiolucencies in the mandible *(A)* and maxilla *(B)*. *C,* Microscopic appearance of a central giant cell granuloma showing the same features as a peripheral giant cell granuloma except for the absence of surface mucosa.

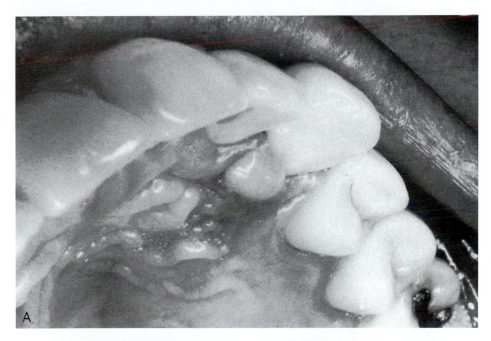

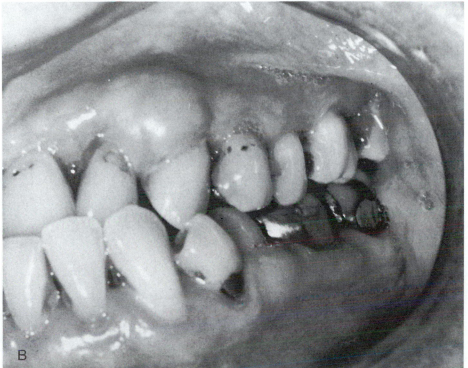

▪ *f* **i g u r e 2–44**   Irritation fibroma. *A,* Gingiva. *B,* The development of fibroma followed by the healing of a periodontal abscess. (Courtesy of Dr. Murray Schwartz.)

Illustration continued on following page

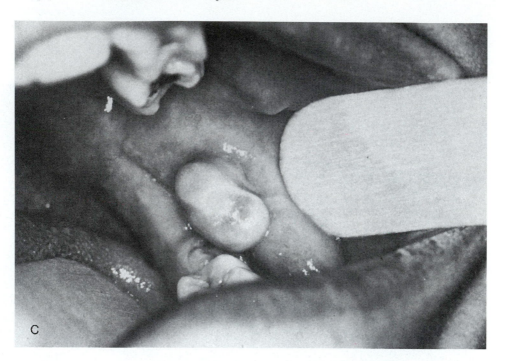

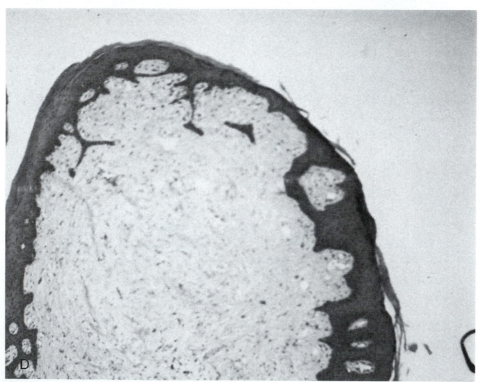

■ *f i g u r e* **2–44**   *Continued C,* Irritation fibroma of the buccal mucosa. *D,* Microscopic appearance of a fibroma.

The **peripheral ossifying fibroma** is a common gingival lesion, the cause of which is not known. It is thought to originate in the periodontal ligament. It is more completely described in Chapter 5.

Denture-induced Fibrous Hyperplasia

Denture-induced fibrous hyperplasia is commonly called **epulis fissuratum** or **inflammatory hyperplasia.** This lesion is caused by an ill-fitting denture and is located in the vestibule along the denture border. It is composed of dense, fibrous connective tissue surfaced by stratified squamous epithelium, the same type of tissue seen in the irritation fibroma. The lesion is usually somewhat larger than the irritation fibroma. It is arranged in elongated folds of tissue into which the denture flange fits (Fig. 2–45). The surface of the lesion is often ulcerated.

Treatment. Since this lesion does not resolve even with prolonged removal of the denture, treatment involves surgical removal of the excess tissue and construction of a new denture.

Papillary Hyperplasia of the Palate

from canida albicans

Papillary hyperplasia of the palate, or **palatal papillomatosis,** is a form of denture stomatitis. It is almost always associated with a removable full or partial denture or an orthodontic appliance. The palatal mucosa, most commonly the vault area, is covered by multiple erythematous papillary projections that give the area a granular or cobblestone appearance (Fig. 2–46; Color Plate 67). Each of the papillary projections consists of fibrous connective tissue, usually chronically inflamed and surfaced by stratified squamous epithelium. The precise cause of this type of hyperplasia is not understood.

Treatment. Surgical removal of the hyperplastic papillary tissue before construction of a new denture is generally necessary.

Gingival Hyperplasia

Gingival hyperplasia is characterized by an increase in the bulk of the free and attached gingiva, especially that involving the interdental papillae (Fig. 2–47). There is no stippling, and the gingival margins are rounded. The tissue consistency may vary from soft to firm, and the appearance may vary from erythematous to a normal pink color, depending on the degree of inflammation. Gingival hyperplasia may be generalized or localized and may vary from mild focal enlargement of interdental papillae to severe generalized gingival enlargement that may cover the crowns of the teeth. The enlarged tissue may appear red, a normal mucosal color, or paler, depending on the amount of inflammation and degree of vascularity.

Most cases are the result of an unusual tissue response to chronic inflammation associated with local irritants such as plaque or calculus. Hormonal changes—for example, those occurring in pregnancy and puberty—and certain drugs such as phenytoin (Dilantin; Color Plate 87), nifedipine (Procardia; Color Plate 88), and cyclosporine can increase the tissue response to local factors. Hereditary forms of gingival fibromatosis occur, beginning in early childhood. In some cases the cause of gingival hyperplasia cannot be identified.

If the tissue is inflamed and bleeds easily, biopsy and histologic examination of the tissue may be necessary to rule out the gingival enlargement that may occur in individuals with leukemia.

Treatment. **Gingivoplasty** (reshaping the gingiva) or **gingivectomy** (removing

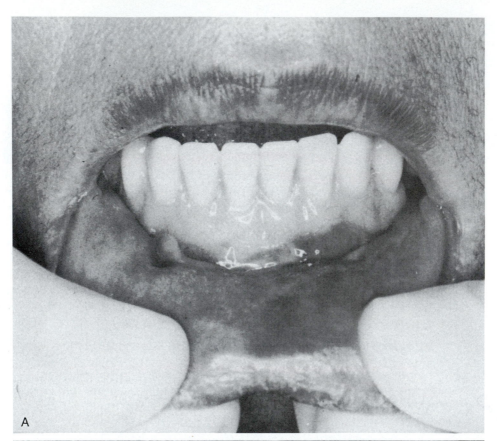

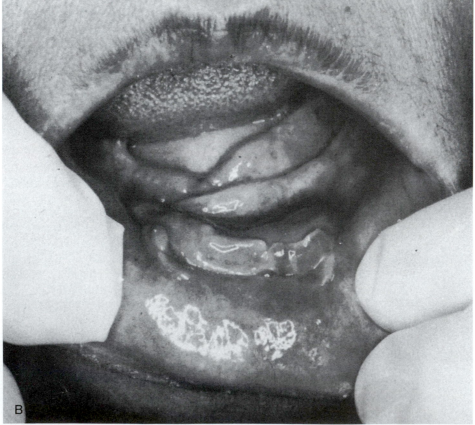

■ *f i g u r e 2–45*   Denture-induced fibrous hyperplasia (epulis fissuratum). *A*, With denture;
B, without denture.

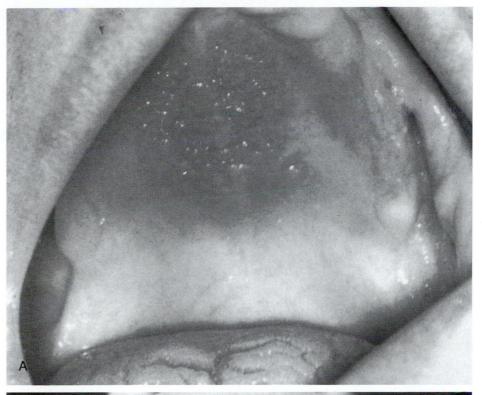

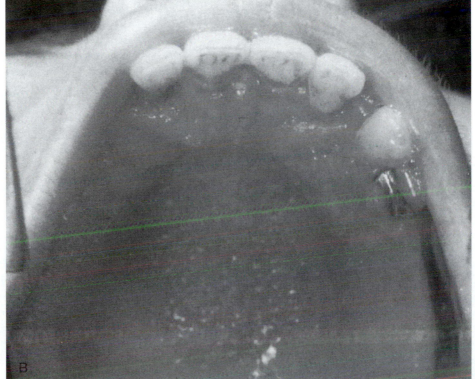

■ *f* i g u r e 2–46   Papillary hyperplasia of the palate. *A*, Full denture. *B*, Partial denture. (*A* and *B*, Courtesy of Dr. Edward V. Zegarelli.)

Illustration continued on following page

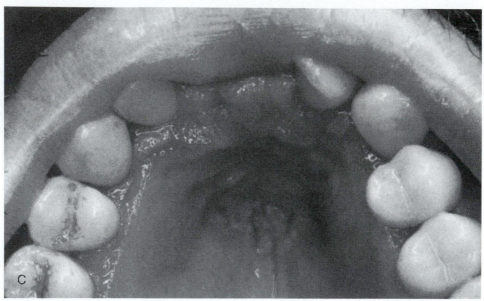

▪ *f i g u r e 2–46*   *Continued C,* Papillary hyperplasia from a "flipper."

gingival tissue) may be necessary to recontour the gingival tissue. Meticulous oral hygiene is helpful in reducing additional hyperplasia.

Periapical Inflammation and Radicular Cyst

Dental caries or trauma to a tooth may result in a variety of responses: inflammation, infection, chronic hyperplastic pulpitis, and necrosis of the dental pulp. The inflammatory process begins in the dental pulp and then extends into the periapical area (the area surrounding the apical portion of the tooth root at the site of the apical foramen). This condition occurs because once the inflammatory process has been established in the dental pulp, the only route it can follow is through the root canal into the periapical area. The presence of accessory canals may lead to areas of inflammation located on the lateral portion of the tooth root.

Chronic Hyperplastic Pulpitis

Chronic hyperplastic pulpitis, or **pulp polyp,** is an excessive proliferation of chronically inflamed dental pulp tissue. It occurs in teeth with large, open carious lesions, in children and young adults, and in primary or permanent molars. Chronic hyperplastic pulpitis appears as a red or pink nodule of tissue that often fills the entire cavity in the tooth, the tissue protruding from the pulp chamber (Fig. 2–48). It is usually asymptomatic, and, because the hyperplastic tissue contains so few nerves, it is usually insensitive to manipulation. The proliferation of pulp tissue rather than pulpal necrosis, which can also result from dental caries, is thought to be related to the large root opening and blood supply of the tooth involved.

The hyperplastic tissue is granulation tissue. Inflammatory cells, primarily lymphocytes and plasma cells and sometimes neutrophils, are commonly present. The tissue is generally surfaced by stratified squamous epithelium. Since there is no epithelium in normal pulp tissue, this epithelium is thought to result from desquamation of the surface oral mucosa.

Treatment.   Chronic hyperplastic pulpitis is treated by either extraction or endodontic treatment of the involved tooth.

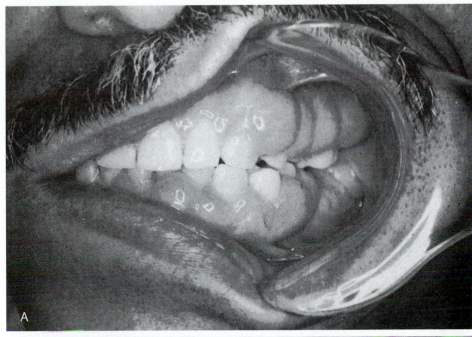

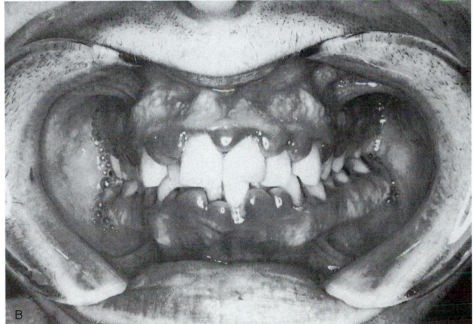

▪ *figure* 2-47   Gingival hyperplasia. *A*, Fibrous; *B*, inflamed.

Periapical Abscess

An acute **periapical abscess** is composed of a purulent exudate, or pus, surrounded by connective tissue containing neutrophils and lymphocytes (Fig. 2–49*A*). The patient with this condition complains of severe pain, which is a result of inflammation causing pressure on nerves because of the exudate and chemical mediators released in the area. The periapical abscess may develop directly from the inflammation in the pulp, but it more commonly develops in an area of previously existing chronic inflammation. The pus that forms seeks a path of least resistance and finds either a channel or a fistula out

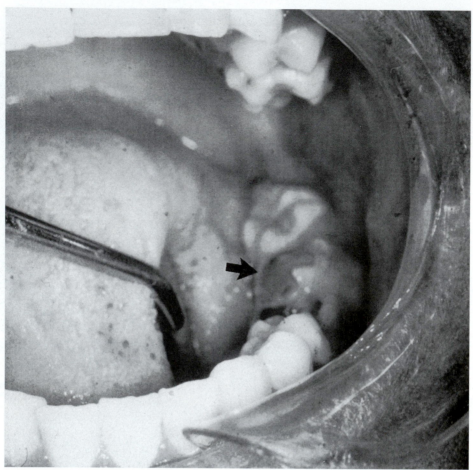

f i g u r e 2-48   Chronic hyperplastic pulpitis (pulp polyp) *(arrow).*

of the tissue, or it spreads to contiguous areas through oral and facial tissue spaces (see Fig. 2–3; Color Plate 80). The tooth associated with the abscess is usually quite painful and may be slightly extruded from its socket. If the acute abscess develops directly from pulpal inflammation, there may be no radiographic changes except for a slight thickening of the apical periodontal ligament space. If the abscess develops in a pre-existing area of periapical chronic inflammation, a distinct radiolucent area is seen at the apex.

Treatment.   A periapical abscess is treated by establishing drainage, either by opening the pulp chamber or by extracting the tooth. If the abscess has extended into adjacent tissue, an incision may be necessary to establish drainage. The patient may also be given antibiotic therapy.

Dental or Periapical Granuloma

A **periapical granuloma** is a localized mass of chronic granulation tissue that forms at the opening of the pulp canal, generally at the apex of a nonvital tooth root (Fig. 2–49B,C). This is a chronic process from the outset. Most cases are completely asymptomatic. Sometimes the tooth is sensitive to pressure and percussion because of the inflammation in the apical area. The tooth may also feel slightly extruded from its socket. The radiographic change may vary from a slight thickening of the periodontal

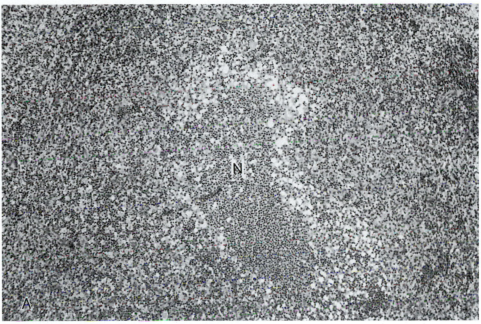

■ **f i g u r e 2-49**   *A,* Periapical abscess.

Illustration continued on following page

ligament space in the area of inflammation to a diffuse radiolucency to a distinct well-circumscribed radiolucency surrounding the root apex.

The periapical granuloma is composed of granulation tissue containing lymphocytes, plasma cells, and macrophages. Dense fibrous connective tissue is often present. The periapical granuloma is different from the granuloma of granulomatous inflammation, which is a distinctive type of inflammation characteristic of certain diseases (e.g., tuberculosis). Epithelial rests of Malassez, which are remnants of tooth-forming tissue, are present in the periapical granuloma.

Treatment.   The periapical granuloma is treated by root canal therapy or extraction of the tooth.

Radicular Cyst (Periapical Cyst)

A **radicular cyst,** or **periapical cyst,** is a true cyst consisting of a pathologic cavity lined by epithelium. It occurs in association with the root of a nonvital tooth (Fig. 2–50). It is the most common cyst occurring in the oral region. The epithelial lining of the cyst develops in a periapical granuloma as a result of proliferation of the epithelial rests of Malassez.

A periapical cyst develops when the epithelium within the inflamed connective tissue of the periapical granuloma proliferates, forming an epithelial mass that increases in size through division of the peripheral cells. The peripheral cells are the equivalent of the basal cell layer of the epithelium. As the cells in the central portion of the mass become more and more separated from the source of nutrition in the connective tissue, they degenerate centrally, forming a cavity (lumen) that is lined by epithelium and filled with fluid. Histologically, the periapical cyst is identical to the periapical granuloma except for cystic space lined by epithelium.

Most periapical cysts are asymptomatic and are discovered on radiographic examination. The radiographic appearance of the radicular cyst is the same as that of the periapical granuloma. It appears as a radiolucency, usually well circumscribed, that is

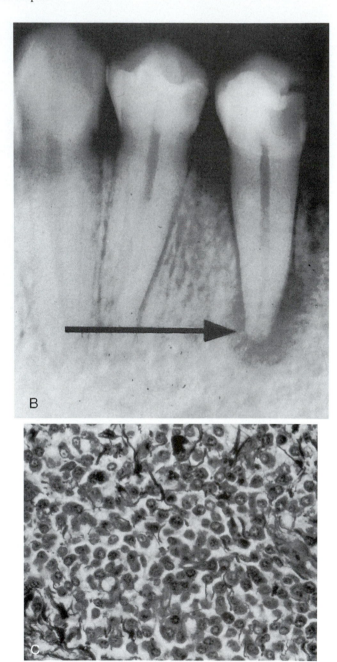

■ *f i g u r e* 2–49

Continued B, Radiograph of a periapical granuloma *(arrow). C*, High magnification shows inflammatory cells. (From Regezi JA, Sciubba JJ: Oral Pathology: Clinical-Pathologic Correlations. Philadelphia, WB Saunders, 1989, p 302.)

attached to a tooth root. It is not possible to differentiate reliably a periapical granuloma from a radicular cyst on the basis of the radiographic appearance alone. A periapical cyst may form in association with any tooth. The cyst may occur lateral to the tooth root rather than at the apex if it is associated with a lateral pulp canal. Other types of cysts can resemble a periapical cyst radiographically, and therefore removal of the cyst and microscopic examination of the tissue are necessary.

Treatment.   The radicular cyst is treated by root canal therapy, apicoectomy, or extraction and curettage of the periapical tissues. A residual cyst forms when the tooth is removed and all or part of a periapical cyst is left behind (Fig. 2–51). Radiographically, a residual cyst is a well-circumscribed radiolucency located at the site of tooth extraction. It is treated by surgical removal of the cyst.

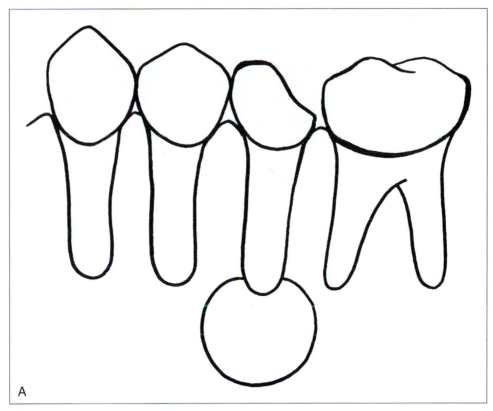

A

■ *f* i g u r e **2–50**   Radicular cyst. *A*, Diagram of a radicular cyst located around the root of an erupted tooth.

Illustration continued on following page

Resorption of Teeth

Tooth structure can be resorbed in the same manner as bone. This occurs normally in the process of exfoliation of deciduous teeth and may also occur in other situations. Resorption of the tooth structure beginning at the outside of the tooth is called external resorption. This usually involves the root of a tooth but can occasionally involve the crown of an impacted tooth.

Just as bone resorption can occur when inflammatory tissue is present, so can tooth resorption. Resorption of the root of a tooth sometimes occurs when a periapical granuloma is present. Bone resorption as a response to pressure allows orthodontic tooth movement to occur. Pressure can also cause resorption of tooth structure. This can occur from excessive occlusal or orthodontic forces and with benign and malignant tumors. When a tooth that has been avulsed is reimplanted, the root is resorbed and replaced by bone. Occasionally, resorption may involve the crown of an impacted tooth or the roots of teeth, and the cause cannot be identified. This is called **idiopathic tooth resorption.**

External root resorption first appears as a slight raggedness or blunting of the root apex and can proceed to severe loss of tooth substance (Fig. 2–52). The condition is not reversible, but progression of the process can be avoided if the cause can be identified and removed. Resorption of impacted teeth can also occur. Generalized root resorption may also occur following orthodontic tooth movement.

Internal tooth resorption can occur in any tooth; usually only a single tooth is involved. In some cases no cause can be identified. However, it is usually associated

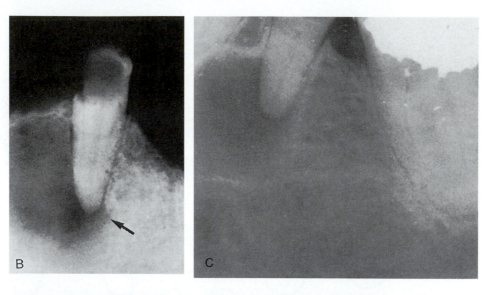

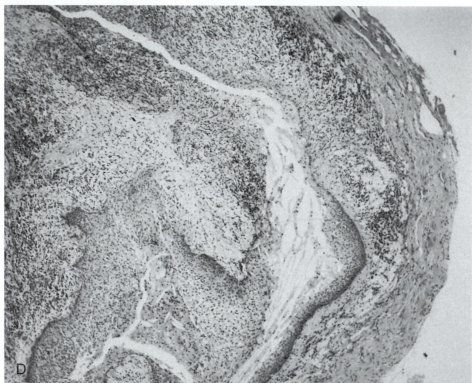

■ **ƒ i g u r e 2–50**   *Continued B* and *C,* Radiograph showing a well-circumscribed radiolucency around the root of a tooth. *D,* Microscopic features of a radicular
cyst.

with an inflammatory response in the pulp. If the process occurs in the coronal part of
the tooth, it may be seen clinically as a pinkish area. The dental hard tissue has
resorbed and is thinner than normal, and the pink color results from the vascular,
inflamed connective tissue that can be seen through the remaining enamel and dentin.
When the process involves the root, it can be seen only radiographically. A round to
ovoid radiolucent area is seen in the central portion of the tooth associated with
the pulp.

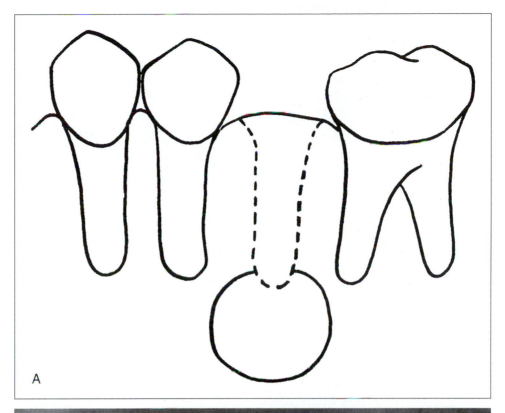

A

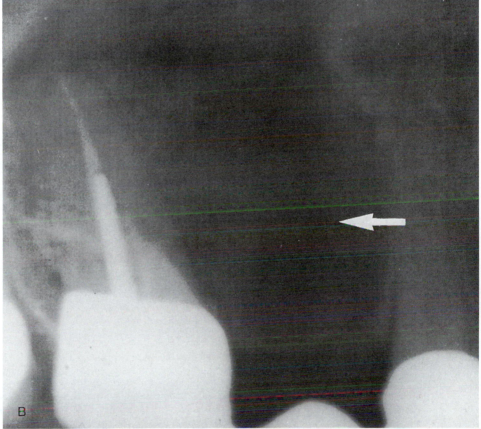

B

━ *f* i g u r e **2–51**   *A,* Diagram of a residual cyst. *B,* Radiograph of a residual cyst showing a
radiolucency at the site of a previously extracted tooth. (Courtesy of Drs.
Paul Freedman and Stanley Kerpel.)

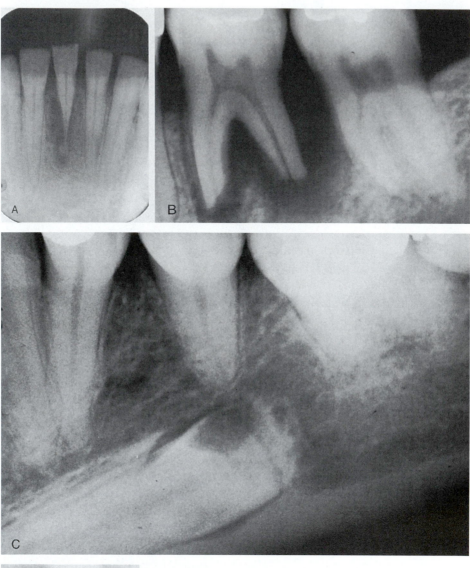

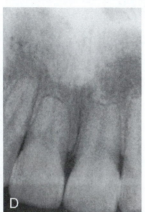

■ *f* i g u r e 2–52

Tooth resorption. *A*, Root resorption of a mandibular anterior tooth associated with chronic inflammation. (Courtesy of Dr. Gerald P. Curatola.) *B*, Resorption of tooth structure and bone due to chronic inflammation. *C*, Idiopathic resorption of an impacted tooth. *D*, Generalized root resorption associated with orthodontic tooth movement.

Treatment. Root canal treatment can be successfully performed if internal resorption is discovered early. If not treated, the process can extend through the dental hard tissue and cause a perforation. After this perforation occurs, the tooth must be extracted.

Focal Sclerosing Osteomyelitis

Focal sclerosing osteomyelitis, also called **condensing osteitis,** is a change in bone near the apices of teeth that is thought to be a reaction to low-grade infection. Radiographically, a radiopaque area is seen extending below the roots of the involved tooth (Fig. 2–53). The tooth most commonly associated with focal sclerosing osteomyelitis is the mandibular first molar. Occasionally, the mandibular second molar and the mandibular premolars may also be involved.

Radiographically, focal sclerosing osteomyelitis appears as a radiopaque area extending below the roots of the tooth. The borders may be diffuse or well defined. Occasionally the periphery of the area is radiolucent, and in other cases a central radiolucency surrounded by radiopacity is seen. Microscopically, it is dense bone with little marrow or connective tissue. There is generally very little inflammation present.

Focal sclerosing osteomyelitis is often associated with a carious or restored tooth. It is generally asymptomatic. However, pain may be associated if pulpal inflammatory disease is present. Focal sclerosing osteomyelitis may be present at any age, but it is typically first seen in young adults.

Diagnosis and Treatment. The diagnosis can usually be made on the basis of the characteristic radiographic appearance. Occasionally, biopsy may be necessary to

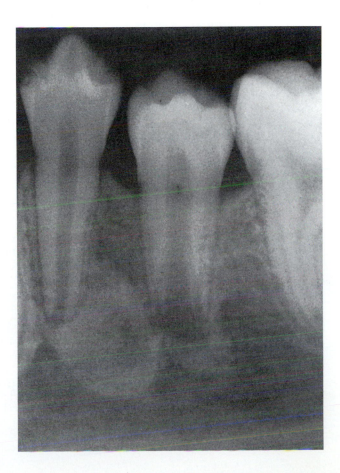

■ *figure* 2-53
Focal sclerosing osteomyelitis.

rule out other radiopaque lesions such as osteoma, complex odontoma, or ossifying fibroma. Treatment is not necessary. The sclerotic bone remains even after treatment of the involved tooth.

Alveolar Osteitis ("Dry Socket")

Alveolar osteitis or **dry socket** is a postoperative complication of tooth extraction. The most frequently affected area is the socket of an extracted mandibular third molar. Following the extraction of the tooth, the blood clot breaks down and is lost before healing has taken place. Pain develops several days after the extraction. On examination the tooth socket appears empty and the bone surfaces exposed. The patient complains of pain, bad odor, and bad taste. Since there is no infection, fever, swelling, and erythema are not present.

Treatment.   Treatment of alveolar osteitis is directed at relief of pain and includes gentle irrigation and insertion of a medicated dressing.

SELECTED REFERENCES

BOOKS

Cotran RS, Kumar V, Robbins SL (eds): Robbins Pathologic Basis of Disease, 5th ed. Philadelphia, WB Saunders, 1994.
Kent TH: Introduction to Disease, 2nd ed. East Norwalk, CT, Appleton-Century-Crofts, 1987.
Peterson LJ (ed): Principles of Oral and Maxillofacial Surgery. Philadelphia, JB Lippincott, 1992.
Peterson LJ, Ellis E III, Hupp JR, Tucker MR (eds): Contemporary Oral and Maxillofacial Surgery. St. Louis, CV Mosby, 1988.
Regezi JA, Sciubba JJ: Oral Pathology: Clinical-Pathologic Correlations, 2nd ed. Philadelphia, WB Saunders, 1993.
Shafer WG, Hine MK, Levy BL: A Textbook of Oral Pathology, 4th ed. Philadelphia, WB Saunders, 1983.
Sittig M: Handbook of Toxic and Hazardous Chemicals. Park Ridge, NJ, Noyes, 1981.
Sonis ST, Fazio RC, Fang L: Principles and Practice of Oral Medicine, 2nd ed. Philadelphia, WB Saunders, 1995.
Trowbridge HO, Emling RC: Inflammation: A Review of the Process, 4th ed. Carol Stream, IL, Quintessence, 1993.

JOURNAL ARTICLES

Inflammation and Repair

Harlan JM: Neutrophil-mediated vascular injury. Acta Med Scand (Suppl) 715:123, 1987.
Ryan G, Majno G: Acute inflammation: A review. Am J Pathol 83:185, 1987.
Sieggreen M: Healing of physical wounds. Nurs Clin North Am 22:439, 1987.

Lesions from Physical and Chemical Injuries of the Teeth

Abrams RA, Ruff JC: Oral signs and symptoms in the diagnosis of bulimia. J Am Dent Assoc 113:761, 1986.
Brady WF: The anorexia nervosa syndrome. Oral Surg Oral Med Oral Pathol 50:509, 1980.
Cash RC: Bruxism in children: Review of the literature. J Pedodontics 12:107, 1988.
Centerwall BS, Armstrong CW, Funkhouser LS, et al: Erosion of dental enamel among competitive swimmers at a gas-chlorinated swimming pool. Am J Epidemiol 123:641, 1986.
Hanemura H, Houston F, Rylander H, et al: Periodontal status and bruxism. A comparative study of patients with periodontal disease and occlusal parafunctions. J Periodontol 58:173, 1987.
Järvinen V, Meurman JH, Hyvarinen H, et al: Dental erosion and upper gastrointestinal disorders. Oral Surg Oral Med Oral Pathol 64:298, 1988.
Pollman L, Berger F, Pollman S: Age and dental abrasion. Gerodontics 3:94, 1987.

Rawlinson A: Case report. Labial cervical abrasion caused by misuse of dental floss. Dent Health 26:3, 1987.

Richmond NL: Update on dental erosion. Office and home treatment for hypersensitive teeth. J Ind Dent Assoc 66:29, 1987.

Roberts MW, Li SH: Oral findings in anorexia nervosa and bulimia nervosa: A study of 47 cases. J Am Dent Assoc 115:497, 1987.

Rugh JD, Harlan J: Nocturnal bruxism and temporomandibular disorders. Adv Neurol 49:329, 1988.

Simmons MS, Thompson DC: Dental erosion secondary to ethanol-induced emesis. Oral Surg Oral Med Oral Pathol 64:731, 1987.

Physical and Chemical Injuries and Reactive Lesions of the Oral Soft Tissues

Axell T, Hedin C: Epidemiologic study of excessive oral melanin pigmentation with special reference to the influence of tobacco habits. Scand J Dent Res 90:432, 1982.

Buchner A, Hansen LS: Amalgam pigmentation (amalgam tattoo) of the oral mucosa. Oral Surg Oral Med Oral Pathol 49:39, 1980.

Gormley MB, Marshall J, Jarrett W, et al: Thermal trauma: A review of 22 electrical burns of the lip. J Oral Surg 30:531, 1972.

Greer RO, Paulsion TC: Oral tissue alterations associated with the use of smokeless tobacco by teenagers. Oral Surg Oral Med Oral Pathol 56:275, 1983.

Needleman HL, Berkowitz RJ: Electric trauma to the oral tissues of children. J Dent Child 41:19, 1974.

Sist T, Green G: Traumatic neuroma of the oral cavity. Oral Surg Oral Med Oral Pathol 51:394, 1981.

Tipton J: The selection of sun blocking topical agents to protect the skin. Plast Reconstr Surg 62:223, 1978.

Tylenda CA, Roberts MW, Elin RJ, et al: Bulimia nervosa: Its effect on salivary chemistry. J Am Dent Assoc 122:37, 1991.

Welsh RA, Donely C: The association between occlusion and attrition. Aust Orthodont J 12:138, 1992.

Westergaard J, Moe D, Pallesen U, Holmen L: Exaggerated abrasion and erosion of human dental enamel surfaces. A case report. Scand J Dent Res 101:265, 1993.

Physical and Chemical Injuries of Teeth

Järvinen V, Rytomaa I, Meurman JH: Location of dental erosion in a referred population. Caries Res 26:391, 1992.

Mitchell-Lewis DA, Phelan JA, Kelly RB, et al: Identifying oral lesions associated with crack cocaine use. J Am Dent Assoc 125:1104, 1994.

Owens BM, Johnson WW, Schuman NJ: Oral amalgam pigmentation (tattoos): A retrospective study. Quintessence International 23:805, 1992.

Owens BM, Schuman NJ, Johnson WW: Oral amalgam tattoos: A diagnostic study. Compendium 14:210, 1993.

Pullinger AG, Seligman DA: The degree to which attrition characterizes differentiated patient groups of temporomandibular disorders. J Orofacial Pain 7:196, 1993.

Rossie KM, Guggenheimer J: Thermally induced 'nicotine' stomatitis. A case report. Oral Surg Oral Med Oral Pathol 70:597, 1990.

Short term changes a surprise with smokeless tobacco oral lesions. J Am Dent Assoc 122:62, 1991.

Zimmers PL, Gobetti JP: Head and neck lesions commonly found in musicians. J Am Dent Assoc 125:1487, 1994.

Reactive Connective Tissue Hyperplasia

Bonetti F, Pelosi G, Martignoni G, et al: Peripheral giant cell granuloma: Evidence for osteoclastic differentiation. Oral Surg Oral Med Oral Pathol 70:471, 1990.

Brown RS, Sein P, Corco R, et al: Nitrendipine-induced gingival hyperplasia: First case report. Oral Surg Oral Med Oral Pathol 70:593, 1990.

Daley TD, Nartey NO, Wysocki GP: Pregnancy tumor: An analysis. Oral Surg Oral Med Oral Pathol 72:196, 1991.

Daley T, Wysocki G, Day C: Clinical and pharmacologic correlations in cyclosporine-induced gingival hyperplasia. Oral Surg Oral Med Oral Pathol 62:417, 1986.

Gould A, Escobar V: Symmetrical gingival fibromatosis. Oral Surg Oral Med Oral Pathol 51:62, 1981.

Keith D: Side-effects of diphenylhydantosis: A review. J Oral Surg 36:206, 1978.

Zain RB, Fei YJ: Fibrous lesions of the gingiva: A histopathologic analysis of 204 cases. Oral Surg Oral Med Oral Pathol 70:466, 1990.

Periapical Inflammation and Radicular Cyst

Harris EF, Butler MI: Patterns of incisor root resorption before and after orthodontic correction in cases
    with anterior open bites. Am J Orthod Dentofacial Orthop 101:112, 1992.
Harris EF, Robinson QC, Woods MA: An analysis of causes of apical root resorption in patients not treated
    orthodontically. Quintessence International 24:417, 1993.

REVIEW QUESTIONS

1. The initial response of the body to injury is always the process of
    (A) Immunity
    (B) Inflammation
    (C) Repair
    (D) Hyperplasia

2. What type of inflammation occurs if the injury is minimal and brief and the source
    is removed from the tissue?
    (A) Fatal
    (B) Acute
    (C) Chronic
    (D) Subacute

3. The first microscopic event of the inflammatory response involving the microcircu-
    lation is
    (A) Dilation
    (B) Increased permeability
    (C) Formation of exudate
    (D) Constriction

4. Which one of the following is an example of chronic inflammation?
    (A) Necrotizing sialometaplasia
    (B) Periapical granuloma
    (C) Acute necrotizing ulcerative gingivitis (ANUG)
    (D) Aspirin burn

5. The directed movement of white blood cells to the area of injury is called
    (A) Pavementing
    (B) Margination
    (C) Phagocytosis
    (D) Chemotaxis

6. Which cells dominate in chronic inflammation?
    (A) Neutrophils
    (B) Macrophages and lymphocytes
    (C) Neutrophils and macrophages
    (D) Neutrophils and lymphocytes

7. The macrophage has many functions. Which is NOT a function of the macro-
    phage?
    (A) Phagocytosis
    (B) Removal of large foreign matter
    (C) Removal of inhaled particles
    (D) Formation of antibodies

8. What term is used to describe blood plasma and proteins leaving the blood vessels and entering the surrounding tissues during inflammation?
   (A) Hyperemia
   (B) Exudate
   (C) Margination
   (D) Erythema

9. The process of phagocytosis directly involves the
   (A) Ingestion of foreign substances by white blood cells
   (B) Plasma fluids and proteins entering the surrounding tissues
   (C) White blood cells displaced to the blood vessel walls
   (D) White blood cells attaching to the blood vessel walls

10. The neutrophil or polymorphonuclear leukocyte is a cell that
    (A) Is derived from the precursor red blood cell
    (B) Contains lysosomal enzymes
    (C) Has an agranular cytoplasm
    (D) Is produced only in infancy

11. During inflammation the second type of white blood cell to emigrate from the blood vessel into the injured tissue is the
    (A) Neutrophil
    (B) Red blood cell
    (C) Lymphocyte
    (D) Monocyte

12. Complement mediates the inflammatory process by
    (A) Decreasing vascular permeability
    (B) Releasing the neutrophil's histamine granules
    (C) Causing cytolysis
    (D) Decreasing phagocytosis

13. Granulation tissue can be described as
    (A) Immature connective tissue
    (B) Exudate
    (C) Keloid
    (D) Healing by tertiary intention

14. Enlarged lymph nodes noted during systemic involvement with inflammation are
    (A) Termed leukocytosis
    (B) Regulated by the hypothalamus
    (C) Due to changes in their lymphocytes
    (D) Palpated along blood vessel drainage routes

15. Which statement concerning repair in the body is TRUE?
    (A) Repair can be completed with the injurious agents present
    (B) Functioning cells and tissue components are always replaced by functioning scar tissue
    (C) Repair is the body's final defense mechanism
    (D) Replacement by live cells and new tissue components is a perfect process

16. It is important for the clot to remain in place during repair because it
    (A) Later becomes granulation tissue
    (B) Serves as a guide for migrating epithelial cells
    (C) Acts as a scaffold for cellular emigration
    (D) Remodels later to become scar tissue

17. Healing by secondary intention refers to healing of an injury when there is
    (A) An incision with clean edges joined by sutures
    (B) Formation of only a small clot
    (C) Increased formation of granulation tissue
    (D) Decreased formation of scar tissue

18. An increase in the size of an organ or tissue resulting from an increase in the number of its cells is termed
    (A) Hyperemia
    (B) Hyperplasia
    (C) Inflammation
    (D) Hypertrophy

19. Normal bone tissue repair can be interrupted by
    (A) Removal of osteoblast-producing tissues
    (B) Decreased movement of bone tissue
    (C) Removal of an area of hemorrhage
    (D) Reduction in amount of tissue infection

20. Which one of the following would appear as a pigmented lesion?
    (A) Amalgam tattoo
    (B) Traumatic ulcer
    (C) Frictional keratosis
    (D) Aspirin burn

21. Which statement is FALSE?
    (A) Attrition is the wearing away of tooth structure during mastication
    (B) Bruxism is the same as mastication
    (C) Erosion is the loss of tooth structure resulting from chemical action
    (D) Abrasion is due to a mechanical, repetitive habit

22. Loss of tooth structure associated with bulimia is due to
    (A) Attrition
    (B) Erosion
    (C) Bruxism
    (D) Abrasion

23. An aspirin burn
    (A) Occurs as a result of an overdose of aspirin
    (B) Is usually painless
    (C) Results from a misuse of aspirin
    (D) Usually takes a few weeks to heal

24. Your patient presents with a generalized white appearance of the palate. Tiny red dots may be seen surrounded by a thickened white to gray area. Overall the palate appears cracked. You may suspect
    (A) Papillary hyperplasia of the palate
    (B) Nicotine stomatitis
    (C) An aspirin burn
    (D) Necrotizing sialometaplasia

25. The primary and most common cause of a mucocele is
    (A) Inflammation
    (B) Tumor formation
    (C) Severing of or trauma to a minor salivary gland duct
    (D) Obstruction of a salivary gland duct

26. A ranula is located on the
    (A) Lower lip
    (B) Buccal mucosa
    (C) Retromolar area
    (D) Floor of the mouth

27. Which one of the following would not occur on the gingiva?
    (A) Irritation fibroma
    (B) Pyogenic granuloma
    (C) Giant cell granuloma
    (D) Epulis fissuratum

28. Generalized loss of tooth structure primarily on the lingual surfaces of teeth is associated with
    (A) Erosion
    (B) Attrition
    (C) Abrasion
    (D) Bruxism

29. External tooth resorption occurs as a result of
    (A) Caries
    (B) Salivary gland dysfunction
    (C) Chronic inflammation
    (D) Medication

30. Which one of the following is considered to be the most likely cause of necrotizing sialometaplasia?
    (A) Blocked salivary gland ducts
    (B) Radiation therapy
    (C) Loss of blood supply
    (D) A sialolith

31. The most common site for a mucocele to occur is the
    (A) Floor of the mouth
    (B) Lower lip
    (C) Buccal mucosa
    (D) Retromolar area

32. The peripheral giant cell granuloma occurs on the
    (A) Gingiva
    (B) Hard palate
    (C) Buccal mucosa
    (D) Floor of the mouth

33. A sialolith is
    (A) Chronic inflammation of a salivary gland
    (B) Acute inflammation of a salivary gland
    (C) A pooling of saliva in the connective tissue
    (D) A salivary gland stone

34. Which statement is FALSE?
    (A) A periapical cyst develops from a periapical granuloma
    (B) A periapical abscess always causes periapical changes
    (C) A periapical granuloma is a circumscribed area of chronically inflamed tissue
    (D) A periapical cyst is also a radicular cyst

35. Epulis fissuratum results from irritation caused by
    (A) The denture flange
    (B) Denture adhesive
    (C) Poor suction from the denture in the palatal vault
    (D) An allergic reaction to the acrylic in the denture

36. Which statement is TRUE?
    (A) A traumatic neuroma is never painful
    (B) Necrotizing sialometaplasia is considered a denture-related lesion
    (C) Chronic hyperplastic pulpitis is the same as gingival hyperplasia
    (D) Gingival hyperplasia may be caused by medication

37. Loss of tooth structure caused by chemical action describes
    (A) Abrasion
    (B) Drug allergy
    (C) Erosion
    (D) Attrition

38. One of the clinical features of this type of cyst is that when the pulp is tested, the tooth involved is *not* vital. It is probably
    (A) Residual
    (B) Radicular
    (C) Dentigerous
    (D) Dermoid

39. Which cyst results from extracting a tooth without removing the cystic sac?
    (A) Radicular
    (B) Primordial
    (C) Residual
    (D) Periodontal

40. The most common cause of the radicular cyst is
    (A) Deep restorations without a base
    (B) Caries
    (C) Occlusal trauma
    (D) Toothbrush abrasion at the cementoenamel junction

41. The wearing away of tooth structure through an abnormal mechanical action defines
    (A) Attrition
    (B) Abrasion
    (C) Erosion
    (D) Gemination

42. Which one of the following is not associated with the etiologic factors for attrition?
    (A) Toothpaste
    (B) Bruxism
    (C) Mastication
    (D) Diet

43. Heavy plaque and calculus, mouth breather, orthodontic appliances, and overhanging restorations best describe some of the etiologic factors for
    (A) Phenytoin (Dilantin) hyperplasia
    (B) A reaction from nifedipine (Procardia)
    (C) Irritation fibromatosis
    (D) Chemical fibromatosis

44. The giant cell granuloma
    (A) May occur on the tongue
    (B) May present as a multilocular radiolucency
    (C) Is histologically the same as a pyogenic granuloma
    (D) Occurs primarily in men older than 60 years of age

45. During examination of the dentition, the dental hygienist notes the presence of active wear facets. This indicates that the patient is
    (A) A bruxer
    (B) Bulimic
    (C) A vegetarian
    (D) Lip biting

46. A patient presents with loss of tooth structure on the labial surfaces of the anterior teeth and reports a high concentration of acidic foods in the diet. You would most likely suspect
    (A) Abrasion
    (B) Erosion
    (C) Bruxism
    (D) Attrition

47. The amalgam tattoo represents amalgam particles in the tissue and is most commonly observed in the oral cavity on the
    (A) Lateral borders of the tongue
    (B) Anterior palate near the rugae
    (C) Floor of the mouth
    (D) Posterior gingiva and edentulous ridge

3

Immunity

MARGARET J. FEHRENBACH

ULLA E. LEMBORN

JOAN A. PHELAN

Objectives

After studying this chapter, the student should be able to:

1. Define each of the words in the vocabulary list for this chapter.
2. Describe the primary difference between the immune response and the inflammatory response.
3. List the two main types of lymphocytes and their origins.
4. List three activities of macrophages.
5. Describe, using the cells involved, the difference between the humoral immune response and the cell-mediated immune response.
6. Describe the difference between active and passive immunity.
7. Give one example of active immunity, and give one example of passive immunity.
8. List and describe four types of hypersensitivity reactions, and give an example of each.
9. Define autoimmunity, and describe how it results in disease.
10. Define immunodeficiency, and describe how it results in disease.
11. Describe and contrast the clinical features of each of the three types of aphthous ulcers.
12. List three systemic diseases associated with aphthous ulcers.
13. Describe and compare the clinical features of urticaria, angioedema, contact mucositis, fixed drug eruption, and erythema multiforme.
14. Describe the clinical and histologic features of lichen planus.
15. List the triad of systemic signs that compose Reiter's syndrome, and describe the oral lesions that occur in this syndrome.
16. Name the three diseases that are traditionally included in the classification of histiocytosis X. State the range of ages affected and the oral manifestations, if any, and the prognosis of each disease. Name the two cells that characterize these diseases histologically.

17. Describe the oral manifestations of each of the following autoimmune diseases:
    Sjögren's syndrome
    Lupus erythematosus
    Pemphigus vulgaris
    Cicatricial pemphigoid
    Behçet's syndrome
18. Describe the clinical features of desquamative gingivitis, and list three diseases in which it may occur.
19. Describe the components of Behçet's syndrome.
20. Describe how infection occurs and the factors involved.
21. Describe the mechanism that allows opportunistic infection to develop.
22. For each of the following infectious diseases, name the organism causing it; list the route or routes of transmission of the organism and the oral manifestations of the disease; and describe how the diagnosis is made:
    Tuberculosis
    Actinomycosis
    Syphilis (primary, secondary, tertiary)
    Verruca vulgaris
    Condyloma acuminatum
    Primary herpetic gingivostomatitis
23. List and describe four forms of oral candidiasis.
24. List two examples of opportunistic infections that can occur in the oral cavity.
25. Describe the clinical features of herpes labialis.
26. Describe the clinical features of intraoral herpes simplex infection, and compare them with the clinical features of minor aphthous ulcers.
27. Describe the clinical characteristics of herpes zoster when it affects the facial area and oral cavity.
28. List two oral infectious diseases for which a cytologic smear may be helpful to the diagnosis.
29. List the four diseases associated with the Epstein-Barr virus that occur in the oral region.

Vocabulary

Acantholysis (ăk″kan-thol′ĭ-sis)   Dissolution of the intercellular bridges of the prickle cell layer of the epithelium

Allergy (al′er-je)   A hypersensitive state acquired through exposure to a particular allergen; re-exposure to the same allergen elicits an exaggerated reaction

Anaphylaxis (an″ah-fĭ-lak′sis)   A type of hypersensitivity or allergic reaction in which the exaggerated immunologic reaction results from the release of vasoactive substances such as histamine; the reaction occurs on re-exposure to a foreign protein or other substance after sensitization

Antibody (an′tĭ-bod″e)   A protein molecule, also called an immunoglobulin, that is produced by plasma cells and reacts with a specific antigen

Antigen (an′tĭ-jen)   Any substance able to induce a specific immune response

Autoantibody (aw″to-an′tĭ-bod″e)   An antibody that reacts against an antigenic constituent of the person's own tissues

Autoimmune disease (aw″to-ĭ-mun′dĭ-zēz′)   A disease characterized by tissue injury caused by a humoral or cell-mediated immune response against constituents of the body's own tissues

B lymphocyte (B lim′fo-sīt)   A lymphocyte, also called a B cell, that matures without passing through the thymus and matures into plasma cells that produce antibodies

Cell-mediated immunity (sel me′de-a″ted ĭ-mu′nĭ-te)   Immunity in which the predominant role is played by T lymphocytes

Granuloma (gran″u-lo′mah)   A tumor-like mass of inflammatory tissue consisting of a central collection of macrophages, often with multinucleated giant cells, surrounded by lymphocytes

Granulomatous disease (gran″u-lom′ah-tus dĭ-zēz′)   A disease characterized by the formation of granulomas

Humoral immunity (hu′mor-l ĭ-mu′-nĭ-te)   Immunity in which antibodies play the predominant role

Hypersensitivity (hi″per-sen″sĭ-tiv′ĭ-te)   A state of altered reactivity in which the body reacts to a foreign agent with an exaggerated immune response

Immune complex (ĭ-mūn′ kom′pleks)   A combination of antibody and antigen

Immunodeficiency (ĭm″u-no-dĕ-fish′en-se)   A deficiency of the immune response resulting from hypoactivity or decreased numbers of lymphoid cells

Immunoglobulin (ĭm″u-no-glob′u-lin)   A protein, also called an antibody, synthesized by plasma cells in response to a specific antigen

LE cell   A cell that is a characteristic of lupus erythematosus and other autoimmune diseases; it is a mature neutrophil that has phagocytized a spherical inclusion derived from another neutrophil

Lymphoid tissue (lim′foid tish′u)   Tissue composed of lymphocytes supported by a meshwork of connective tissue

Macrophage (mak′ro-fāj)   A large mononuclear phagocyte derived from monocytes;

macrophages become mobile when stimulated by inflammation and interact with lymphocytes in an immune response

Mucositis (mu″ko-sī′tis) Mucosal inflammation

Natural killer cell (NK cell) A lymphocyte that circulates in the blood and primarily protects against viral infections

Nicolsky's sign (nĭ-kol′skēz sīn) In some bullous diseases, such as pemphigus vulgaris and bullous pemphigus, the superficial epithelium separates easily from the basal layer on exertion of firm, sliding manual pressure *NK Cells*

Opportunistic infection (op″or-tu-nis′tik in-fek′shun) A disease caused by a microorganism that does not ordinarily cause disease but becomes pathogenic under certain circumstances

Parenteral (pah-ren′ter-al) Administered by injection

Pathogenic microorganism (path-o-jen′ik mi″kro-or′gan-izm) A microorganism that causes disease

Rheumatoid factor (roo′mah-toid fak′tor) A protein, immunoglobulin M (IgM), found in serum and detectable on laboratory tests; it is associated with rheumatoid arthritis and other autoimmune diseases

T lymphocyte (T lim′fo-sīt) A lymphocyte that passes through the thymus before migrating to tissues; the T lymphocyte, also called a T cell, is responsible for cell-mediated immunity *Memory*

Thymus (thī′mus) A lymphoid organ situated in the chest; it reaches maximal development at about puberty and then undergoes gradual involution

Whitlow (hwit′lo) An infection involving the distal phalanx of a finger

Xerophthalmia (ze″rof-thal′me-ah) Abnormal dryness of the eyes

Xerostomia (ze″ro-sto′me-ah) Dryness of the mouth caused by decreased salivary flow

---

The acute inflammatory response, which is described in Chapter 2, is a rapid first line of defense against tissue injury and disease-producing microorganisms. The immune response, described in this chapter, occurs after the inflammatory response and is generally necessary for complete recovery. This chapter begins with a description of the immune response and includes both infectious diseases and those oral diseases that result from harmful effects of the immune response. Surveillance against neoplastic cells also requires the immune response. The neoplastic process is described in Chapter 5.

THE IMMUNE RESPONSE

The immune response, like the inflammatory response, defends the body against injury, particularly from foreign substances like microorganisms. The immune response differs from the inflammatory response in that it has the capacity to remember and responds more quickly to a foreign substance that enters the body a second time. It works amid the background of an already activated inflammatory response and a working repair process and involves a complex network of white blood cells, primarily lymphocytes, and their products.

ANTIGENS

Antigens are the foreign substances against which the immune system defends the body. These substances are mainly proteins and are often microorganisms and their toxins. Transformed human cells, such as tumor cells or cells infected by viruses, can be antigens. Human tissue, as in the case of an organ transplant, tissue graft, or incompatible blood transfusion, can be an antigen. In diseases called **autoimmune diseases,** parts of an individual's own body become antigens.

CELLS INVOLVED IN THE IMMUNE RESPONSE

The cells involved in the immune response are the following:

- B lymphocytes (plasma cells)
- T lymphocytes
- Macrophages
- Eosinophils
- Mast cells
- Natural killer (NK) cells

Lymphocytes

The primary white blood cells involved in the immune response are **lymphocytes.** These cells are able to recognize and respond to an antigen. Lymphocytes, like other white blood cells, are derived from a precursor cell called the **stem cell,** which is located in the bone marrow. Lymphocytes constitute 20% to 25% of the white blood cell population. They are antigen-sensitive cells that are long-lived and able to move. Different types of lymphocytes have different functions. The two main types of lymphocytes are called **B lymphocytes** (B cells) and **T lymphocytes** (T cells) (Fig. 3–1). A third type of lymphocyte is called the **natural killer (NK) cell.** This type of lymphocyte is not identified as either a B or a T lymphocyte. NK cells have the ability to destroy cells that they recognize as foreign. They primarily protect against viral infections. Macrophages are also involved in the immune response.

B Lymphocytes

After developing from the stem cell in the bone marrow, the B lymphocyte matures and resides in lymphoid tissue, which is found in lymph nodes and many other body locations. Pharyngeal tonsils are also composed of lymphoid tissue. When lymphocytes are stimulated by an antigen, they travel to the site of injury. There are two main types of B lymphocytes. One type becomes the **plasma cell** when stimulated by antigen. The plasma cells produce the specific antibody needed to fight the antigen. The other type of B lymphocyte is the B memory cell. This type of B lymphocyte retains the memory of previously encountered antigens. In the presence of an antigen, this cell duplicates itself. All the newly formed cells retain the capacity to remember the previously encountered antigen.

Plasma cells produce proteins called **antibodies**. Antibodies, also called **immuno-globulins,** are carried in blood serum. Specific antibodies are produced in response to specific antigens. A diagram of the basic structure of an antibody is illustrated in Figure

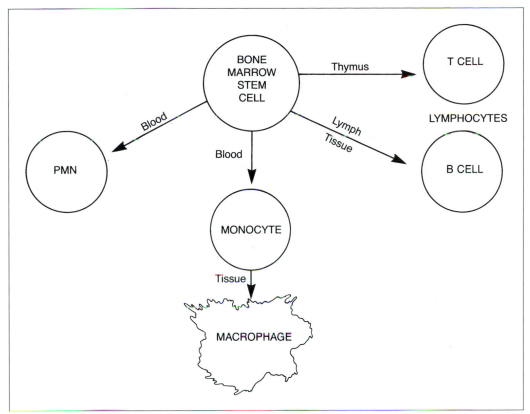

𝑓 i g u r e 3–1   The differentiation of B and T lymphocytes. The primary cell of the immune response is the lymphocyte. The two main types of lymphocytes are the B lymphocyte and the T lymphocyte. Lymphocytes, like other white blood cells, are derived from a stem cell in the bone marrow. PMN = polymorphonuclear leukocytes or neutrophils.

3–2. There are five different types of antibodies produced—IgG (immunoglobulin G), IgM (immunoglobulin M), IgE (immunoglobulin E), IgA (immunoglobulin A), and IgD (immunoglobulin D). They all have the same basic structure; however, in each type of antibody, this structure is arranged differently. The different antibodies also have different functions. Figure 3–3 illustrates the arrangement of the basic antibody structure in the five types of antibodies.

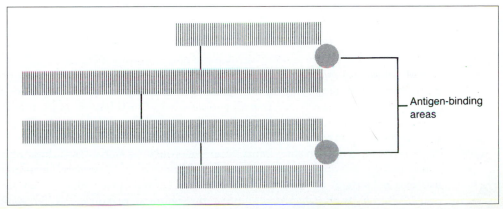

𝑓 i g u r e 3–2   The basic structure of an antibody includes four protein chains and an antigen-binding area.

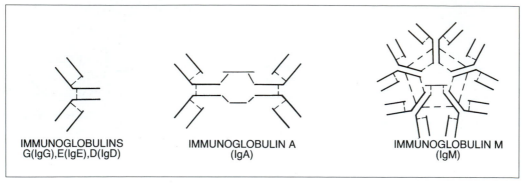

IMMUNOGLOBULINS
G(IgG),E(IgE),D(IgD)

IMMUNOGLOBULIN A
(IgA)

IMMUNOGLOBULIN M
(IgM)

■ *f i g u r e 3–3*   The five types of antibodies have the same basic structure but are arranged differently. This variation in structure allows them to function differently.

Antibodies combine with antigen, forming an **immune complex** called an antigen-
antibody complex. The formation of an antigen-antibody complex renders the antigen
inactive. The level of a specific antibody in the blood is called the **antibody titer**
and can be measured by laboratory tests. This is helpful in the diagnosis of some
infectious diseases.

T Lymphocytes

After they develop from the bone marrow stem cell, the T lymphocytes travel to
the thymus, in which they mature. The thymus is located in the superior mediastinum
between the sternum and the great vessels in the chest and is a major organ of lymphoid
development. It is quite large in infants and shrinks as an individual matures. The T
lymphocytes take their name from this association with the thymus. Different types of
T lymphocytes have different functions. Some are memory cells. Some, called **T-
helper cells,** increase the functioning of the B lymphocytes and enhance the antibody
response (Fig. 3–4). Others, called **T-suppressor cells,** suppress the functioning of the
B lymphocytes and T-killer cells that are active in surveillance against virally infected
cells or tumor cells. Products of lymphocytes are called **lymphokines.** Different
lymphokines have different functions (Table 3–1). They can help in changing monocytes to macrophages. They also inhibit migration of macrophages so that they stay in
the area of injury. They activate macrophages, and they enhance the ability of macrophages to destroy foreign cells. T lymphocytes may inhibit the migration of neutrophils
and stimulate the activity of fibroblasts to enhance repair.

Macrophages

Macrophages are involved in the immune response to an antigen. They are present
in the connective tissue during inflammation (see Chapter 2). Macrophages are active
in phagocytosis of foreign substances and also help the B lymphocytes and T lymphocytes. After phagocytosis of an antigen at the injury site, the macrophages process and
present the antigen to the lymphocytes. This stimulates the lymphocytes to travel from
the lymphoid tissue to the injury site. Macrophages serve as a link between the
inflammatory and immune responses. In addition to phagocytosis, macrophages can
also act as antigen-presenting cells. When activated, macrophages can function in
many different ways, always amplifying the immune response. Unlike lymphocytes,
macrophages do not remember the encountered antigen and need to be reactivated
during each encounter.

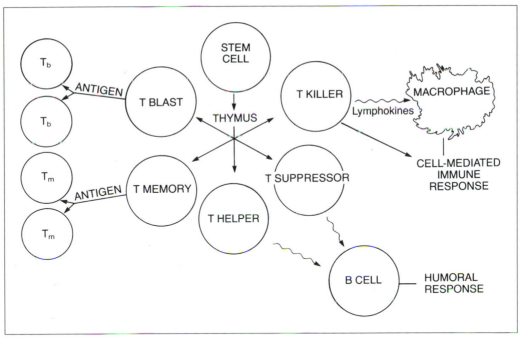

▪ *f* i g u r e 3–4   The various types of T lymphocytes and their involvement in the immune response.

MAJOR DIVISIONS OF THE IMMUNE RESPONSE

The immune response to an antigen can take one of two forms (Fig. 3–5). One form is called the **humoral response,** and the other is called the **cell-mediated response.** The humoral response involves the production of antibodies. The B lymphocytes are the primary cells of the humoral response. The immune system's other main mechanism, the cell-mediated immune response (cell-mediated immunity; CMI), involves lymphocytes working alone (usually T lymphocytes) or assisted by macrophages. Both major responses are regulated by the cell-mediated portion of the immune system, and humoral and cell-mediated responses are interrelated.

MEMORY AND IMMUNITY

Memory is an important function of the immune system. The inflammatory response is not capable of memory; however, some lymphocytes retain the memory of

TABLE 3–1 Lymphokines and Their Functions During the Immune Response	
Lymphokine	**Function**
Interleukins	Stimulation of white blood cell population growth in addition to other functions
Leukocyte-derived chemotactic factor (CTX)	Moves macrophages to the site of injury
Migration inhibitory factor (MIF)	Retains or inhibits macrophages
Macrophage-activating factor (MAF)	Activates macrophages to produce and secrete lysosomal enzymes
Lymphotoxin (LT)	Destruction of fibroblasts
Interferons	Antiviral activities in addition to other functions

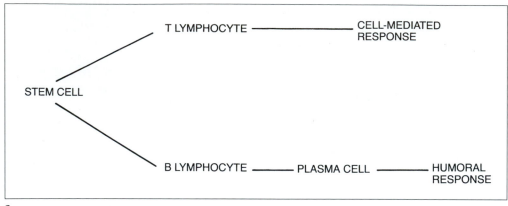

▪ *f i g u r e* **3-5**   The major divisions of the immune response.

an antigen after an initial encounter. For this reason, the immune response to that antigen is much faster the next time it enters the body. The increased responsiveness that results from the retained memory of an already encountered antigen is called **immunity**. Subsequent responses of the immune system to an antigen are faster and stronger.

TYPES OF IMMUNITY

Active Immunity

There are two types of immunity, active and passive. **Active immunity** can occur naturally or can be acquired. It occurs naturally when a disease is caused by a microorganism. Protection against further attack by that microorganism is conferred to the individual if the body recovers from the disease. A less risky way of achieving active immunity is by an acquired or artificial means. A person is injected with or ingests either altered pathogenic microorganisms or products of those microorganisms. This is called a **vaccine,** and the process is called **vaccination.** When the pathogenic microorganism is encountered after vaccination, the immune system produces a stronger, faster response and prevents development of the disease. This production of acquired immunity is called **immunization.** Immunization lowers the risk of an antigen causing disease because it safely prepares the immune system to fight future attacks by the disease-causing microorganism. In some cases more than one exposure to the antigen is needed to ensure adequate immunity. A repeated exposure is called a **booster.** Immunization by vaccination is used to protect children and adults against many diseases. Dental personnel should be vaccinated against the hepatitis B virus because of their high risk of occupational exposure to that virus.

Passive Immunity

Using antibodies produced by another person to protect an individual against infectious disease is called **passive immunity.** This type of immunity can occur naturally, or it can be acquired. Natural passive immunity occurs when antibodies from a mother pass through the placenta to the developing fetus. These antibodies protect a newborn infant from disease until the immune system matures. Passive immunity can be acquired through an injection of antibodies against a microorganism to which the person has not previously developed antibodies. Acquired passive immunity is used to confer immediate protection against the disease caused by that microorganism. These antibodies are collected from individuals who have already had the disease and have naturally produced antibodies to the disease-causing microorganism. This type of passive immunity is short-lived but can act immediately. It is used because the unprepared immune system of an individual takes longer to produce antibodies, and in the meantime the disease may develop. Acquired passive immunity, using hepatitis B immunoglobulin (HBIg), is provided to dental personnel following needle-stick accidents with a used needle or puncture wounds from other instruments if they do not have immunity to hepatitis B.

IMMUNOPATHOLOGY

Immunopathology is the study of immune reactions involved in disease. The immune response helps defend the body against disease-producing antigens, but it can also malfunction and cause tissue damage. Immunopathology includes those diseases caused by malfunctioning of the immune system. Hypersensitivity reactions and autoimmune diseases are examples of conditions in which damage is caused by the immune response.

Hypersensitivity

Hypersensitivity reactions are also called **allergic reactions** and comprise the same types of reactions that occur when the immune response is fighting microorganisms and protecting the body against disease. However, hypersensitivity reactions are exaggerated responses, and tissue destruction occurs as a result of the immune response. There are four main types of hypersensitivity reactions, and they are classified by the nature of the immune response that causes the disease (Table 3–2).

Type I Hypersensitivity (Anaphylaxis)

Type I hypersensitivity is a reaction that occurs immediately (within minutes) after exposure to a previously encountered antigen (e.g., penicillin). Plasma cells produce IgE as a response to the antigen. IgE causes mast cells to release their granules containing histamine, which results in increased dilation and permeability of blood vessels and constricting smooth muscle in the bronchioles of the lungs. This type of hypersensitivity, also called **anaphylaxis**, can be life threatening because the individual may not be able to breathe as a result of the tissue swelling and constriction of the bronchioles.

TABLE 3–2 Hypersensitivity Reactions	
Type of Reaction	**Examples**
Type I (anaphylactic type)	Hay fever
	Anaphylaxis
	Asthma
Type II (cytotoxic type)	Autoimmune hemolytic anemia
Type III (immune complex type)	Autoimmune disease
Type IV (cell-mediated type)	Granulomatous disease, e.g., tuberculosis

Type II Hypersensitivity

In **type II hypersensitivity,** antibody combines with an antigen bound to the surface of tissue cells. Activated complement components in blood participate in this type of hypersensitivity reaction. The result is the destruction of the tissue that has the antigen on the surface of its cells. This type of reaction occurs in incompatible blood transfusions and in **Rhesus incompatibility** (Rh incompatibility). In this condition, the mother's antibodies cross the placenta and destroy the newborn's red blood cells.

Type III Hypersensitivity — Serum Sickness (Penicillin etc.)

In **type III hypersensitivity,** immune complexes are formed between microorganisms and antibody in the circulating blood. The complexes leave the blood and are deposited in various body tissues or in a localized area. In either case the deposition results in the initiation of an acute inflammatory response. Neutrophils are attracted to the tissues in which the complexes have been deposited. As a result of phagocytosis and death of the neutrophils, lysosomal enzymes are released, causing tissue destruction. This type of hypersensitivity occurs in autoimmune diseases such as systemic lupus erythematosus (discussed later).

Type IV Hypersensitivity

Type IV hypersensitivity, also called **delayed hypersensitivity,** involves a cell-mediated immune response rather than a humoral (antibody) response. T lymphocytes that have previously been introduced to an antigen cause damage to the tissue cells themselves or they recruit other cells. This type of hypersensitivity reaction is put to use in the tuberculin test, called a PPD (discussed later), used to diagnose tuberculosis. A skin reaction occurs if the individual tested has previously been exposed to the organism that causes tuberculosis. This type of hypersensitivity is responsible for the rejection of tissue grafts and transplanted organs.

Hypersensitivity to Drugs

Know*

Drugs can act as antigens and cause an immunologically induced inflammatory response. Many factors influence the risk of an allergic (hypersensitivity) reaction to a drug. The route of administration influences how the reaction will be manifested and the severity of the reaction. Topical administration may cause a greater number of reactions than oral and parenteral (administered by injection) routes of administration. However, when a reaction occurs following parenteral administration, it may be more widespread and severe because the allergen (the antigen eliciting the response) can be carried quickly to many parts of the body in the blood stream. The presence of infection may increase the risk of an allergic reaction. Patients with multiple allergies are more likely to have allergic reactions to drugs, and patients with autoimmune diseases (e.g., lupus erythematosus) commonly have adverse reactions to medication. Children are less likely than adults to have an allergic reaction to a drug.

Drugs can cause any of the previously described hypersensitivity reactions. Type I allergy to a drug includes anaphylaxis, urticaria, and angioedema. A systemic anaphylactic reaction is more likely to occur with an injected drug but can also occur with a drug administered orally. Systemic anaphylaxis can be fatal. For example, penicillin can cause a systemic anaphylactic reaction in approximately 1 in 10,000 patients. It causes about 300 deaths a year in the United States, though the overall toxicity of penicillin in all patients is low.

Type II allergy involves IgG and IgM antibodies and is complement dependent.

The antigen combines with antibody and complement and becomes attached to a particular target cell, usually a circulating red blood cell. This causes the cell to be destroyed and results in a type of anemia called **hemolytic anemia.**

Type III allergy results in a complement-dependent vasculitis, producing inflammation and destruction of the blood vessel wall. A classic example is **serum sickness.** This name was given to a reaction that occurred frequently when patients were given large amounts of horse antitoxin serum to provide passive immunity in the treatment of diphtheria and tetanus. This reaction can occur in response to other foreign agents as well. Penicillin is the single most common cause of serum sickness. However, other drugs, such as barbiturates, can cause this reaction as well. The symptoms of serum sickness include fever, painful swelling of the joints (arthritis), renal disturbance or failure, edema around the eyes, carditis, and skin lesions.

Drugs can also cause a type IV hypersensitivity reaction. This cell-mediated allergic reaction can occur in response to topically applied substances and can produce contact dermatitis and mucositis.

Autoimmune Diseases

The immune system learns early to differentiate between itself and foreign substances. This recognition and the nonresponsiveness of the immune system to the body's own cells and tissues is called **immunologic tolerance.** In **autoimmune diseases,** also called **connective tissue diseases,** certain body cells are no longer tolerated, and the immune system treats them as antigens. An autoimmune disease may involve a single cell type or a single organ or may be even more extensive, involving multiple organs. Tissues and even entire organs may be damaged. Genetic factors may play a role in the predisposition of an individual to autoimmune disease, and viral infection may be involved. Several autoimmune diseases have oral manifestations, which are described later in this chapter.

Immunodeficiency

Immunodeficiency is a type of immunopathologic condition that involves a deficiency in number, function, or interrelationships of the involved white blood cells and their products. This condition may be congenital (present at birth) or acquired (develops after birth). Immunodeficiency may be genetically inherited or can be caused by numerous other factors. When a person's immune system is not functioning adequately, opportunistic infections and tumors may develop. Acquired immunodeficiency syndrome (AIDS), which is discussed in Chapter 7, is an example of an immunodeficiency that has numerous oral manifestations.

ORAL DISEASES WITH IMMUNOLOGIC PATHOGENESIS

Aphthous Ulcers

Aphthous ulcers, also known as **canker sores** or **aphthous stomatitis,** are painful oral ulcers for which the cause remains unclear. They frequently recur in episodes. There are three forms of recurrent aphthous ulceration: minor, major, and herpetiform.

The three forms differ in the size and duration of the ulcers. Aphthous ulcers are the more common ulcers in the oral cavity, occurring in about 20% of the general population. However, there is a dramatic variation in occurrence, from as high as 57% of a professional school population to 5% of patients studied in a large inner-city hospital. The first episode of these ulcers usually occurs in adolescence, and they are somewhat more common in females than in males. The clinical appearance and location are important in establishing the diagnosis.

Trauma is the most commonly reported precipitating factor in the development of aphthous ulcers. They are often reported to occur following trauma to the oral mucosa during dental procedures—for example, in the area of film placement or at the site of injection of local anesthetics. Some patients may experience aphthous ulcers as a result of manipulation of oral tissues during dental hygiene treatment. Emotional stress has also been suggested as a contributing factor. Some patients associate the initiation of aphthous ulcers with eating certain foods such as citrus fruits. However, it is possible that patients perceive these foods as causative because of the sensitivity of the ulcers to foods with a high acid content. The recurrence of aphthous ulcers has been associated with menstruation, whereas pregnancy has been found to produce a decrease in the episodes. These ulcers occur in association with certain systemic diseases, such as

- Behçet's syndrome
- Crohn's disease
- Ulcerative colitis
- Cyclic neutropenia
- Sprue (gluten intolerance)
- Intestinal lymphoma

There is substantial evidence that aphthous ulcers have an immunologic pathogenesis. Patients in whom aphthous ulcers develop have slightly elevated levels of antibodies to oral mucous membranes. Histologically, an infiltrate of lymphocytes is present in the lesion, suggesting that cell-mediated immunity may be important in development of the ulcers. The infiltrate contains primarily T-helper cells in the prodromal stage, T-cytotoxic cells in the ulcerative phase, and T-helper cells again in the healing stage. The T-cytotoxic cells are probably responsible for the ulceration. However, the specific antigen they are responding to has not yet been identified.

Minor Aphthous Ulcers

Minor aphthous ulcers are the most commonly occurring type. They appear as discrete, round to oval ulcers that are up to 1 cm in diameter and are surfaced by a yellowish-white fibrin covering surrounded by a halo of erythema (Fig. 3–6; Color Plate 27). The ulcers occur on the movable mucosa of the oral cavity (the mucosa not covering bone) and occasionally extend onto the gingiva. They occur on the labial and buccal mucosa, the maxillary and mandibular vestibular mucosa, the ventral and lateral borders of the tongue, and the soft palate and oropharynx. Minor aphthous ulcers are more common in the anterior part than the posterior part of the mouth. The ulcers often have a prodromal period of 1 to 2 days, which is characterized by a burning sensation or soreness in the area in which the ulcer will form. Aphthous ulcers are exquisitely painful. Single or multiple lesions may be present. The ulcers heal spontaneously in 7 to 10 days.

Major Aphthous Ulcers

Major aphthous ulcers (Sutton's disease, periadenitis mucosa necrotica recurrens) are larger than 1 cm in diameter and are deeper and last longer than minor aphthous

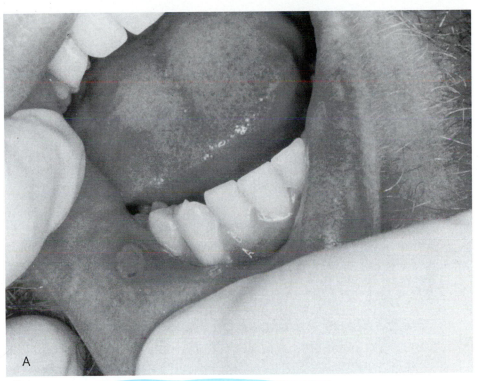

A

figure 3–6   *A*, Example of a minor aphthous ulcer.

Illustration continued on following page

ulcers (Fig. 3–7; Color Plate 28). They are also painful and often occur in the posterior part of the mouth. Major aphthous ulcers may require biopsy for diagnosis to rule out other causes of ulceration. They can take several weeks to heal and frequently result in scarring. Ulcers that resemble major apthous ulcers have been reported to occur in association with human immunodeficiency virus (HIV) infection and AIDS (see Chapter 7).

looks like squamous cell carcinoma 6wks.

Herpetiform Aphthous Ulcers

Herpetiform aphthous ulcers are very tiny (1 to 2 mm) (Fig. 3–8). They are called herpetiform because they resemble ulcers caused by the herpes simplex virus. They are painful, may develop anywhere in the oral cavity, and generally occur in groups.

not caused by virus – vesicles are herpetic
– history – no grapes, a bubble, fluid filled ulcers do not, herpetic do.

Diagnosis

The diagnosis of minor aphthous ulcers is made on the basis of their distinctive clinical appearance, the location of the lesions, and a complete patient history. Table 3–3 summarizes the clinical features of each of the three types of aphthous ulcers. Laboratory results are not specific for any form of aphthous ulcer.

The location of the ulcers is important in differentiating between recurrent aphthous ulcers and recurrent intraoral ulceration caused by the herpes simplex virus (Table 3–4). When they occur intraorally, ulcers resulting from the herpes simplex virus appear on mucosa fixed to bone, that is, the palate and gingiva.

A biopsy is frequently necessary for diagnosing major aphthous ulcers because they may clinically resemble squamous cell carcinoma or deep fungal infections.

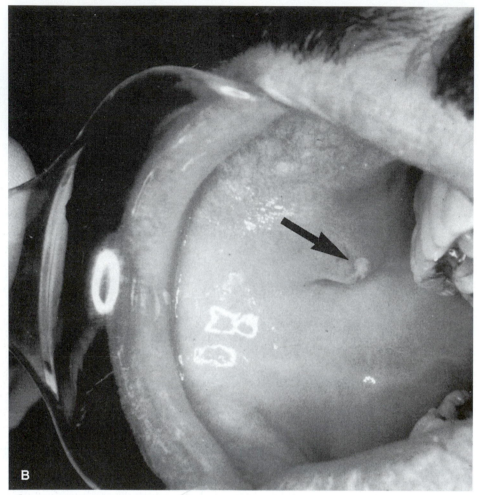

■ f i g u r e 3–6   *Continued B*, Minor aphthous ulcer *(arrow)* on the buccal mucosa on the papilla of Stenson's duct.

Herpetiform aphthous ulcers may be difficult to distinguish clinically from primary herpetic gingivostomatitis. However, there are no systemic signs or symptoms as in primary herpes simplex infection. Herpetiform aphthous ulcers have been reported to respond to topical application of liquid tetracycline. This response may be helpful in confirming the diagnosis of herpetiform aphthous ulcers because true herpes simplex ulceration does not respond to this treatment.

Treatment

The local application of topical steroids is helpful in the treatment of minor aphthous ulcers. Topical steroids are most effective when applied during the prodromal period. Occasionally, systemic steroids may be necessary for managing patients with major aphthous ulcers. Topical application of liquid tetracycline is also helpful, particularly in herpetiform ulceration for which the diagnosis is not clear. The use of topical steroids is contraindicated for viral ulcers, and therefore accurate diagnosis is important. Topical anesthetics can be helpful in decreasing the pain of aphthous ulcers.

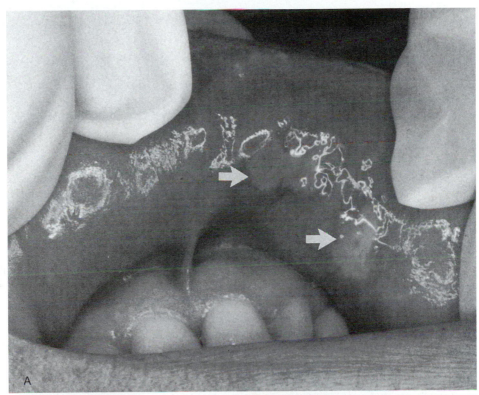

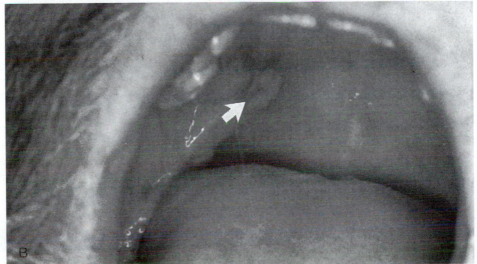

▪ *f i g u r e* 3–7   *A* and *B,* Two examples of major aphthous ulcers *(arrows).*

Illustration continued on following page

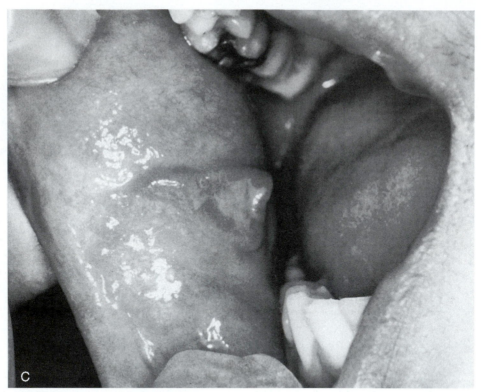

ƒ i g u r e 3–7   *Continued C,* Major aphthous ulcer on the buccal mucosa.

Urticaria and Angioedema

Urticaria and angioedema are similar lesions. **Urticaria,** also called **hives** (Fig. 3–9) appears as multiple areas of well-demarcated swelling of the skin usually accompanied by itching (pruritus). The lesions are caused by localized areas of vascular permeability in the superficial connective tissue beneath the epithelium. **Angioedema** (Fig. 3–10; Color Plate 6) is a similar lesion that appears as a diffuse swelling of tissue caused by permeability of deeper blood vessels. The skin covering the swelling appears normal, and angioedema is usually not accompanied by itching. Urticaria and angioedema may both occur in acute self-limited episodes. Chronic or recurrent forms may occasionally occur.

In most cases of urticaria and angioedema, the cause cannot be identified. Infection, trauma, emotional stress, and certain systemic diseases have been reported to cause these lesions. Ingested allergens are frequent causes of urticaria.

TABLE 3–3 Clinical Features of the Three Types of Recurrent Aphthous Ulcers			
Feature	**Minor**	**Major**	**Herpetiform**
Size	Small, 3–5 mm	Large, 5–10 mm	Very small, 1–2 mm
Location	Unattached mucosa	Unattached mucosa	Unattached mucosa
Most common area	Anterior	Posterior	Anywhere
Number	1–5	1–10	1–100
Scarring	No	Yes	No
Pain	Yes	Yes	Yes
Appearance	Shallow	Deep	Ulcers coalesce

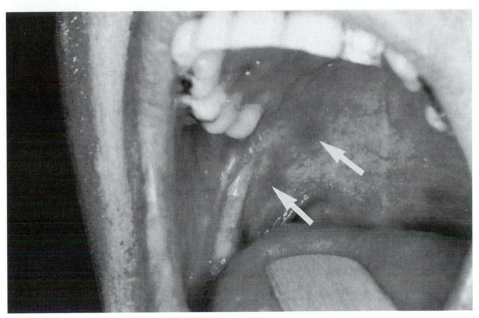

▪ *f i g u r e* 3–8 Herpetiform aphthous ulcers (*arrows*).

Several mechanisms are capable of causing the increased vascular permeability that results in urticaria and angioedema, including the release of the chemical mediator histamine from mast cells stimulated by IgE antibodies (type I hypersensitivity) and the activation of IgG or IgM antibodies along with trauma, causing vascular permeability. Acetylsalicylic acid (aspirin) and nonsteroidal anti-inflammatory drugs such as ibuprofen can produce a nonspecific effect that can cause vascular permeability. There is also a rare hereditary form of angioedema in which there is uncontrolled activation of the complement cascade, resulting in prolonged vascular permeability. *Antihistamine*

The diagnoses of urticaria and angioedema are based on the clinical appearance *Benadryl.* of the lesions and the histories.

Treatment

Avoidance of the causative agent, if identified, is important in managing patients with recurring urticaria and angioedema. Immediate treatment is essential. Antihistaminic drugs are the principal method of treatment. Angioedema involving the larynx and pharynx can cause asphyxiation and therefore may be fatal.

TABLE 3–4 Comparison of the Clinical Features of Recurrent Minor Aphthous Ulcers and Recurrent Herpes Simplex Ulceration

Feature	Aphthous Ulcer	Herpes Simplex Ulceration
Location	Nonkeratinized mucosa	Keratinized mucosa
Number	One to several	Multiple (crops)
Vesicle precedes ulcer	No	Yes
Pain	Yes	Yes
Size	<1 cm	1–2 mm
Borders	Round to oval	Crops of ulcers coalesce to form a large irregular ulcer
Recurrent	Yes	Yes

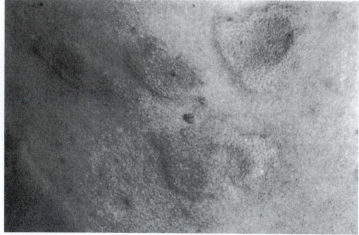

figure 3–9   Urticaria. (From Bork K, Brauninger W: Diagnosis and Therapy of Common Skin Diseases. Philadelphia, WB Saunders, 1988, p 13.)

Contact Mucositis and Dermatitis

Contact mucositis and **dermatitis** are lesions that result from the direct contact of an allergen with the skin or mucosa. The development of these conditions involves cell-mediated immunity and is an example of type IV hypersensitivity. The exact underlying immunologic basis is not always clear.

In contact mucositis, the mucosa becomes erythematous and edematous, often accompanied by burning and pruritus (Fig. 3–11). The mucositis occurs at the point at which the offending agent has contacted the mucosa, giving it a smooth, shiny appearance that is firm to palpation. Small vesicles and ulcers may appear in the affected

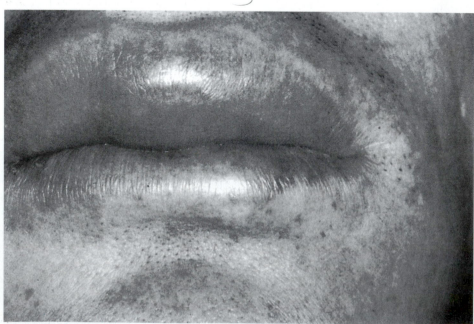

figure 3–10   Angioedema. (Courtesy of Dr. Edward V. Zegarelli.)

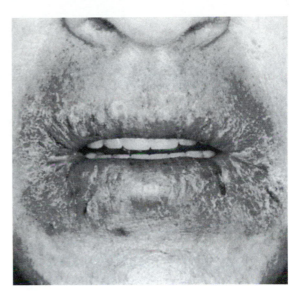

■ **f i g u r e 3–11**
Contact cheilitis. (From Arnold HL, Odom RB,
James W: Andrew's Diseases of the Skin, 8th ed.
Philadelphia, WB Saunders, 1990, p 15.)

areas. In contact dermatitis, the initial lesion may be erythematous, with swelling and vesicles. Later the area becomes encrusted with a scaly, white epidermis.

Topical antibiotics, antihistamines, preservatives in local anesthetics, and components of topical medication are common causes of allergic reactions. Acrylics, metal-based alloys, epoxy resins, and the flavoring agents in dentifrices have all been reported to cause contact mucositis.

Contact dermatitis, particularly that affecting the hands, may occur in response to the materials used in dentistry. Gloves have decreased the incidence of this dermatitis, but gloves and glove powder have also been responsible for contact dermatitis in some individuals.

Treatment

Skin testing for sensitivity to a particular substance can help in confirming the agent that caused the lesion. However, first the substance has to be identified. Topical and systemic corticosteroids may be used in the management of some patients.

Fixed Drug Eruptions

Fixed drug eruptions are lesions that appear in the same site each time a drug is introduced. The lesions generally appear suddenly after a latent period of several days and subside when the drug is discontinued. They appear again when the drug is reintroduced, usually with greater intensity. Clinically, there may be single or multiple slightly raised reddish patches or clusters of macules on the skin or, rarely, the mucous membranes. Pain and pruritus may be associated with these lesions.

The fixed drug eruption is a type of allergic reaction (type III hypersensitivity) in which immune complexes are deposited along the endothelial wall of blood vessels. The ensuing inflammatory reaction causes vasculitis and subsequent damage to the vessel wall, giving rise to erythema and edema of the superficial layers of the skin or mucosa.

Treatment

If possible, the drug causing the reaction should be identified and its use discontinued.

Erythema Multiforme

Erythema multiforme is an acute, self-limited disease that affects the skin and mucous membranes. The cause is not clear, but there is some evidence that it is a hypersensitivity reaction.

Erythema multiforme most commonly occurs in young adults and affects men more commonly than women. The characteristic skin lesion is called a **target, iris,** or **bull's eye lesion** and consists of concentric rings of erythema alternating with normal skin color. The color is darkest at the center of the lesion (Fig. 3–12). The term erythema multiforme refers to the variety of skin lesions that can occur, which range from macules to plaques to bullae. Erythema multiforme can affect the oral cavity either alone or in association with skin lesions. Skin lesions can occur without oral lesions. The oral lesions are usually ulcers (Fig. 3–13; Color Plates 9 and 45). However, erythematous areas may also occur. The ulcers frequently form on the lateral borders of the tongue. Crusted and bleeding lips are frequently seen in erythema multiforme, and gingival involvement is rare. The disease usually has an explosive onset, and systemic symptoms are mild or lacking. The disease may be chronic on occasion, or there may be recurrent acute episodes. The most severe form of erythema multiforme is called Stevens-Johnson syndrome (Fig. 3–13C). Mucosal lesions are more extensive and painful; genital mucosa and the mucosa of the eyes may be involved; and lips are generally encrusted and bloody.

Although the cause of erythema multiforme is not clear, triggering factors can be identified in some cases. Infections such as herpes simplex, tuberculosis, and histoplasmosis have been associated with episodes of erythema multiforme, as have malignant tumors and drugs such as barbiturates and sulfonamides.

Diagnosis

The diagnosis of erythema multiforme is made on the basis of the clinical features and the exclusion of other diseases. The microscopic appearance is nonspecific. Biopsy and histologic examinations are sometimes helpful in excluding other diseases with similar clinical features but more distinctive histologic features.

Treatment and Prognosis

Topical corticosteroids may be helpful in mild cases of erythema multiforme, but systemic corticosteroid treatment is usually needed. Eye lesions in Stevens-Johnson syndrome may lead to scarring and blindness.

Lichen Planus

Lichen planus is a benign, chronic disease affecting the skin and oral mucosa. In some patients this disease may affect both the skin and the oral mucosa. In others either oral mucosa or skin alone may be affected. The lesions have a characteristic pattern of interconnecting lines called **striae,** resembling the pattern of the plant lichen as it grows on rocks and trees.

The classic appearance of lichen planus affecting the oral mucosa is an arrangement of interconnecting white lines and circles (Fig. 3–14; Color Plates 22 and 46). The slender white lines are called **Wickham's striae.** The fundamental lesion is a small papule—a pinhead-sized domed or hemispheric glistening white nodule on the mucosa. The clinical appearance depends on the arrangement of these minute papules and

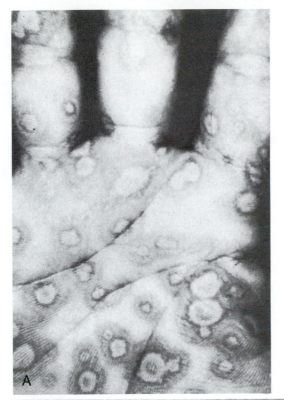

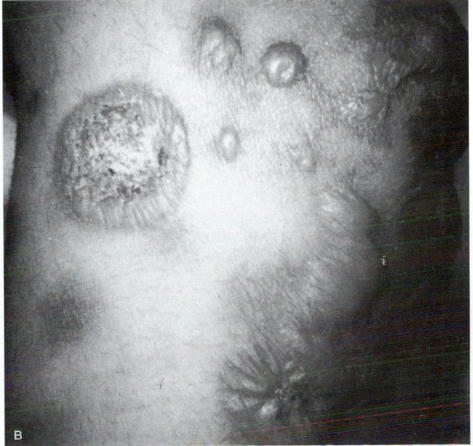

f i g u r e 3–12 Skin lesions of erythema multiforme. *A*, Target lesion. (From Shafer WG, Hine MG, Levy BM: A Textbook of Oral Pathology, 4th ed. Philadelphia, WB Saunders, 1983, p 817.) *B*, Bullae.

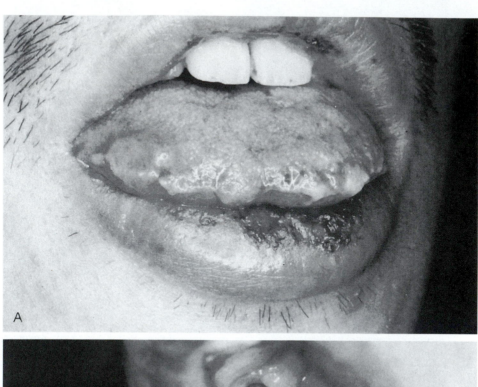

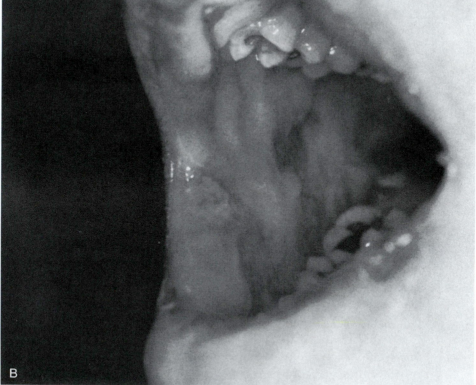

▪ *f* i g u r e **3–13**   Oral lesions of erythema multiforme. *A,* Crusted lip lesions with edema, ulceration, and erythema. *B,* Erythematous and ulcerated lesions of the buccal mucosa.

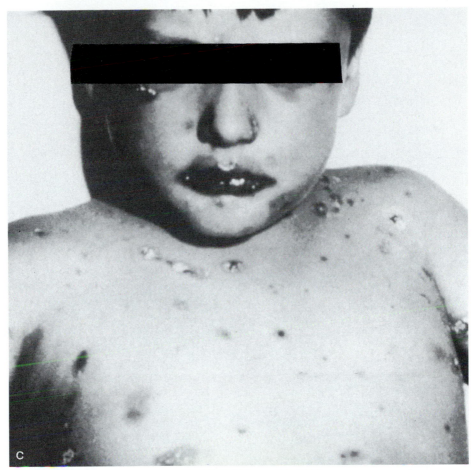

f **i g u r e 3–13** *Continued C,* Stevens-Johnson syndrome. (*C,* Courtesy of Dr. Sidney Eisig.)

striae. The most common location is the buccal mucosa. However, lichen planus also occurs on the tongue, lips, floor of the mouth, and gingiva. Lesions of lichen planus are usually distributed symmetrically in the oral cavity.

The prevalence of lichen planus in the general population of the United States has been reported to be about 1%. In one study of 100 cases, the age of individuals affected ranged from 13 to 78 years. However, the disease is most common in middle age. A slight female predominance has been suggested. In another reported study of 200 cases, most were found to be asymptomatic and were discovered on routine oral examination.

Many factors have been implicated in lichen planus; however, the cause remains unknown. Erosive lesions do tend to worsen with emotional stress. Many drugs and chemicals have been shown to produce lichenoid lesions. If a drug can be identified as the causative agent, discontinuation of the drug should cause the lesions to disappear. At times, however, it is not possible to discontinue the drug.

Types of Lichen Planus

Several forms of lichen planus have been described. Those in which the epithelium separates from the connective tissue and erosions or bullae or ulcers form are called **erosive** and **bullous lichen planus** (Fig. 3–15; Color Plate 22). Another type of lichen

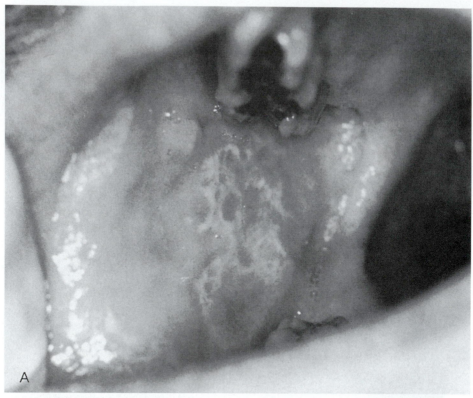

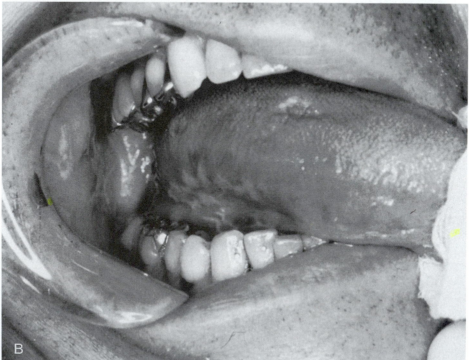

■ *f i g u r e 3–14*   *A* and *B*, Two examples of the oral lesions of lichen planus.

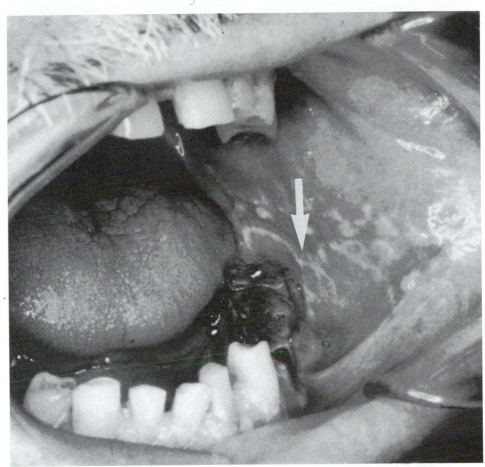

▪ *f i g u r e 3–15*   Lichen planus. Erosion of the mucosa appears as erythema adjacent to white striae *(arrow)*.

planus is described as a white, slightly raised plaque-like lesion that may have a reticular pattern at its periphery.

Gingival lesions clinically described as **desquamative gingivitis** can also be caused by lichen planus (Fig. 3–16). In addition to the gingival lesions, there are generally striated lesions elsewhere.

The skin lesions of lichen planus are 2- to 4-mm papules. Wickham's striae may also be present, as may pruritus (Fig. 3–17). Lesions can occur anywhere on the skin, but the most common sites are the lumbar region, the flexor surfaces of the wrist, and the anterior surface of the ankles. Some patients have only skin lesions, some have only oral lesions, and others have both skin and oral lesions.

Diagnosis

The diagnosis of lichen planus is made on the basis of the distinctive clinical appearance and the histologic appearance of biopsy tissue (Fig. 3–18). The epithelium is generally parakeratotic and may be hyperplastic or atrophic. The characteristic microscopic features include degeneration of the basal cell layer of the epithelium in small to extensive areas, saw-tooth–shaped rete ridges, and a broad band of lymphocytes in the connective tissue immediately subjacent to the epithelium. In erosive areas the

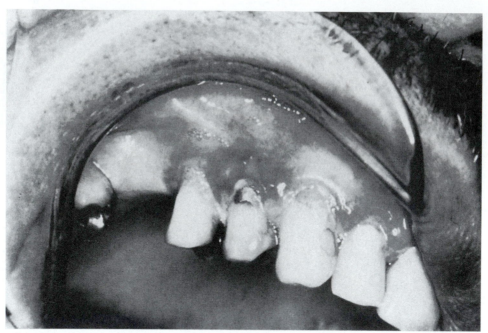

▪ *f* i g u r e **3–16**   Lichen planus. The gingival lesions of lichen planus are described clinically as desquamative gingivitis.

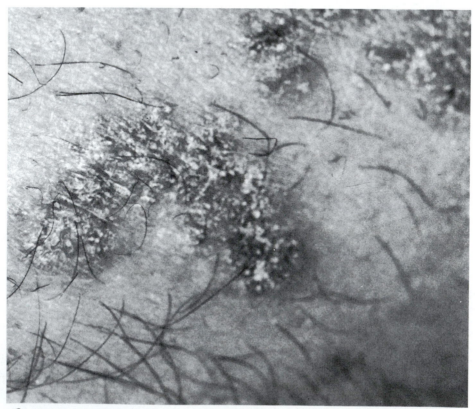

▪ *f* i g u r e **3–17**   Skin lesions of lichen planus.

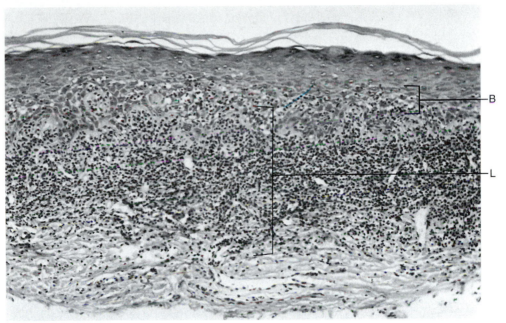

f i g u r e 3–18   Lichen planus seen by low-power microscopy. Note the degeneration of the basal cell layer of the epithelium (B) and the band-like infiltrate of lymphocytes (L).

separation of the epithelium from the connective tissue occurs at the interface of the epithelium and connective tissue. Epithelial atypia and dysplasia may also occur in lesions that appear clinically as lichen planus, and it has been suggested that these lesions may be premalignant.

Treatment and Prognosis

Lichen planus is a chronic disease. Treatment is indicated only when lesions are symptomatic. Erosive lesions usually respond quickly when topical corticosteroid medication is applied. Improvement of gingival lesions with meticulous oral hygiene has been reported.

Studies have been reported that suggest that patients with lichen planus may be at increased risk for the development of squamous cell carcinoma. Therefore, regular oral soft tissue examination and biopsy of any lesions not consistent with lichen planus are recommended.

Reiter's Syndrome

Reiter's syndrome comprises the triad of arthritis, urethritis, and conjunctivitis. The cause of this syndrome is unknown. (A syndrome is a group of signs and symptoms that occur together. Other syndromes are described elsewhere in this text.) An antigenic marker called **HLA-B27** is present in most patients with Reiter's syndrome, suggesting a genetic influence. An abnormal immune response to a microbial antigen is considered the most likely mechanism of occurrence. Reiter's syndrome is far more prevalent (10 to 15:1) in men than in women.

Reiter's syndrome characteristically develops 1 to 4 weeks after venereal or gastrointestinal infection. The syndrome is usually benign and self-limited.

The arthritis of Reiter's syndrome usually involves the joints of the lower extremities (knees and ankles). It may be asymmetric and migratory, chronic and recurrent.

Radiographically, a periosteal proliferation can be detected on the heels, ankles, metatarsals, phalanges, knees, and elbows. Fever, malaise, and weight loss may be associated with the arthritis. The urethritis usually precedes the other lesions. No infectious organisms can be identified. The conjunctivitis is usually mild, but some individuals experience iritis (inflammation of the iris).

Skin and mucous membrane lesions are seen in many patients with Reiter's syndrome. Oral lesions occur almost anywhere in the oral cavity (Fig. 3–19). Aphthous-like ulcers, erythematous lesions, and geographic tongue–like lesions have been described in patients with Reiter's syndrome.

Diagnosis

The diagnosis of Reiter's syndrome is made on the basis of the clinical signs and symptoms. There are no laboratory tests that confirm the diagnosis.

Treatment and Prognosis

The disease lasts from weeks to months. The patient may experience spontaneous remission, but recurrent attacks are common. Aspirin or other nonsteroidal anti-inflammatory drugs are generally used for treatment.

Histiocytosis X

Idiopathic histiocytosis and Langerhans cell granulomatosis are other names for **histiocytosis X.** Three entities have traditionally been grouped under the category of histiocytosis X: Letterer-Siwe disease, Hand-Schüller-Christian disease, and solitary eosinophilic granuloma. Histologically, all are characterized by a combination of macrophages (also called histiocytes and Langerhans cells) and eosinophils (Fig. 3–20).

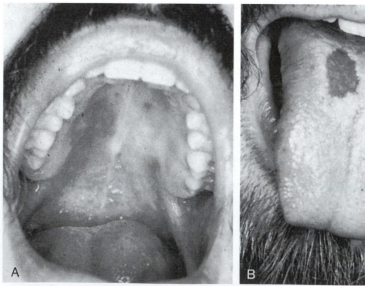

■ *f i g u r e 3–19*   *A* and *B*, Lesions are present on the palate and tongue in this patient with Reiter's syndrome.

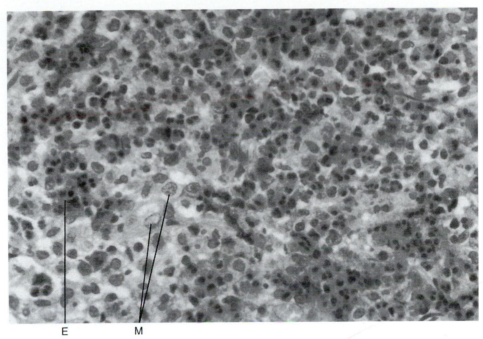

f i g u r e 3–20   Histiocytosis X seen by high-power microscopy. E = eosinophils; M = macrophages.

unknown etiology - but immune deficiency

However, in all three diseases the proliferating cell is the macrophage. The presence of eosinophils is thought to result from the production of an eosinophilic chemotactic factor produced by the macrophage.

The Langerhans cell (a type of macrophage that proliferates in these three conditions) is an immunologically competent cell of the mononuclear phagocyte series and participates in cell-mediated immunity. The cause and pathogenesis of the diseases classified as histiocytosis X remain unclear. They are included in this chapter because they appear to be immunologic diseases. A reactive process, a primary immunodeficiency disease, and a neoplastic process have all been suggested. Although considered together, the prognosis of the three diseases is different, and they may not truly be variants of the same disease.

Letterer-Siwe Disease

Letterer-Siwe disease (acute disseminated histiocytosis) is an acute fulminating disorder that usually affects children younger than 3 years of age. The course of the disease is usually so rapid that significant oral involvement does not often occur. The disease resembles a lymphoma in that it generally has a rapidly fatal course that sometimes responds to chemotherapy.

Hand-Schüller-Christian Disease

Hand-Schüller-Christian disease (also called **multifocal eosinophilic granuloma** and **chronic disseminated histiocytosis**) occurs in children, usually less than 5 years of age. A classic triad is seen in about 25% of patients. All changes are due to localized collections of macrophages (Langerhans cells). The triad includes single to multiple well-defined or "punched-out" radiolucent areas in the skull (may also occur

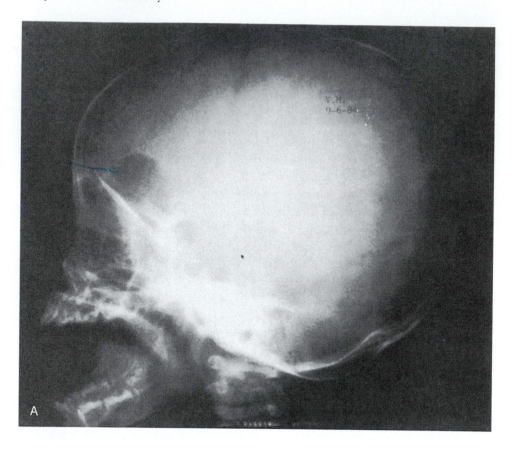

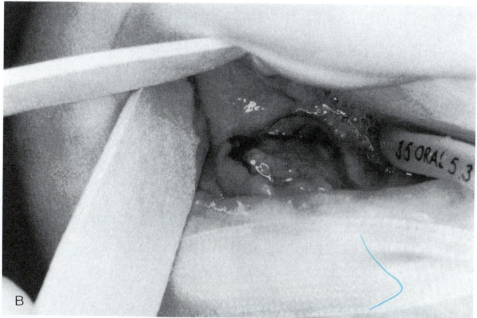

▪ *f* i g u r e **3–21**   Hand-Schüller-Christian disease. *A,* Skull radiograph. *B,* Ulcerated lesion of the mandible. (Courtesy of Dr. Sidney Eisig.)

in the jawbones), unilateral or bilateral exophthalmos, and diabetes insipidus that is due to collections of macrophages in the sella turcica area, affecting the pituitary gland.

Oral manifestations of Hand-Schüller-Christian disease include sore mouth with or without ulcerative lesions, halitosis, gingivitis, unpleasant taste, loose and sore teeth, early exfoliation of teeth, and nonhealing extraction sites. There is a characteristic loss of supporting alveolar bone that mimics advanced periodontal disease (Fig. 3–21).

Eosinophilic Granuloma

Eosinophilic granuloma primarily affects older children and young adults. Males are affected twice as commonly as females. The skull and mandible are commonly involved with eosinophilic granuloma. The radiographic appearance varies, and the lesion may resemble periodontal disease or periapical inflammatory disease or may appear as a well-circumscribed radiolucency with or without a sclerotic border (Fig. 3–22). Cases of multifocal eosinophilic granuloma have also been reported.

Treatment. Eosinophilic granuloma is treated by conservative surgical excision; recurrence is rare. Low-dosage radiation therapy may also be used for treatment.

AUTOIMMUNE DISEASES THAT AFFECT THE ORAL CAVITY

Several autoimmune diseases affect the oral cavity (Table 3–5). In this type of disease, tissue damage occurs because the immune system treats the person's own cells

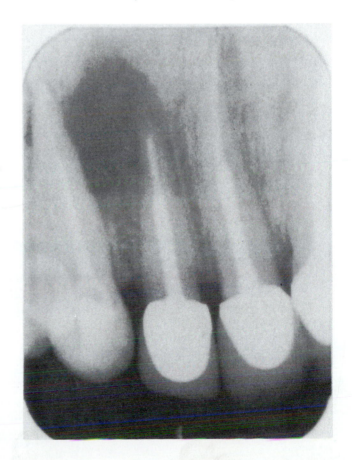

f i g u r e **3-22**

Radiograph of eosinophilic granuloma. (Courtesy of Drs. Paul Freedman and Stanley Kerpel.)

TABLE 3-5 Autoimmune Diseases That Affect the Oral Region	
Disease	**Oral Manifestation**
Sjögren's syndrome	Xerostomia
Lupus erythematosus	White, erosive lesions of the oral mucosa
Pemphigus vulgaris	Mucosal ulceration, bullae
Benign mucous membrane pemphigoid	Mucosal ulceration, desquamative gingivitis
Behçet's syndrome	Aphthous ulcers
Pernicious anemia*	Mucosal atrophy, mucosal ulceration, loss of filiform and fungiform papillae

*Described in Chapter 7.

and tissues as antigens. An individual with one autoimmune disease has an increased risk of another autoimmune disease developing. Although these are systemic diseases, they are included in this chapter because of their relationship to immunity.

Sjögren's Syndrome

Sjögren's syndrome is an autoimmune disease that affects the salivary and lacrimal glands, resulting in a decrease in the amount of saliva and tears. This combination of dry mouth and dry eyes is sometimes called **sicca** (dry) **syndrome.** Decreased salivary flow results in dry mouth **(xerostomia),** and decreased lacrimal flow results in dry eyes **(xerophthalmia).** The eye damage that occurs in Sjögren's syndrome is called **keratoconjunctivitis sicca.** Other secretory glands, such as sweat glands and glands that lubricate the vagina, can also be affected. The specific cause of Sjögren's syndrome is not known. Both cellular immunity and humoral immunity are involved.

In some patients only the mouth and eyes are involved. In others the autoimmune process can be more extensive. Many patients (about 50%) with Sjögren's syndrome have another autoimmune disease, such as rheumatoid arthritis or systemic lupus erythematosus. Lacrimal and salivary gland involvement without the presence of another autoimmune disease is called **primary Sjögren's syndrome.** When another autoimmune disease accompanies salivary and lacrimal gland involvement, the combination is called **secondary Sjögren's syndrome.**

The oral manifestation of Sjögren's syndrome is xerostomia (dry mouth), which occurs as a result of decreased salivary flow and causes the mucosa to become erythematous. Patients complain of oral discomfort. Lack of saliva causes the mouth to feel sticky. Lips are cracked and dry, and there is a generalized loss of filiform and fungiform papillae on the dorsum of the tongue (Fig. 3–23). Patients with xerostomia are at high risk for the development of caries, periodontal disease, and oral candidiasis.

Both major and minor salivary glands are affected. Parotid gland enlargement, usually bilateral and symmetric, occurs in about 50% of patients (Fig. 3–24). The characteristic histologic appearance of these enlarged glands consists of replacement of the glands by lymphocytes and the presence of islands of epithelium called **epimyoepithelial islands.** Biopsy of the minor salivary glands is often performed to confirm a diagnosis of Sjögren's syndrome. The minor glands show aggregates of lymphocytes surrounding the salivary gland ducts (Fig. 3–25).

In addition to the oral findings, patients with decreased lacrimal flow that results in xerophthalmia complain of burning and itching of the eyes and photophobia (abnormal visual intolerance to light). Severe eye involvement may lead to ulceration and opacification of the cornea. Twenty percent of patients with Sjögren's syndrome also have Raynaud's phenomenon, which is a disorder affecting the fingers and toes. Cold

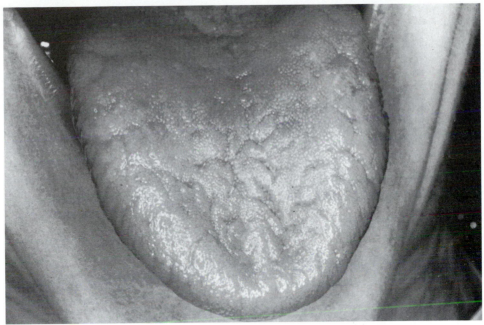

f i g u r e 3–23   Sjögren's syndrome. This patient had severe xerostomia. The filiform papillae are lacking.

and emotional stress trigger the reaction, which is characterized by an initial pallor of the skin that results from vasoconstriction and reduced blood flow. The initial pallor is followed by cyanosis, which occurs because of the decreased blood flow. When the skin is rewarmed, the blood vessels dilate and the hyperemia results in a reddening of the skin. Finally, in minutes to hours, the color returns to normal. Raynaud's phenomenon

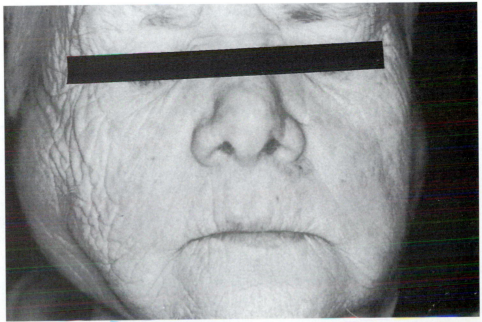

f i g u r e 3–24   Bilateral parotid gland swelling seen in Sjögren's syndrome. (Courtesy of Dr. Louis Mandel.)

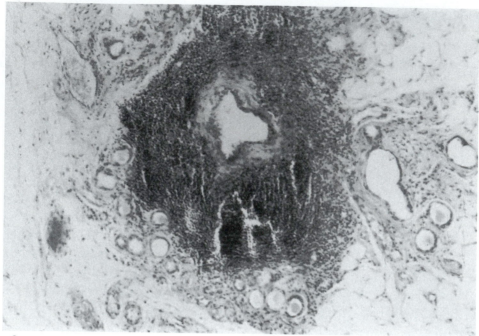

f i g u r e 3–25 Microscopy of a minor salivary gland from a patient with Sjögren's syndrome. (Courtesy of Dr. Harry Lumerman.)

can occur alone or in association with other autoimmune diseases, as well as in Sjögren's syndrome. Patients with Sjögren's syndrome might also complain of myalgia, arthralgia, and chronic fatigue.

Laboratory abnormalities are commonly found in patients with this syndrome. Ninety percent of patients with Sjögren's syndrome have a positive reaction to rheumatoid factor, which is an antibody to IgG that is present in serum. It is an antibody to an antibody. Patients with other autoimmune diseases, such as rheumatoid arthritis, also react positively to rheumatoid factor. Other autoantibodies, called **anti–Sjögren's syndrome A (SS-A)** and **anti–Sjögren's syndrome B (SS-B)**, are also found in patients with Sjögren's syndrome. Other laboratory abnormalities include mild anemia, a decreased white blood cell count, an elevated erythrocyte sedimentation rate, and a diffuse elevation of serum immunoglobulins.

Diagnosis and Management

The diagnosis of Sjögren's syndrome is made when at least two of its three components are present: xerostomia, keratoconjunctivitis sicca, and rheumatoid arthritis or another autoimmune disease. Xerostomia can result from conditions other than autoimmune disease. Measurement of stimulated and unstimulated salivary flow and biopsy of minor salivary glands can be helpful in the diagnosis of Sjögren's syndrome. A characteristic pattern is seen in a parotid sialogram (Fig. 3–26). The pattern reflects the lack of functioning glandular elements.

Keratoconjunctivitis is confirmed by eye examination. Lacrimal flow is measured using filter paper. Special examination techniques are necessary to demonstrate the corneal erosions.

The course of the disease for the majority of patients is chronic and benign. However, patients with Sjögren's syndrome are at risk for the development of other, more serious autoimmune diseases, lymphoma, and Waldenström's macroglobulinemia

long term Steroids will mask infections + compromise immunity. Heal more slowly.

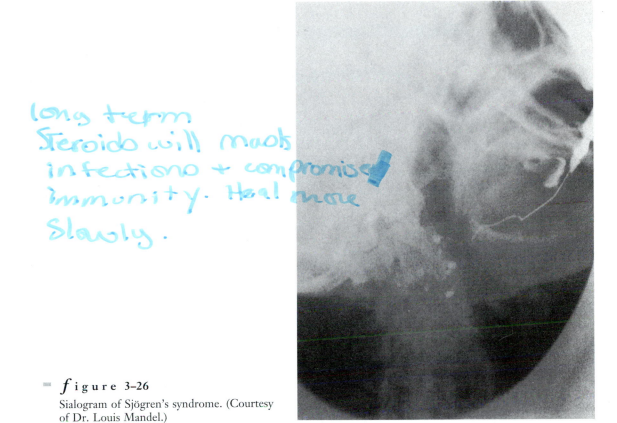

■ **f i g u r e 3–26**
Sialogram of Sjögren's syndrome. (Courtesy of Dr. Louis Mandel.)

(a disorder characterized by a high concentration of IgM in serum) and should therefore be followed by a physician.

Treatment

Sjögren's syndrome is usually treated symptomatically. Nonsteroidal anti-inflammatory agents are used for the arthritis. In severe cases corticosteroids and other immunosuppressive drugs may be necessary. Saliva substitutes are helpful, and the use of a humidifier at night makes the xerostomia more tolerable. Sugarless gum or lozenges may be used to stimulate saliva production. However, the greater the destruction of salivary gland tissue, the less saliva will be stimulated. An "artificial tears" formula containing methylcellulose helps to protect the eye from the drying effects of the disease. Glasses provide shielding and are helpful to minimize the drying effects of wind. Pilocarpine may also be used in some patients to increase salivary flow.

The effects of xerostomia can be minimized by maintaining good oral hygiene and using fluoride toothpaste with daily fluoride rinses. The interval between recall appointments should be sufficiently short to ensure early detection and treatment of root caries. The toothbrush and other oral hygiene aids may need modification if arthritis affects the movement of hands and arms.

Systemic Lupus Erythematosus

Systemic lupus erythematosus (SLE) is an acute and chronic inflammatory autoimmune disease of unknown cause. The disorder affects women eight times more frequently than it does men, predominantly during the childbearing years. It occurs three times more frequently in black women than in white women. SLE is a syndrome rather than a specific disease entity and includes a wide spectrum of disease activity and signs and symptoms that range from lesions confined to the skin (discoid lupus erythematosus) to a widespread, debilitating, life-threatening disease with multiple organ involvement. SLE is usually chronic and progressive with periods of remission and exacerbation.

Both cellular immunity and humoral immunity are impaired in SLE. It has been suggested that cellular immunity is primarily affected, resulting in deregulation of the humoral response. Antigen-antibody complexes are deposited in various organs and stimulate an inflammatory response, which may be responsible for the tissue damage that occurs in SLE. Autoantibodies to the patient's deoxyribonucleic acid (DNA) (antinuclear antibodies) are present in serum. These circulating antibodies are responsible for the positive antinuclear antibody (ANA) and lupus erythematosus (LE) laboratory test results. Production of these antibodies is enhanced by estrogen. Antibodies to lymphocytes are present in some patients. There is evidence for a genetic component in the pathogenesis of SLE.

Clinical Features   *Premed-*

Skin lesions are among the most common signs of the disease, occurring in 85% of individuals (Fig. 3–27). The most common skin lesion is an erythematous rash involving areas of the body exposed to sunlight. The classic "butterfly" rash occurs over the bridge of the nose, and there may be erythematous lesions on the fingertips. The lesions can heal with scarring in the center as they continue to spread at the periphery. The skin lesions tend to worsen when exposed to sunlight. Atrophy and hypo- or hyperpigmentation can follow these lesions. Other skin lesions—such as bullae, purpura, a discoid rash, vitiligo, or subcutaneous nodules—can also occur.

Arthritis and arthralgia are common manifestations of SLE. Any joint can be involved, and symptoms resemble rheumatoid arthritis but without severe deformities. Raynaud's phenomenon occurs in 15% of patients. Myalgia and myositis also occur. A retinal vasculitis causes degeneration of the nerve fiber layer of the retina and can cause

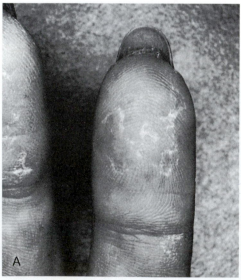 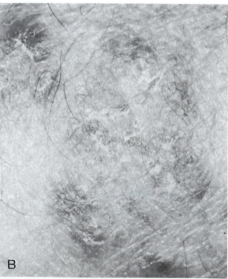

■ *figure 3–27*   *A* and *B*, Two examples of skin lesions in lupus erythematosus.

loss of vision. Thrombocytopenia can occur. Psychoses and depression are signs of central nervous system involvement, and seizures can be present. Involvement of the pleura may cause shortness of breath and chest pain. Pericarditis, cardiac arrhythmias, and endocarditis may be seen late in the disease. Kidney involvement is common.

Oral lesions accompany skin lesions in about 25% of patients with discoid lupus erythematosus, which is the mildest form of lupus erythematosus. Oral lesions appear as erythematous plaques or erosions. White striae radiating from the center of the lesion are usually present. The lesions may resemble lichen planus but are less symmetric in their distribution. The involvement of the oral mucosa in this disease is usually mild and is similar to that seen in discoid lupus erythematosus (Fig. 3–28). Petechiae and gingival bleeding may be present in patients with severe thrombocytopenia. Sjögren's syndrome may be present in some patients with SLE.

Diagnosis

The diagnosis of SLE is usually based on the classic multiorgan involvement and the presence of antinuclear antibodies in serum. The diagnosis of SLE is difficult if the onset is slow and insidious. The histologic appearance of oral lesions resembles that of lichen planus. Microscopically, destruction of the basal cells is seen, as in lichen planus. However, the inflammatory infiltrate is distributed around blood vessels in the connective tissue rather than in a subepithelial band. Direct immunofluorescence and immunohistochemical testing of skin and mucosal lesions shows granular and linear deposits of immunoglobulins along the basement membrane zone.

Treatment and Prognosis

Once the diagnosis of SLE is made, the decision as to whether treatment is indicated depends on the degree of disease activity. This once-fatal disease is now managed with several drugs. Aspirin and nonsteroidal anti-inflammatory agents are used for mild signs and symptoms. Hydroxychloroquine, an antimalarial agent, and corticosteroids combined with other immunosuppressive agents, such as azathioprine and cyclophosphamide, are also used. If the course of the disease is mild and only a few organs are involved, the prognosis is excellent. The disease can also be fatal. Kidney involvement can be associated with severe hypertension and rapid onset of renal failure, which is a cause of death in patients with SLE. Other common causes of death include hemorrhage secondary to thrombocytopenia, nervous system involvement, and infection.

SLE is an extremely complex disease. A consultation with the patient's physician should take place before initiating dental treatment. Antibiotic prophylaxis to prevent bacterial endocarditis may be necessary. The extent of systemic involvement and the drugs being used for treatment should be clarified.

Pemphigus Vulgaris

Pemphigus vulgaris is a severe, progressive autoimmune disease that affects the skin and mucous membranes. It is characterized by intraepithelial blister formation that results from breakdown of the cellular adhesion between epithelial cells. This type of epithelial cell separation is called **acantholysis.** The patient with pemphigus vulgaris has circulating autoantibodies that are reactive against components of the epithelial cell attachment mechanism. The higher the titer of circulating antibodies, the greater the epithelial destruction. These autoantibodies are also found in surrounding epithelial cells. Pemphigus vulgaris is the type of pemphigus seen most frequently. There are

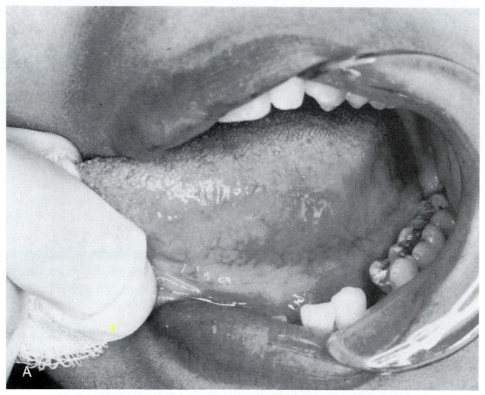

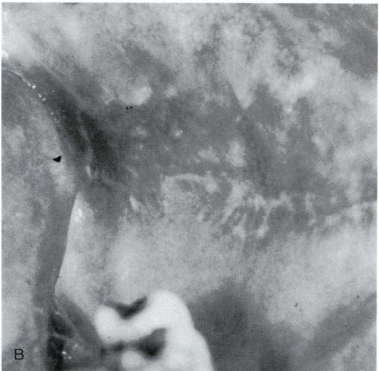

■ *f i g u r e* **3–28** *A* and *B*, Oral lesions in lupus erythematosus.

three other forms of pemphigus: pemphigus vegetans, pemphigus foliaceus, and pemphigus erythematosus. These are much rarer conditions, but all are characterized by epithelial acantholysis. There is no sex predilection. A broad age range has been reported, including both children and elderly individuals. Most cases occur in the fourth and fifth decades of life. Genetic and ethnic factors have been reported. Although it is a relatively rare condition, pemphigus vulgaris is often seen in Ashkenazic Jews.

In more than 50% of cases of pemphigus vulgaris, the first signs of disease occur in the oral cavity. Oral lesions can precede cutaneous lesions by many months. The appearance of oral lesions ranges from shallow ulcers to fragile vesicles or bullae. Because the bullae are so fragile, they rupture soon after they form, and the detached epithelium remains as a gray membrane (Fig. 3–29). Ulcers are painful and range in size from small to very large. Gentle finger pressure with movement on clinically normal mucosa can produce a cleavage in the epithelium and result in the formation of a bulla. This is called **Nikolsky's sign.**

Skin lesions in pemphigus vulgaris include erythema, vesicles, bullae, erosions, and ulcers.

Microscopic examination of tissue shows an intact basal layer of epithelium attached to the underlying connective tissue (Fig. 3–30). The loss of attachment between the epithelial cells results in detached cells that appear rounded. These rounded cells are called **acantholytic cells** or Tzanck cells and are present in the area of separation. Tzanck cells may also be seen on cytologic smear, but the diagnosis must be confirmed by biopsy.

Diagnosis

The diagnosis of pemphigus vulgaris is made by biopsy and microscopic examinations and direct or indirect immunofluorescence. Direct immunofluorescence is performed on biopsy tissue and identifies autoantibodies present in the tissue. The tissue is viewed through a special microscope, and in pemphigus vulgaris fluorescence is seen

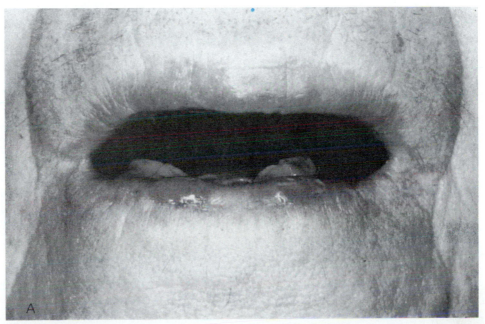

f i g u r e 3–29 *A,* Example of oral lesions in pemphigus vulgaris.

Illustration continued on following page

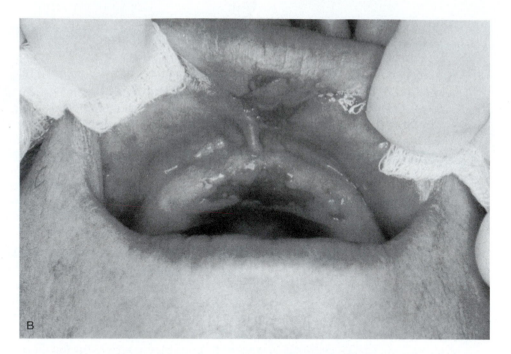

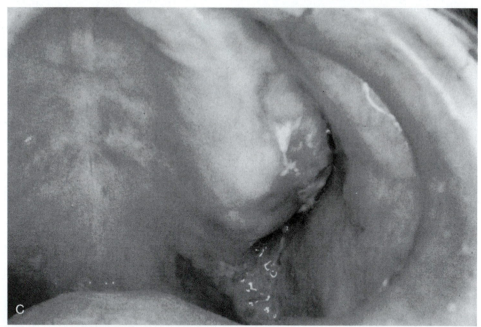

▪ *figure 3–29*   *Continued B* and *C,* Examples of oral lesions in pemphigus vulgaris. (*B* and *C,* Courtesy of Dr. Fariba Younai.)

surrounding the cells in the prickle cell layer. In indirect immunofluorescence, the patient's serum is used to detect the presence of circulating autoantibodies. Eighty percent of patients with pemphigus vulgaris have the identifiable circulating autoantibodies.

Treatment and Prognosis

Treatment generally involves high doses of corticosteroids. Other immunosuppressive drugs, such as azathioprine and methotrexate, are often used in addition to systemic

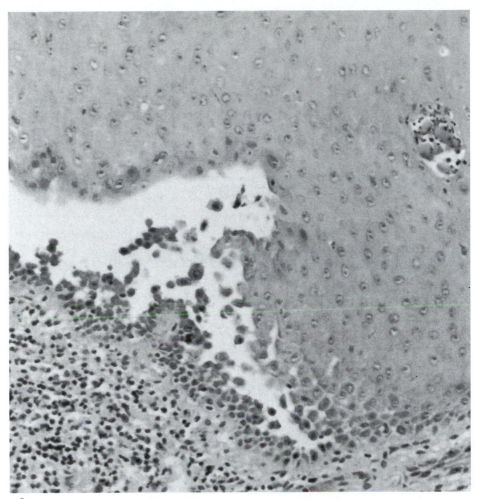

■ *f i g u r e* **3–30**   Pemphigus vulgaris seen by microscopy.

corticosteroids. The amount of autoantibodies present in the patient's serum correlates with the severity of lesions, and therefore this concentration of autoantibodies is used to monitor the success of drug treatment. Pemphigus vulgaris was at one time a life-threatening disease. Today the mortality rate is about 8% to 10% in 5 years and is related to the complications of corticosteroid treatment rather than to the disease itself.

Other autoimmune diseases may occur in association with pemphigus vulgaris. Among them are lupus erythematosus, rheumatoid arthritis, and Sjögren's syndrome.

Cicatricial Pemphigoid

Cicatricial pemphigoid is also called **mucosal pemphigoid** and **benign mucous membrane pemphigoid.** It is a chronic autoimmune disease that affects the oral mucosa, conjunctiva, genital mucosa, and skin. It is not as severe as pemphigus vulgaris. Lesions may heal with scarring. The term cicatricial pemphigoid refers to this healing with scarring. Autoantibodies and complement components have been identified at the basement membrane of the epithelium. The lesions occur as a result of cleavage of the epithelium from the underlying connective tissue in this area. The most common site for cicatricial pemphigoid lesions is the gingiva. The appearance ranges from erythema to ulceration and involves both the free and the attached gingiva. The gingival lesions have been called <mark>desquamative gingivitis</mark> (Fig. 3–31; Color Plate 85). However, desquamative gingivitis is a clinical and descriptive term, and similar lesions can be seen in lichen planus and pemphigus vulgaris. Nikolsky's sign can be produced on normal-appearing tissue. Bullae, erosions, and ulcers can also occur in other locations in the oral cavity. Bullae are thick walled and much less fragile than those of pemphigus vulgaris, and they may persist for 24 to 48 hours.

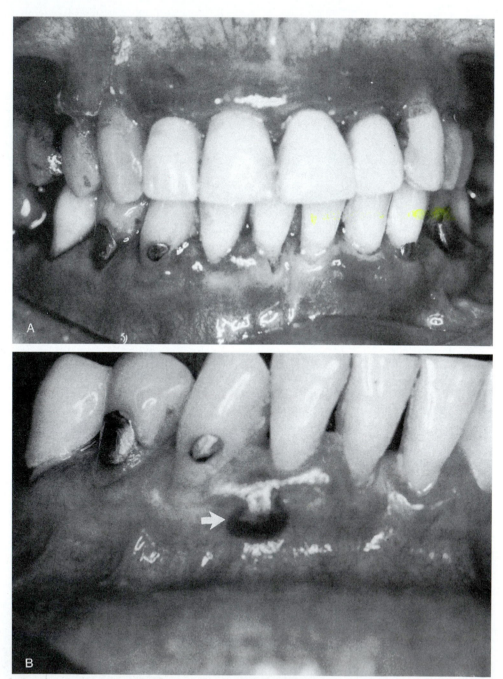

■ *f i g u r e* **3–31**   *A* and *B*, Cicatricial pemphigoid (desquamative gingivitis). (Courtesy of Dr. Victor M. Sternberg.)

Diagnosis

The diagnosis of cicatricial pemphigoid is made by biopsy and histologic examination. On microscopic examination, the epithelium appears to detach from the connective tissue at the basement membrane (Fig. 3–32). There is no degeneration of the epithelium. An inflammatory infiltrate, usually with prominent plasma cells and eosinophils, is seen in the connective tissue. Direct immunofluorescence shows a linear pattern of fluorescence at the basement membrane. Indirect immunofluorescence (identifying autoantibodies in serum) is usually not helpful in the diagnosis of cicatricial pemphigoid.

Treatment and Prognosis

Cicatricial pemphigoid is a chronic disease that follows a benign course. Gingival involvement can occur alone, or more extensive lesions can be present. Topical corticosteroid application is helpful in the management of mild cases. In more severe cases, high doses of systemic corticosteroids may be necessary. The disease may be difficult to control and slow to respond to therapy. Patients may experience episodes of exacerbation followed by periods of remission. If eye lesions are present, severe damage to the cornea, conjunctiva, and eyelid can occur.

Bullous Pemphigoid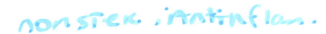

Some investigators have suggested that bullous and cicatricial pemphigoid are variants of a single disease. However, there are differences between the two diseases that make this questionable. Eighty percent of patients with bullous pemphigoid are older than 60 years of age, and there is no sex predilection. Unlike cicatricial pemphigoid, circulating autoantibodies are usually detectable but do not correlate with disease activity. Oral lesions are less common in bullous pemphigoid than in cicatricial pemphigoid, occurring in only about one third of patients. When they occur, the gingival lesions are very similar to those of cicatricial pemphigoid, and other mucosal lesions are more extensive and painful.

As in cicatricial pemphigoid, the microscopic appearance of bullous pemphigoid shows a cleavage of the epithelium from the connective tissue at the basement membrane.

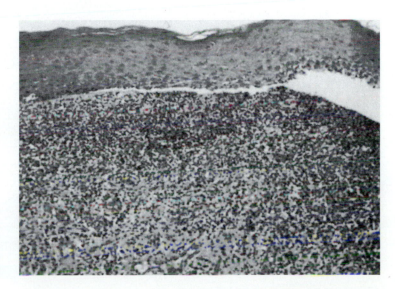

■ *f* i g u r e **3–32**
Cicatricial pemphigoid seen by microscopy.

Treatment and Prognosis

High doses of systemic corticosteroids and nonsteroidal anti-inflammatory drugs are used in the management of bullous pemphigoid. The disease is chronic with periods of remission and is usually not life threatening.

Behçet's Syndrome   *P. 96 in.*

Behçet's syndrome is a chronic, recurrent autoimmune disease consisting primarily of oral ulcers, genital ulcers, and ocular inflammation. There is no sex predilection, and the mean age of onset is 30 years. Evidence for an autoimmune pathogenesis includes the identification of antibodies to human mucosa in patients with Behçet's syndrome.

The oral ulcers that occur in Behçet's syndrome are very similar in appearance to aphthous ulcers (Fig. 3–33). They are painful and recurrent. The lesions range in size from a few millimeters to several centimeters. The genital ulcers are usually small and are located on the scrotum or base of the penis and on the labia majora. The ocular lesions usually begin with photophobia and can develop into conjunctivitis and uveitis. The skin lesions show a papular pattern of pustules and are most common on the trunk and limbs.

Diagnosis

The diagnosis of Behçet's syndrome requires that two of the principal manifestations (oral, genital, ocular) be present. A pustular lesion that develops after a needle puncture is highly suggestive of Behçet's syndrome.

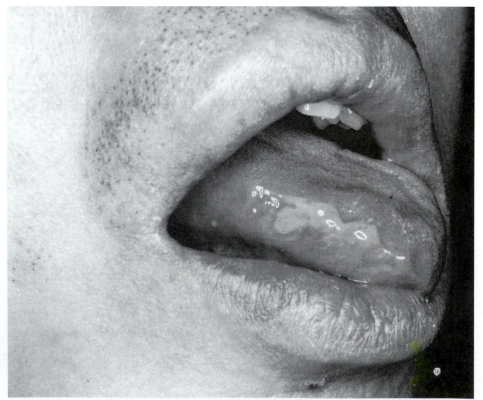

▪ *figure* 3–33   Oral lesion seen in Behçet's syndrome. Aphthous-like oral mucosal ulcer.

Treatment and Prognosis

Systemic and topical corticosteroids are used in the management of Behçet's syndrome. Chlorambucil is used for the ocular lesions. Occasionally, other immunosuppressive drugs are needed.

INFECTIOUS DISEASES

Human beings are surrounded and inhabited by an incredible number of microorganisms. The ability of these organisms to cause disease depends on both the microorganism and the state of the body's defenses. Although these microorganisms are traditionally divided into those that produce disease (pathogenic) and those that do not (nonpathogenic), many of the usually nonpathogenic microorganisms can proliferate and cause disease in an immunologically weakened individual.

Numerous infectious diseases can affect the tissues of the oral cavity. Bacterial, fungal, and viral infections are the most common, but even protozoan and helminthic infections, though extremely rare, have been reported. Infection occurs when the body's defenses are not sufficient to prevent microorganisms from causing disease.

The oral cavity contains numerous microorganisms that make up the normal oral flora. Changes such as a decrease in salivary flow, antibiotic administration, and immune system alterations affect the oral flora so that organisms that are usually nonpathogenic are able to cause disease. This type of infection is called an **opportunistic infection.**

The oral cavity can be the primary site of involvement of an infectious disease, or a systemic infection can have oral manifestations. These infections are usually transmitted from one individual to another by several different routes. Organisms can be transferred through the air on dust particles or water droplets. Some organisms require intimate and direct contact to be transferred. Some can be transferred on hands and objects, and others, such as hepatitis B, must be transferred from one person to another in blood or other body fluids.

Microorganisms initially invading the oral tissues can cause a local infection, systemic infection, or both. Microorganisms circulating in the blood stream can cause lesions in the oral cavity, and microorganisms causing infection in the lungs can be transferred to oral tissues when they are present in sputum.

The first line of defense against infectious disease is the inflammatory response (see Chapter 2). Bacteria penetrating epithelial surfaces act as foreign bodies and stimulate the inflammatory response. The accumulation of a large number of phagocytic cells at the inflammatory site is of primary importance in ingestion and destruction of invading bacteria.

The inflammatory response is a nonspecific response. However, the responses of the immune system are highly specific. Specific antibodies are formed in response to specific antigens. Microorganisms are antigens. Humoral immunity (antibodies) is an effective defense against some microorganisms, and cellular immunity is the primary defense against others, such as intracellular bacteria (tuberculosis), viruses, and fungi.

Microbial infections are responsible for many more diseases than those included in this chapter. The diseases discussed here are the most common, cause specific oral lesions, and help to illustrate principles of infectious disease. Dental caries and periodontal disease are clearly important to dental hygienists. However, they are not included in this text because they are usually studied in courses other than oral pathology. The dental hygienist frequently encounters oral infectious diseases and must be able to recognize their clinical features and significance for control of infection.

Bacterial Infections

Tuberculosis

Tuberculosis is an infectious chronic granulomatous disease usually caused by the organism *Mycobacterium tuberculosis*. The chief form of the disease is a primary infection of the lung. Inhaled droplets containing bacteria lodge in the alveoli of the lungs. After undergoing phagocytosis by macrophages, the organisms are resistant to destruction and multiply in the macrophages. They then disseminate in the blood stream. After a few weeks dissemination ceases. The signs and symptoms of this lung infection include fever, chills, fatigue and malaise, weight loss, and persistent cough. The bacteria can be carried to widespread areas of the body and cause involvement of organs such as the kidneys and liver. This is called **miliary tuberculosis.** Involvement of the submandibular and cervical lymph nodes causes enlargement of those nodes and is called **scrofula** or **tuberculous lymphadenitis.** The lung infection can occur at any age. Most commonly, it becomes completely walled off and heals by fibrosis and calcification. A reactivation of the primary lesion can occur years after the initial infection.

Oral lesions associated with tuberculosis occur but are rare. They most likely appear when organisms are carried from the lungs in sputum and are transmitted to the oral mucosa (Fig. 3–34). The tongue and palate are the most common sites for oral lesions of tuberculosis, but they may occur anywhere in the oral cavity, even in bone as in osteomyelitis. Oral lesions appear as painful, nonhealing, slowly enlarging ulcers that can be either superficial or deep.

Diagnosis

Oral lesions of tuberculosis are identified by biopsy and microscopic examination of the tissue. They are chronic granulomatous inflammatory lesions composed of areas of necrosis surrounded by lymphocytes, macrophages, and multinucleated giant cells.

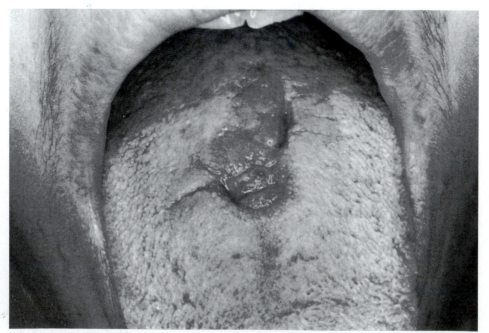

figure 3–34   Ulcer on tongue seen in tuberculosis.

Similar lesions occur in sarcoidosis, deep fungal infections, and foreign body reactions. Staining the tissue to be examined microscopically with a special stain may reveal the organisms. Tissue culture to diagnose tuberculosis requires a specialized laboratory.

A skin test is used to determine if an individual has been exposed and infected with *Mycobacterium tuberculosis*. An antigen called **purified protein derivative (PPD)** is injected into the skin. If the individual's cell-mediated immune system has previously encountered the antigen, a positive inflammatory skin reaction occurs—a type IV hypersensitivity reaction. This skin reaction indicates previous infection with the bacteria but not necessarily active disease. A positive skin test result is generally followed by chest radiographs to determine if active disease is present.

Tuberculosis is an infectious disease that can be occupationally transmitted to dental health care personnel. Until recently, the prevalence of tuberculosis was steadily declining. However, recently there has been a dramatic increase in new cases, particularly in densely populated urban areas. It has been suggested that this increase is related to HIV infection. Since cases of tuberculosis are increasing in prevalence, routine use of universal precautions, including eye protection, mask, or facial shield, is important in preventing the transmission of airborne droplet infections such as tuberculosis.

Treatment and Prognosis

Oral lesions resolve with treatment of the patient's primary (usually pulmonary) disease. Several different combination medications, including isoniazid (INH) and rifampin, are used to treat tuberculosis. Treatment continues for many months and may continue for as long as 2 years. Patients become noninfectious shortly after treatment begins. Consultation with the patient's physician should confirm that treatment is ongoing and the patient is no longer infectious.

Actinomycosis

Actinomycosis is an infection caused by a filamentous bacterium called *Actinomyces israelii* (Fig. 3–35). These organisms were at one time thought to be fungi and therefore the name ends in the suffix "mycosis," which usually indicates a fungal infection.

The most characteristic form of the disease is the formation of abscesses that tend to drain by the formation of sinus tracts (see Fig. 3–35). The colonies or organisms

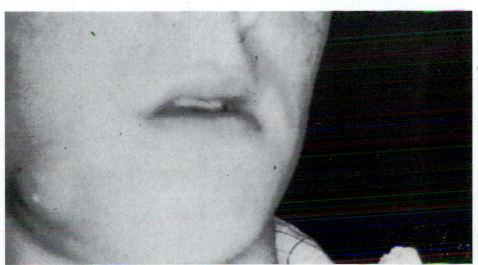

figure 3–35 Actinomycosis. (Courtesy of Dr. Edward V. Zegarelli.)

appear in the pus as tiny bright-yellow grains and are called **sulfur granules** because of their yellow color. These organisms are common inhabitants of the oral cavity. It is not clear why these organisms only occasionally cause disease. Predisposing factors have not been identified. The infection is often preceded by tooth extraction or an abrasion of the mucosa.

Diagnosis and Treatment

The diagnosis of actinomycosis is generally made by identifying the colonies in the tissue from the lesion. Actinomycosis is treated with high doses of antibiotics for a long-term period.

Syphilis

Syphilis is a disease caused by the spirochete *Treponema pallidum*. The organism is transmitted from one person to another by direct contact. The spirochete, a corkscrew-like organism, can penetrate mucous membranes but requires a break in the continuity of the skin surface in order to invade through the skin. The organisms die quickly when exposed to air and changes in temperature. Syphilis is usually transmitted through sexual contact with a partner who has active lesions. It can also be transmitted by transfusion of infected blood or by transplacental inoculation of a fetus from an infected mother.

The disease occurs in three stages: primary, secondary, and tertiary (Table 3–6). The lesion of the primary stage, called the **chancre,** is highly infectious and forms at the site at which the spirochete enters the body (Fig. 3–36; Color Plate 42). Regional lymphadenopathy accompanies the chancre. The lesion heals spontaneously after several weeks without treatment, and the disease enters a latent period.

The secondary stage occurs about 6 weeks after the primary lesion appears. In the secondary stage, there are diffuse eruptions of the skin and mucous membranes. The skin lesions have many forms. The oral lesions are called **mucous patches** and appear as multiple, painless, grayish-white plaques covering ulcerated mucosa. The lesions of secondary syphilis are the most infectious. They undergo spontaneous remission but can recur for months or years. Following remission the disease may remain latent for many years.

The tertiary lesions occur years after the initial infection if treatment for the infection has not been given. They chiefly involve the cardiovascular system and the central nervous system. The localized tertiary lesion is called a **gumma** and is noninfectious. A gumma can occur in the oral cavity; the most common sites are the tongue and palate. The lesion appears as a firm mass that eventually becomes an ulcer. The gumma is a destructive lesion and can lead to perforation of the palatal bone.

Congenital Syphilis

Syphilis can be transmitted from an infected mother to the fetus because the organism can cross the placenta and enter the fetal circulation. Congenital syphilis

TABLE 3–6 Stages of Syphilis	
Stage	**Oral Lesion**
Primary	Chancre
Secondary	Mucous patch
Latent	None
Tertiary	Gumma

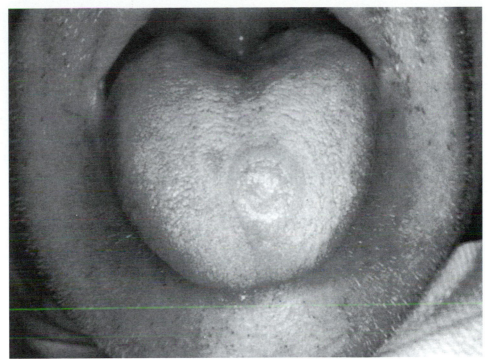

figure 3–36   Chancre on tongue seen in primary syphilis. (Courtesy of Dr. Norman Trieger.)

mulberry molars, deformity on bridge of nose

often causes serious and irreversible damage to the child (e.g., facial and dental abnormalities). These developmental disorders are described in Chapter 4.

Diagnosis and Treatment

The diagnosis of syphilitic lesions occurring on skin can be made using a special microscopic technique called a **dark-field examination** to identify the spirochetes. However, other spirochetes are present in the oral cavity, and therefore this examination is not reliable for oral lesions. Two serologic (blood) tests are commonly used to confirm the diagnosis of syphilis, the VDRL (Venereal Disease Research Laboratory) test and the FTA-ABS (fluorescent treponemal antibody absorption) test. These tests may produce negative results in primary syphilis because sufficient antibodies may not have formed for the test result to be positive.

Syphilis is generally treated with penicillin. The VDRL test is used again to evaluate the success of treatment. The antibody titer decreases if treatment has been successful.

Acute Necrotizing Ulcerative Gingivitis

Opportunistic

Acute necrotizing ulcerative gingivitis, also called **ANUG,** is a painful erythematous gingivitis in which there is necrosis of the interdental papillae (Fig. 3–37; Color Plate 76). ANUG is most likely caused by both a fusiform bacillus and a spirochete (*Borrelia vincentii*) and is associated with decreased resistance to infection.

The gingiva is painful and erythematous, with necrosis of the interdental papillae generally accompanied by a foul odor and metallic taste. The necrosis results in cratering of the interdental papillae area. Sloughing of the necrotic tissue presents as a

always in proximal

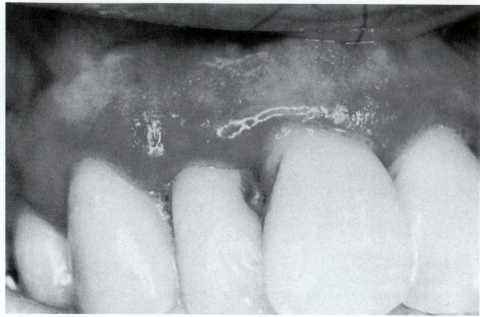

ƒigure 3–37   Acute necrotizing ulcerative gingivitis.

pseudomembrane over the tissues. Systemic manifestations of infection, such as fever and cervical lymphadenopathy, may be present. ANUG can readily be distinguished from acute marginal gingivitis (Color Plate 78).

Pericoronitis

— most common on 3rd molars

Pericoronitis is an inflammation of the mucosa around the crown of a partially erupted, impacted tooth. The soft tissue around the mandibular third molar is the most common location for pericoronitis. The inflammation is usually due to infection by bacteria that are part of the normal oral flora, which proliferate in the pocket between the soft tissue and the crown of the tooth. Compromised host defenses, ranging from minor illnesses to immunodeficiency, are associated with an increased risk of pericoronitis. Trauma from an opposing molar and impaction of food under the soft tissue flap (operculum) covering the distal portion of the third molar may also precipitate pericoronitis.

Diagnosis

The diagnosis of pericoronitis is made on the basis of the clinical presentation. The tissue around the crown of a partially erupted tooth is swollen, erythematous, and painful.

Treatment and Prognosis

Treatment of pericoronitis includes mechanical débridement and irrigation of the pocket and systemic antibiotics. Extraction of the impacted molar is usually necessary to prevent recurrence.

Acute Osteomyelitis

Acute osteomyelitis involves acute inflammation of the bone and bone marrow (Fig. 3–38*A*). Acute osteomyelitis of the jaws is most commonly a result of the extension

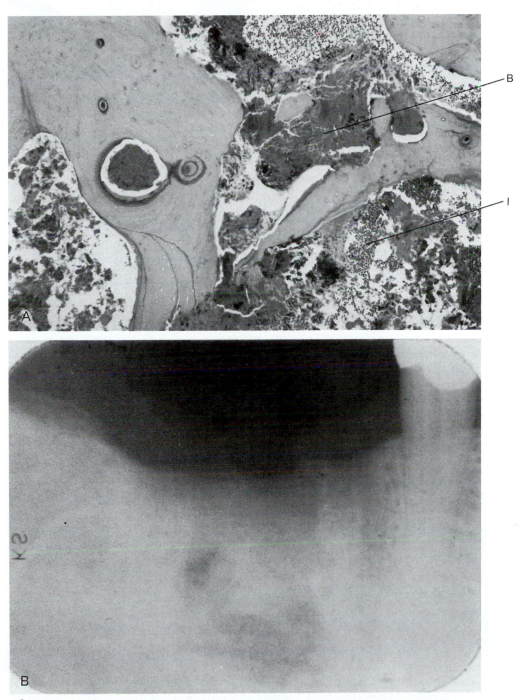

A, Low-power microscopy of acute osteomyelitis showing nonviable bone. Bacterial colonies (B) and inflammatory cells (I) are seen between trabeculae of bone. *B,* Chronic osteomyelitis as seen radiographically.

of a periapical abscess. It may follow fracture of the bone or surgery and may also result from bacteremia.

Diagnosis

The diagnosis of the specific organisms that cause acute osteomyelitis is made on the basis of culture results, and treatment is based on antibiotic sensitivity testing. Microscopic examination shows nonviable bone, necrotic debris, acute inflammation, and bacterial colonies in the marrow spaces. No change is seen on the radiograph unless the disease has been present for more than a week.

Treatment and Prognosis

The treatment of acute osteomyelitis involves drainage of the area and the use of appropriate antibiotics.

Chronic Osteomyelitis

Chronic osteomyelitis is a long-standing inflammation of bone. It may follow inadequately treated acute osteomyelitis, long-term inflammation with no recognized acute phase, Paget's disease, sickle cell disease, or bone irradiation that results in decreased vascularity. The involved bone is painful and swollen, and radiographic examination reveals a diffuse and irregular radiolucency that can eventually become radiopaque (Fig. 3–38B). When radiopacity develops, the condition is called **chronic sclerosing osteomyelitis.**

Diagnosis

The diagnosis of chronic osteomyelitis is based on biopsy results and the histologic examination, which shows chronic inflammation of bone and marrow. Bacterial culture may be helpful, but bacteria may be difficult to identify.

Treatment

Treatment of chronic osteomyelitis involves débridement and administration of systemic antibiotics. In some patients, the use of hyperbaric oxygen may be needed to successfully treat this lesion.

Fungal Infections

Candidiasis

Candidiasis, also called **moniliasis** and **thrush,** occurs as a result of an overgrowth of the yeast-like fungus *Candida albicans.* It is the most common oral fungal infection. This fungus is part of the normal flora in many individuals, particularly those who wear dentures. Overgrowth of *Candida albicans* can result from many different conditions. Some of these include

- Antibiotic therapy
- Cancer chemotherapy
- Corticosteroid therapy
- Dentures
- Diabetes mellitus

- HIV infection
- Hypoparathyroidism
- Infancy (newborn)
- Multiple myeloma
- Primary T-lymphocyte deficiency
- Xerostomia

Newborn infants are particularly susceptible to an overgrowth of this fungus because they do not have either an established oral flora or a fully developed immune system. Pregnant women often have *Candida* vaginitis, and the infant is infected while passing through the birth canal. Antibiotics can alter the bacteria of the oral flora, which can allow the overgrowth of *Candida albicans*. Systemic and topical corticosteroids, diabetes, and cell-mediated immune system deficiency are other factors that allow the overgrowth of this fungus. Candidiasis is one of the most common oral lesions that occurs in association with immunodeficiency (see Chapter 7). Candidiasis generally affects the superficial layers of the epithelium; therefore, when it is present, the proliferating organisms are easily identified in a scraping (smear) of the lesion.

Types of Oral Candidiasis

There are several forms of oral candidiasis, and recognition of their clinical features is important so that candidiasis is included in the differential diagnosis of a variety of clinical presentations. The types of oral candidiasis are

- Pseudomembranous
- Erythematous (acute atrophic)
- Chronic atrophic (denture stomatitis)
- Chronic hyperplastic (*Candida* leukoplakia)
- Angular cheilitis

Pseudomembranous Candidiasis. A white curd-like material is present on the mucosal surface in **pseudomembranous candidiasis** (Fig. 3–39; Color Plate 68). The underlying mucosa is erythematous. There is sometimes a burning sensation, and the patient may complain of a metallic taste.

Erythematous or Acute Atrophic Candidiasis. An erythematous, often painful, mucosa is the presenting complaint in **erythematous** or **acute atrophic candidiasis** (Fig. 3–40; Color Plate 65). This type of candidiasis may be localized to one area of the oral mucosa or may be more generalized.

Chronic Atrophic Candidiasis. The most common type of candidiasis affecting the oral mucosa is called **chronic atrophic candidiasis** (Fig. 3–41). It is also known as **denture stomatitis.** This type of candidiasis also presents as erythematous mucosa, but the erythematous change is limited to the mucosa covered by a full or partial denture. The lesions may vary from petechiae-like to more generalized and granular. It is most common on the palate and maxillary alveolar ridge and is usually asymptomatic, being discovered on examination by the dental hygienist or dentist.

Chronic Hyperplastic Candidiasis. Candidal leukoplakia and **hypertrophic candidiasis** are other names for **chronic hyperplastic candidiasis** (Fig. 3–42). It appears as a white lesion that does not wipe off. An important diagnostic feature of this type of candidiasis is its response to antifungal medication: when leukoplakia is caused by candidiasis, it disappears when treated with antifungal medication.

Angular Cheilitis. *Candida* organisms often cause **angular cheilitis** (Fig. 3–43; Color Plate 3). It appears as erythema or fissuring at the labial commissures. Angular cheilitis may be due to other factors, such as nutritional deficiency; however, it most

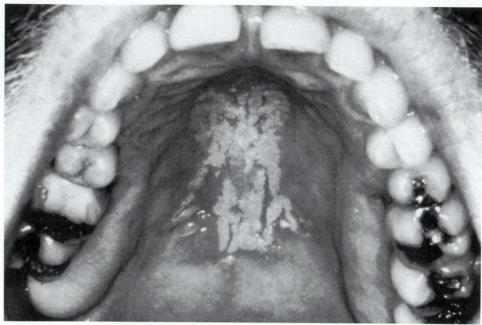

■ *figure* 3–39   Pseudomembranous candidiasis.

commonly results from *Candida* infection. Angular cheilitis frequently accompanies intraoral candidiasis.

Median Rhomboid Glossitis. Several studies have reported an association between **median rhomboid glossitis** (Fig. 3–44; Color Plate 39) and candidiasis. It appears as an erythematous, often rhombus-shaped flat to raised area on the midline of the posterior dorsal tongue. *Candida* organisms have been identified in some lesions, and some lesions disappear with antifungal treatment. However, the response to antifungal treatment is not consistent; therefore, though this lesion has been associated with candidiasis, the cause is not yet clear.

Chronic Mucocutaneous Candidiasis. A severe form of candidiasis that usually occurs in patients who are severely immunocompromised is called **chronic mucocutaneous candidiasis.** There are many immunodeficiency syndromes that include mucocutaneous candidiasis. The patient presents with chronic oral and genital mucosal candidiasis and has skin lesions as well. The skin lesions usually involve the nails and skin folds.

Diagnosis and Treatment

Since *Candida* is part of the oral flora in many individuals, the use of a culture for diagnosis is not particularly helpful. A positive culture result indicates that the organisms are present but not that they are causing infection. The use of the smear (Fig. 3–45) is much more helpful. The surface of the lesion is vigorously scraped with a tongue blade, and the scrapings are spread on a glass slide and fixed with alcohol. The slide is then sent to an oral pathology laboratory for staining and examination. In addition to the smear, the response of the lesion to antifungal treatment is important in confirming the diagnosis of candidiasis. Lesions caused by *Candida* should resolve with antifungal treatment. Both topical and systemic medications are used for candidiasis. However, in some patients, particularly those who are immunocompromised, candidiasis is persistent and recurrent.

Although the final diagnosis and management of a patient with oral candidiasis

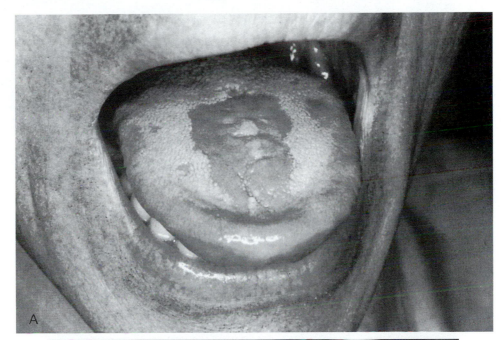

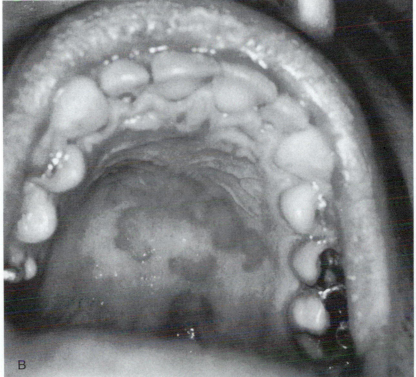

▪ *f* **i g u r e 3–40**   Erythematous candidiasis. *A,* Recent onset and erythematous lesions elsewhere in the oral cavity differentiate this from median rhomboid glossitis.
B, Response to antifungal treatment confirmed the diagnosis of oral candidiasis in this patient.

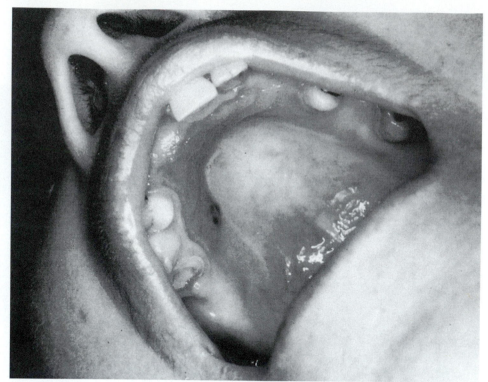

figure 3-41   Chronic atrophic candidiasis (denture stomatitis).

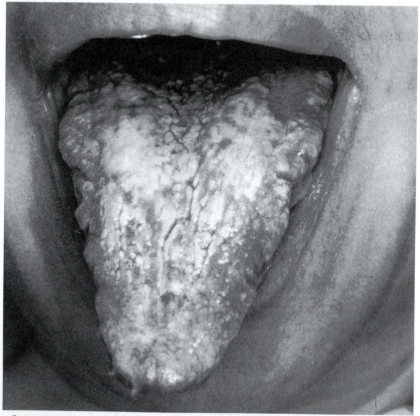

figure 3-42   Chronic hyperplastic candidiasis. The white appearance of the tongue did not wipe off, and it disappeared with antifungal treatment.

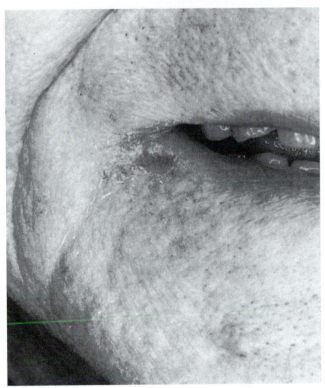

▪ *f i g u r e* **3–43**   Angular cheilitis.

will be handled by the dentist, dental hygienists are often the first to recognize the oral changes characteristic of this condition. Recurrent oral candidiasis may be an early sign of a severe underlying medical problem.

Deep Fungal Infections

Oral lesions occur in some deep fungal infections, for example, histoplasmosis, coccidioidomycosis, blastomycosis, and cryptococcosis. They are all characterized by primary involvement of the lungs. Oral lesions are due to implantation of the organism carried by sputum from the lungs to the oral mucosa.

Infections caused by some of these organisms are more common in certain areas of the United States than in others. Histoplasmosis is widespread in the midwestern United States, and coccidioidomycosis is more prevalent in parts of the western United States, particularly the San Joaquin Valley of California. Blastomycosis is common in the Ohio-Mississippi river basin area. Therefore, oral lesions caused by these organisms are most likely seen in areas of the country in which the infection is most common. Cryptococcosis is transmitted through inhalation of organisms contained in dust from bird droppings, particularly from pigeons. In addition to the regional distribution of these infections, reactivation, including the development of oral lesions, can also occur in patients who are immunocompromised.

Diagnosis

The initial signs and symptoms of these deep fungal infections are usually related to the primary lung infection. Oral lesions are preceded by pulmonary involvement. These oral lesions are chronic, nonhealing ulcers that can resemble squamous cell

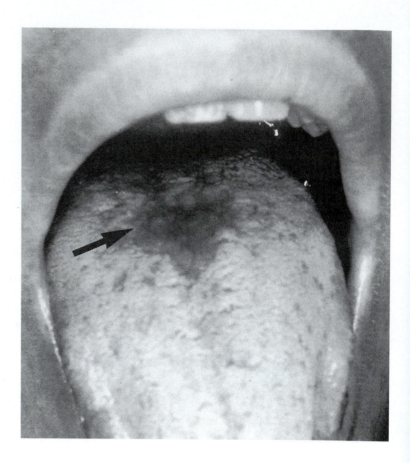

■ *f* i g u r e 3–44
Median rhomboid glossitis *(arrow)*.

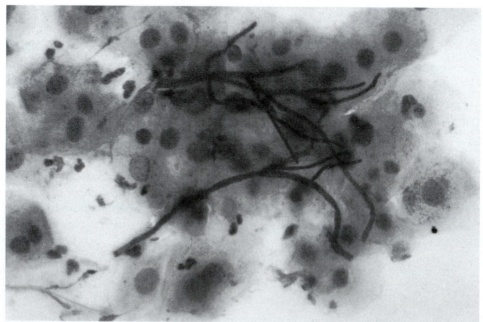

■ *f* i g u r e 3–45 Photomicrograph of a smear showing epithelial cells and *Candida* organisms.

carcinoma. Diagnosis is made by biopsy and microscopic examination. Special staining of the tissue reveals the organisms, which can be identified by their microscopic appearance. Culture of the tissue can also be done and is useful in establishing the diagnosis.

Treatment

Antifungal medications, such as amphotericin B or ketoconazole, are used to treat these infections. However, latent infections may remain even after treatment and may reappear if the individual's immune system becomes deficient.

Mucormycosis

Mucormycosis, also called **phycomycosis,** is a rare fungal infection. The organism is a common inhabitant of soil and is usually nonpathogenic. However, infection with this organism occurs in diabetic and debilitated patients. The disease often involves the nasal cavity, maxillary sinus, and hard palate and can present as a proliferating mass in the maxilla. The diagnosis is made by biopsy and identification of the organisms in the tissue.

Viral Infections

Papillomavirus Infection

Many types of papillomaviruses have been identified. Several have been identified in oral lesions, and some have been identified in normal oral mucosa.

Verruca Vulgaris

The **verruca vulgaris,** or **common wart,** is a papillary oral lesion caused by a papillomavirus. It is a common skin lesion. Oral lesions are less common than skin lesions, but they do occur. The virus is inoculated by direct contact and may be transmitted from skin to oral mucosa. The lips are one of the most common intraoral sites for this lesion. Autoinoculation occurs through finger sucking or fingernail biting in patients with verrucae on the hands or fingers (Fig. 3–46). The verruca vulgaris is usually a white, papillary, exophytic lesion (Fig. 3–47) that closely resembles the benign tumor of squamous epithelium called the **papilloma** (see Chapter 5).

Histologically, the verruca vulgaris consists of finger-like projections of markedly keratotic, stratified squamous epithelium that exhibits a prominent granular cell layer, and numerous cells with clear cytoplasm are present in the upper spinous layer of the epithelium. These cells contain the viral particles that are visible by electron microscopic examination. Each of the projections contains a central core of fibrous connective tissue containing many blood vessels. The vacuolated cells in the epithelium contain the viral particles.

Diagnosis. Biopsy and histologic examination reveal the light microscopic features of this lesion. Immunologic staining is also useful in identifying these viruses.

Treatment and Prognosis. Conservative surgical excision is the treatment of choice for verruca vulgaris. These lesions may recur. In addition, patients with skin lesions should be instructed to refrain from finger sucking or fingernail biting to prevent reinoculation and development of new lesions.

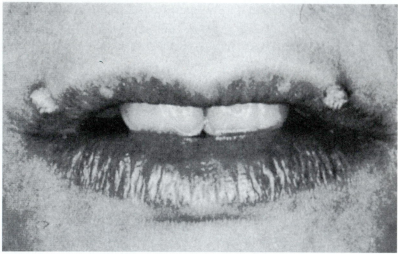

ƒ i g u r e 3–46   Verruca vulgaris on the lips of a girl with similar lesions
on her fingers. (From Shafer WG, Hine MG, Levy BM:
A Textbook of Oral Pathology, 4th ed. Philadelphia, WB
Saunders, 1983, p 88.)

Condyloma Acuminatum

The **condyloma acuminatum** is a benign papillary lesion that is caused by
another papillomavirus. The virus is generally transmitted by sexual contact and is
most common in the anogenital region. It is transmitted to the oral cavity through
oral-genital contact or self-inoculation. *finger nail biting*

Oral condylomas appear as papillary, bulbous masses and can occur anywhere in
the oral mucosa (Fig. 3–48; Color Plate 17). Multiple lesions may be present. They
have been reported to occur on the tongue, buccal mucosa, palate, gingiva, and alveolar

ANAL/ORAL SEX   looks like papilloma but is PINK + more vascular. NOT keratinized.

p.103

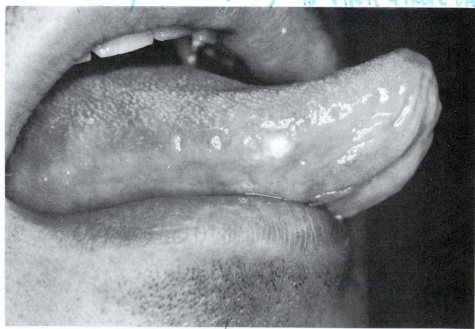

ƒ i g u r e 3–47   Verruca vulgaris.

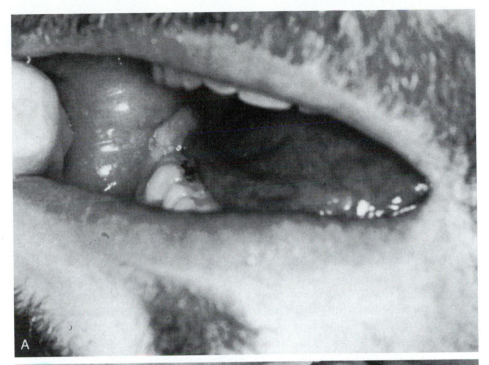

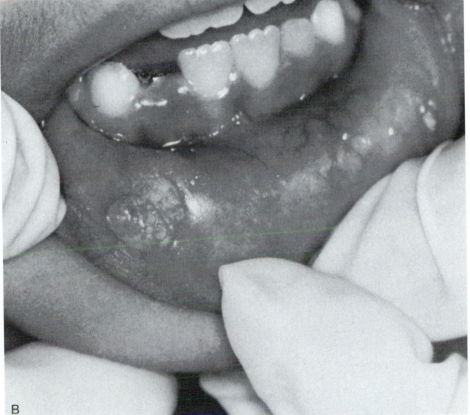

▪ *f* i g u r e **3–48**   Condyloma acuminatum. *A*, Retromolar area. *B*, The presence of condyloma acuminatum in a child is strongly suggestive of sexual abuse. (Courtesy of Dr. Sidney Eisig.)

ridge. The oral condyloma tends to be more diffuse than the papilloma or verruca vulgaris and is generally not as well keratinized as the verruca vulgaris, which is often white; the condyloma is pink.

Histologically, the condyloma acuminatum is composed of finger-like (papillary) projections of epithelium covering cores of connective tissue. The epithelium is thickened, and cells with clear cytoplasm are seen throughout the epithelium. These clear cells contain viral particles that can be identified through immunologic staining.

Treatment and Prognosis. When the condyloma acuminatum occurs in the oral cavity, it is generally treated by conservative surgical excision. However, recurrence is common, and multiple lesions make management difficult. Patients should be instructed to avoid oral-genital contact with an infected partner to prevent reinoculation.

Focal Epithelial Hyperplasia

Focal epithelial hyperplasia, also called **Heck's disease,** is characterized by the presence of multiple whitish to pale-pink nodules distributed throughout the oral mucosa (Fig. 3–49). The disease is most common in children and was first described in Native Americans but has since been described in many different areas of the world. There is evidence that this disease is caused by another human papillomavirus. The lesions are generally asymptomatic and do not require treatment. They resolve spontaneously within a few weeks. Histologically, the lesions show thickened epithelium with broad, connected rete ridges. Cells in the epithelium have clear cytoplasm, which is a common finding in lesions caused by human papillomaviruses.

Herpes Simplex Infection

There are two major forms of the herpes simplex virus—type 1 and type 2. Oral infections are generally caused by type 1, and genital infections are most commonly caused by type 2. Oral infection with the herpes simplex virus occurs in an initial (primary) form and a recurrent (secondary) form. The herpes simplex virus is one of a

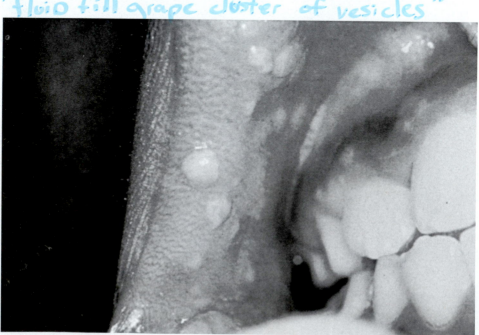

f i g u r e **3–49**   Focal epithelial hyperplasia. (Courtesy of Dr. Stanley Kerpel.)

group of viruses called herpesviruses. Other herpesviruses are varicella-zoster virus, Epstein-Barr virus, and cytomegalovirus. Herpes simplex viruses have the ability to persist in an individual in a clinically quiescent or latent state. The primary infection undergoes remission without the virus being completely eliminated.

(CMV)

Primary Herpetic Gingivostomatitis

The oral disease caused by initial infection with the herpes simplex virus is called **primary herpetic gingivostomatitis** (Fig. 3–50; Color Plate 43). It is characterized by painful, erythematous, and swollen gingiva and multiple tiny vesicles on the perioral skin, vermilion border of the lips, and oral mucosa. They progress to form ulcers. Systemic symptoms such as fever, malaise, and cervical lymphadenopathy generally occur first, followed by gingival involvement and the appearance of mucosal vesicles and ulcers. The disease most commonly occurs in children between the ages of 6 months and 6 years. However, it may occur at any age if an individual who has not been previously exposed to the virus comes into contact with it or if a sufficient level of antibodies has not developed to confer protection against reinfection. Since there are many more individuals with antibodies to herpes simplex than there are who have a history of the disease, the majority of infections are thought to be subclinical. The disease is usually self-limited. The lesions heal spontaneously in 1 to 2 weeks.

HIV - reoccur more often as HIV worsens

Recurrent Herpes Simplex Infection

The herpes simplex virus tends to persist in a latent state, usually in the nerve tissue of the trigeminal ganglion, and causes localized recurrent infections. It has been estimated that one third to one half of the population of the United States experiences recurrent herpes simplex infection. The most common type of recurrent oral herpes simplex infection occurs on the vermilion border of the lips and is called **herpes labialis** (Fig. 3–51; Color Plate 4), which is also called a **cold sore** or **fever blister.** Recurrent infections often occur following certain stimuli, such as sunlight, menstrua-

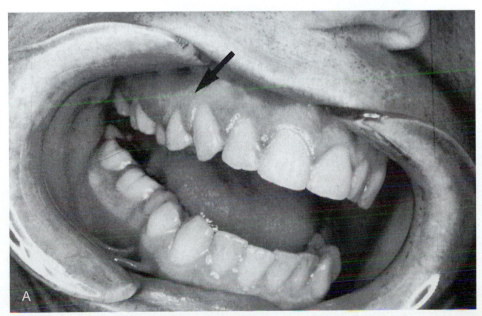

f i g u r e **3–50**   *A*, Example of primary herpetic gingivostomatitis.
Illustration continued on following page

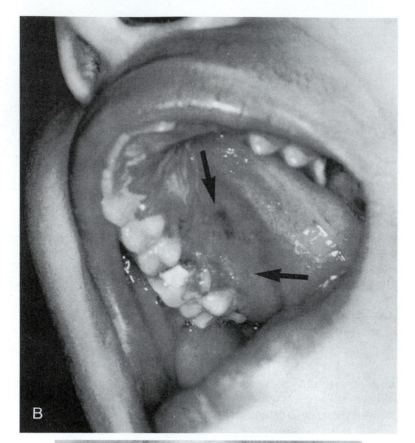

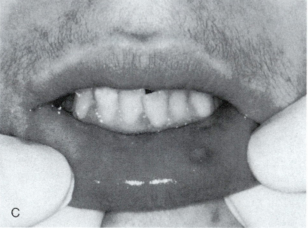

■ *f* i g u r e 3–50   *Continued B* and *C,* Two examples of primary herpetic gingivostomatitis.

tion, fatigue, fever, and emotional stress. These stimuli are thought to trigger the viral replication and immunologic changes that result in clinical lesions. Recurrent herpes simplex infection can also occur intraorally (Fig. 3–52). The appearance and location of these lesions are important to distinguish them from aphthous ulcers (see Table 3–3). Recurrent intraoral herpes simplex occurs on keratinized mucosa that is fixed to bone, most commonly the hard palate and gingiva. The lesions appear as painful crops of tiny vesicles or ulcers that can coalesce to form a single ulcer with an irregular border. There are usually prodromal symptoms such as pain, burning, or tingling in

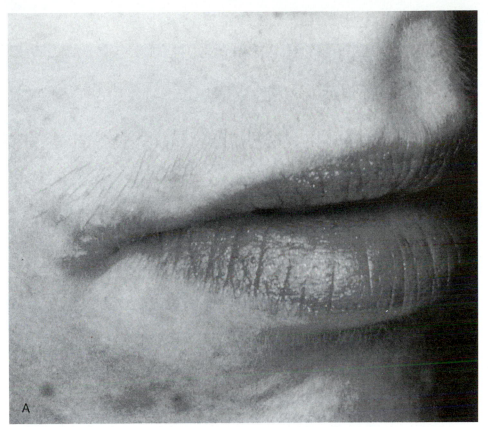

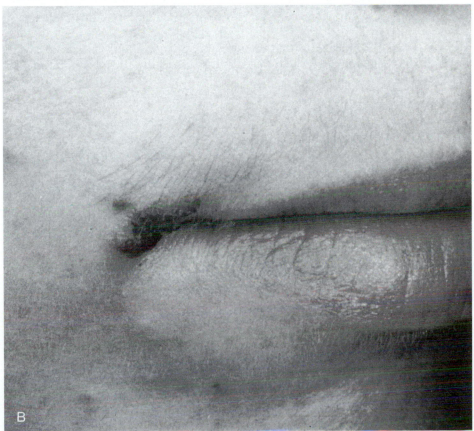

f i g u r e 3-51   Herpes labialis. *A*, Twelve hours after onset. *B*, Forty-eight hours after onset.

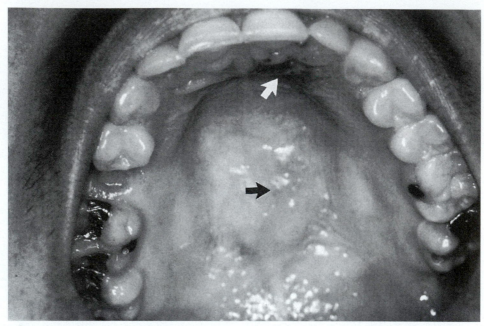

▪ *figure* 3–52   Recurrent intraoral herpes simplex *(arrows)*.

the area in which the vesicles develop. The lesions heal without scarring in 1 to 2 weeks. Episodes of recurrence vary from once a month in some individuals to once a year in others.

Herpes simplex virus is transmitted by direct contact with an infected individual, and the lesions of the primary infection occur at the site of inoculation. The herpes

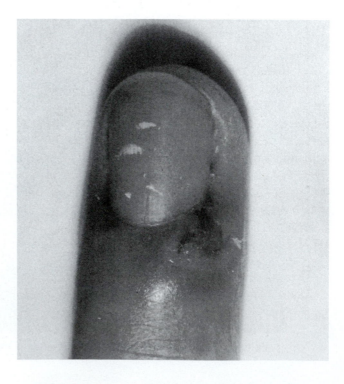

▪ *figure* 3–53
Herpetic whitlow in a dental hygienist.
(Courtesy of Susan Rod Graham.)

simplex virus can be isolated from both primary and recurrent lesions. The amount of virus present is highest in the vesicle stage. There is also evidence that the virus is present in the oral cavity in some individuals when no lesions are present. Herpes simplex virus can cause a painful infection of the fingers, called **herpetic whitlow**, in dentists and dental hygienists (Fig. 3–53). Herpetic whitlow can be either a primary or a recurrent infection. Herpes simplex can also cause eye infection (Fig. 3–54). Routine barrier infection-control procedures (mask, eye protection, and gloves) are important in preventing the transmission of the herpes simplex virus to dental health care workers.

Diagnosis

The diagnosis of herpes simplex infection, both primary and recurrent, is generally made on the basis of the clinical characteristics of the disease (see Table 3–4). In immunocompromised patients the characteristic clinical features may be lacking (see Chapter 7). A viral culture can be performed to confirm the diagnosis. However, this procedure requires a special culture medium and at least 2 days before results are available. Herpes simplex virus causes changes in epithelial cells that can be seen microscopically. These virally altered cells can be seen in tissue obtained by biopsy or on a smear taken by scraping the basal cells of the lesion and spreading them on a glass slide, fixing with alcohol, and submitting them to a pathology laboratory for staining and examination (Fig. 3–55). Smears of herpes simplex ulceration have been reported to be positive for virally altered cells only about 50% of the time.

Treatment

Antiviral drugs, such as acyclovir, are available for the treatment of herpes simplex infection and are used for treating genital herpes simplex infection. Antiviral drugs have not been consistently shown to be effective in treating the oral lesions of herpes simplex infection except in immunocompromised patients. Prevention of herpes labialis may involve the use of sunscreens.

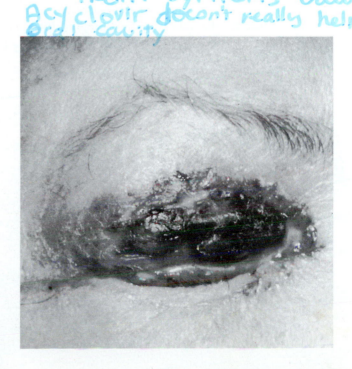

f i g u r e **3-54**

Herpetic eye infection. (Courtesy of Dr. Sidney Eisig.)

Varicella-Zoster Virus

The varicella-zoster virus causes both chickenpox (varicella) and shingles (herpes zoster).

Chickenpox

Chickenpox is a highly contagious disease that causes vesicular and pustular eruptions of the skin and mucous membranes, along with systemic symptoms such as headache, fever, and malaise (Fig. 3–56; Color Plate 82). Chickenpox usually occurs in children, and though there are oral lesions, they generally do not cause severe discomfort. Usually an individual has only a single episode of chickenpox, but second, milder forms have also been described. Recovery generally occurs in 2 to 3 weeks.

Herpes Zoster

Although chickenpox has been described in adults, the virus usually causes a different form of disease in this population, which is called **herpes zoster or shingles.** It is characterized by a unilateral, painful eruption of vesicles along the distribution of a sensory nerve (Fig. 3–57). Whether or not the varicella-zoster virus is harbored in the sensory ganglia during the interval between chickenpox and herpes zoster, in a manner similar to that of the herpes simplex virus, is not clear. However, herpes zoster often occurs in association with immunodeficiency or certain malignancies such as Hodgkin's disease and leukemia. The depression of cell-mediated immunity appears to be important in the development of herpes zoster, which is characterized by the unilateral distribution of vesicles and ulcers. Any of the three branches of the trigeminal nerve may be affected—the ophthalmic branch, the maxillary branch, or the mandibular branch (Fig. 3–58). Oral lesions occur when the maxillary or mandibular branches are affected (Fig. 3–59). The oral lesions, like the skin lesions, are characterized by their unilateral distribution. Prodromal symptoms of pain, burning, or paresthesia often precede the development of vesicles. Oral lesions are painful and begin as vesicles that progress to ulcers. The disease usually lasts for several weeks, and in some patients neuralgia that takes months to resolve may follow the resolution of the lesions.

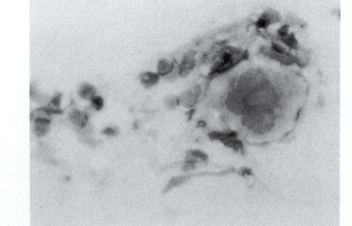

figure 3–55

Smear of virally altered cells resulting from herpes simplex. (Courtesy of Dr. Harry Lumerman.)

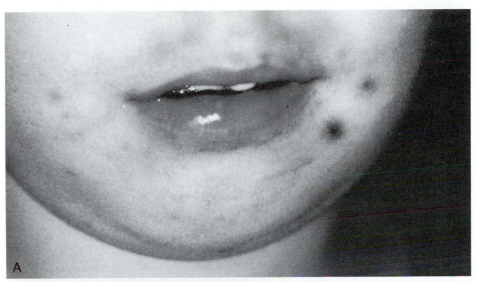

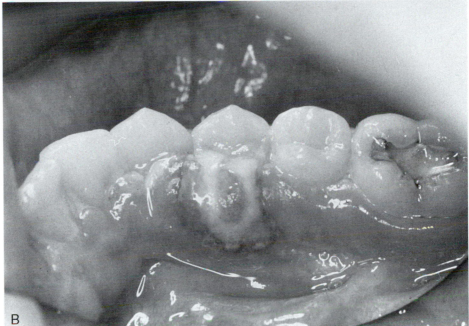

f i g u r e 3–56   Chickenpox. *A*, Skin lesions. *B*, Gingival lesion. (Courtesy of Dr. Roger S. Kitzes.)

Varicella-zoster virus is transmitted primarily by contaminated droplets. The incubation period is about 2 weeks. Both chickenpox and herpes zoster are contagious.

Diagnosis

The diagnosis of varicella and herpes zoster is generally made on the basis of the clinical features. Biopsy or a smear of the lesion may show the same type of virally altered epithelial cells that are seen in herpes simplex infection. Viral cultures may take weeks to grow.

Treatment

Varicella generally requires only supportive treatment. Antiviral drugs are used for immunocompromised patients and for patients with herpes zoster. In some patients

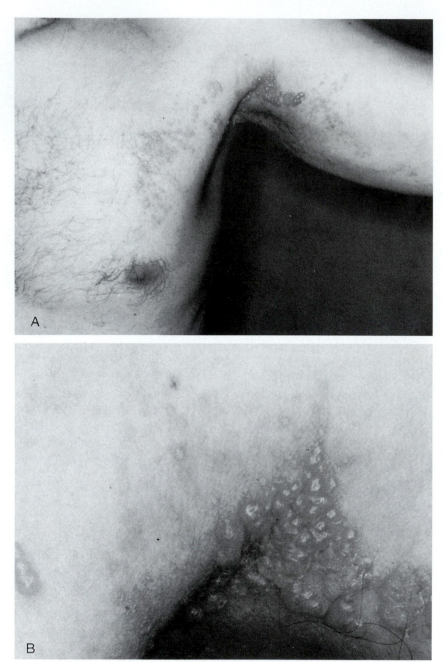

■ *f* i g u r e 3–57   Herpes zoster. *A*, Unilateral distribution of vesicles along the distribution of a sensory nerve. *B*, Many vesicles coalesce to form large lesions.

corticosteroids have been used in an attempt to prevent the pain of postherpetic neuralgia.

Coxsackievirus

The **coxsackievirus,** named for the town in New York where it was first discovered, causes several different infectious diseases, some of which have oral lesions.

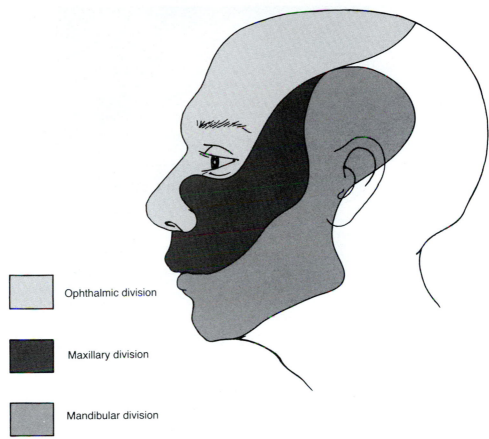

☐ Ophthalmic division

■ Maxillary division

▨ Mandibular division

▪ *f* i g u r e **3–58**   Diagram of the divisions of the trigeminal nerve.

Herpangina

(wHT/GRAY lesion that ulcerates)

Herpangina is caused by a coxsackievirus. Characteristically, vesicles appear on the soft palate (Fig. 3–60), along with fever, malaise, sore throat, and difficulty swallowing (dysphagia). An erythematous pharyngitis is also present. The disease is usually mild to moderate and resolves in less than a week without treatment.

roof of mouth – CRANKY

Hand-Foot-and-Mouth Disease

THIRD

viral

Hand-foot-and-mouth disease is caused by a different coxsackievirus and usually occurs in epidemics in children less than 5 years of age. Oral lesions are generally painful vesicles and ulcers that can occur anywhere in the mouth. Multiple macules or papules occur on the skin, typically on the feet, toes, hands, and fingers. Lesions resolve spontaneously within 2 weeks.

Diagnosis. Although the oral lesions may resemble herpes simplex infection, the distribution of the skin lesions and the mild systemic symptoms usually help to differentiate the two conditions. Viral culture and measurement of circulating antibodies to the type of coxsackievirus that causes hand-foot-and-mouth disease may help to confirm the diagnosis.

Treatment. The disease is generally mild and of short duration. Treatment is generally not required.

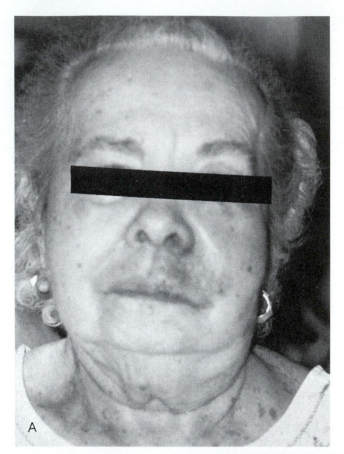

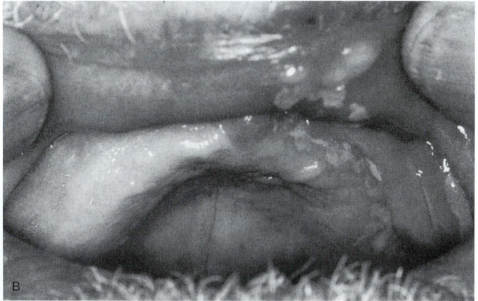

▪ *f* **i g u r e 3–59**   Oral lesions of herpes zoster. *A,* Unilateral facial lesions occurring along
the distribution of the maxillary branch of the trigeminal nerve. *B,* In-
traoral lesions illustrate the unilateral distribution of herpes zoster.

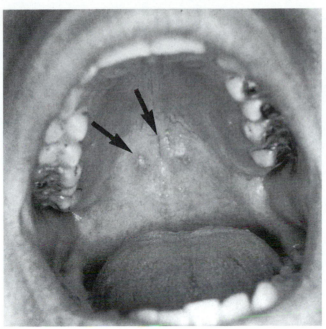

f i g u r e 3–60   Herpangina *(arrows)*.

Other Viral Infections That May Have Oral Manifestations

Measles

[handwritten: Koplick spots]

Measles is a highly contagious disease causing systemic symptoms and a skin rash that results from a type of virus called a **paramyxovirus.** Early in the disease, Koplik's spots, which are small erythematous macules with white necrotic centers, may occur in the oral cavity.

[handwritten: before disease actually sets in.]

Mumps

Mumps, or **epidemic parotitis,** is a viral infection of the salivary glands that is also caused by a paramyxovirus. The disease is characterized by painful swelling of the salivary glands, most commonly bilateral swelling of the parotid glands. *[handwritten: of parotid]*

[handwritten: (orchitis-inflam of Testicles)]

Epstein-Barr Virus

The **Epstein-Barr virus** has been implicated in several diseases that occur in the oral region, including infectious mononucleosis, nasopharyngeal carcinoma, Burkitt's lymphoma, and hairy leukoplakia. Nasopharyngeal carcinoma and Burkitt's lymphoma are rare malignant neoplasms. Infectious mononucleosis and hairy leukoplakia are discussed here.

[handwritten: ADNOPATHY / long duration]

Infectious mononucleosis is an infectious disease caused by the Epstein-Barr virus. It is characterized by sore throat, fever, generalized lymphadenopathy, enlarged spleen, malaise, and fatigue. Palatal petechiae occur in **infectious mononucleosis,** usually appearing early in the course of the disease. The mechanism for the development of these petechiae is unclear. The diagnosis is confirmed by the identification in the blood of mononucleosis cells, which are atypical activated T lymphocytes. Severe complications such as hepatitis occur in some patients. In developed countries infectious

[handwritten vertical note in left margin: CMV - 100% in HIV males - swelling in parotid - uni or bilateral]

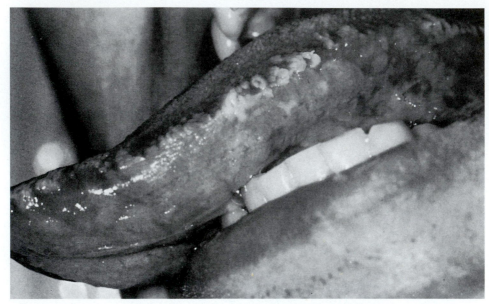

▪ *f i g u r e* **3–61**   Hairy leukoplakia.

mononucleosis occurs principally in late adolescents and young adults in upper socio-economic classes. The virus is transmitted by close contact. Contact with saliva during kissing is a frequent route of transmission of Epstein-Barr virus. In most patients infectious mononucleosis is a benign, self-limited disease that resolves within 4 to 6 weeks. In some patients fatigue lasts much longer.

Hairy Leukoplakia. This irregular, corrugated, white lesion most commonly occurs on the lateral border of the tongue (Fig. 3–61; Color Plate 47). Although hairy leukoplakia was first identified in patients infected with HIV and occurs most commonly in those patients (see Chapter 7), it has also been reported in patients not infected with HIV. Epstein-Barr virus has been identified in the epithelial cells of hairy leukoplakia and is considered to be the cause of the lesion.

Human Immunodeficiency Virus

In addition to hairy leukoplakia, many oral lesions are manifestations of infection with HIV. These are opportunistic infections and develop because of the immunodeficiency that results from HIV infection. The oral manifestations of this infection and its most serious sequela, AIDS, are described in Chapter 7.

SELECTED REFERENCES

BOOKS

Barrett JT: Textbook of Immunology, 5th ed. St. Louis, CV Mosby, 1988.
Bellanti JA: Immunology: Basic Process, 2nd ed. Philadelphia, WB Saunders, 1985.
Cotran RS, Kumar V, Robbins SL, Schoen FJ: Robbins Pathologic Basis of Disease, 5th ed. Philadelphia, WB Saunders, 1994.
Regezi JA, Sciubba JJ: Oral Pathology. Clinical-Pathologic Correlations. Philadelphia, WB Saunders, 1989.
Robbins S, Kumar V: Basic Pathology, 4th ed. Philadelphia, WB Saunders, 1987.
Shafer WG, Hine MK, Levy BM: A Textbook of Oral Pathology, 4th ed. Philadelphia, WB Saunders, 1983.
Sonis ST, Fazio RC, Fang L: Principles and Practice of Oral Medicine, 2nd ed. Philadelphia, WB Saunders, 1995.

Stites DP, Stobo JD, Wells JV: Basic and Clinical Immunology, 5th ed. Los Altos, Lange Medical, 1984.

Trowbridge HO, Emling RC: Inflammation: A Review of the Process, 4th ed. Chicago, Quintessence, 1993.

Wood NK, Goaz PW: Differential Diagnosis of Oral Lesions. St. Louis, CV Mosby, 1985.

JOURNAL ARTICLES

Allen CM: Diagnosing and managing oral candidiasis. J Am Dent Assoc 123:77, 1992.

Anderson KE, Benezra C, Burrows D, et al: Contact dermatitis: A review. Contact Dermatitis 16:55, 1987.

Antoon JW, Miller RL: Aphthous ulcers—a review of the literature of etiology, pathogenesis, diagnosis and treatment. J Am Dent Assoc 101:803, 1980.

Atkinson JC, Fox PC: Sjögren's syndrome: Oral and dental considerations. J Am Dent Assoc 124:74, 1993.

Barnard NA, Scully C, Eveson JW, et al: Oral cancer development in patients with oral lichen planus. J Oral Pathol Med 22:241, 1993.

Barrett AW, Scully CM, Eveson JW: Erythema multiforme involving gingiva. J Periodontol 64:910, 1993.

Baudet-Pommel M, Albuisson E, Kemeny JL, et al: Early dental loss in Sjögren's syndrome. Oral Surg Oral Med Oral Pathol 78:181, 1994.

Challacombe SJ: Immunologic aspects of oral candidiasis. Oral Surg Oral Med Oral Pathol 78:202, 1994.

Cooper MD: B lymphocytes: Normal development and function. N Engl J Med 317:1452, 1987.

Coskey RJ: Fixed drug eruption due to penicillin. Arch Dermatol 111:791, 1975.

Davis LE, Redman JC, Skipper BJ, McLaren LC: Natural history of frequent recurrences of herpes simplex labialis. Oral Surg Oral Med Oral Pathol 66:558, 1988.

Dinarello C, Mier J: Lymphokines. N Engl J Med 317:940, 1987.

Eisenberg E: Lichen planus and oral cancer: Is there a connection between the two? J Am Dent Assoc 123:104, 1992.

Embil JA: Prevalence of recurrent herpes labialis and aphthous ulcers among young adults on six continents. Can Med Assoc J 113:627, 1975.

Eversole LR: Immunopathology of oral mucosal ulcerative, desquamative, and bullous diseases. Oral Surg Oral Med Oral Pathol 77:555, 1994.

Fotos PG, Vincent SD, Hellstein JW: Oral candidiasis: Clinical, historical, and therapeutic features of 100 cases. Oral Surg Oral Med Oral Pathol 74:41, 1992.

Fowler CB, Rees TD, Smith BR: Squamous cell carcinoma on the dorsum of the tongue arising in a long-standing lesion of erosive lichen planus. J Am Dent Assoc 115:707, 710, 1987.

Gabriel SA, Jensen AB, Hartmann D, et al: Lichen planus: Possible mechanisms of pathogenesis. J Oral Med 40:56, 1985.

Gallina G, Cumbo V, Messina P, et al: HLA-A, B, C, DR, MT, and MB antigens in recurrent aphthous stomatitis. Oral Surg Oral Med Oral Pathol 59:364, 1985.

Gawkrodger DJ, Stephenson TJ, Thomas SE: Squamous cell carcinoma complicating lichen planus: A clinico-pathological study of three cases. Dermatology 188:36, 1994.

Greenspan JS: Infections and non-neoplastic diseases of the oral mucosa. J Oral Pathol 12:139, 1983.

Harlan JM: Neutrophil-mediated vascular injury. Acta Med Scand (Suppl) 715:123, 1987.

Harris AM, Van Wyk CW: Heck's disease (focal epithelial hyperplasia): A longitudinal study. Community Dent Oral Epidemiol 21:82, 1993.

Holmstrup P, Schiotz AW, Westergaard J: Effect of dental plaque control on gingival lichen planus. Oral Surg Oral Med Oral Pathol 69:585, 1990.

Iacopino AM, Wathen WF: Oral candidal infection and denture stomatitis: A comprehensive review. J Am Dent Assoc 123:46, 1992.

Itin PH: Oral hairy leukoplakia—10 years on. Dermatology 187:159, 1993.

Jorizzo JL, Salisbury PL, Rogers RS III, et al: Oral lesions in systemic lupus erythematosus. Do ulcerative lesions represent a necrotizing vasculitis? J Am Acad Dermatol 27:389, 1992.

Katz RW, Brahim JS, Travis WD: Oral squamous cell carcinoma arising in a patient with long-standing lichen planus: A case report. Oral Surg Oral Med Oral Pathol 70:282, 1990.

Koorbusch GF, Fotos P, Terhark K: Retrospective assessment of osteomyelitis. Oral Surg Oral Med Oral Pathol 74:149, 1992.

Krippaehne JA, Montgomery MT: Erythema multiforme: A literature review and case report. Special Care Dent 12:125, 1992.

Lacy MF, Reade PC, Hay KD: Lichen planus: A theory of pathogenesis. Oral Surg Oral Med Oral Pathol 56:521, 1983.

Loh HS, Quah TC: Histiocytosis X (Langerhans-cell histiocytosis) of the palate. Case report. Aust Dent J 35:117, 1990.

Lozada-Nur F, Gorsky M, Silverman S Jr: Oral erythema multiforme: Clinical observations and treatment of 95 patients. Oral Surg Oral Med Oral Pathol 67:36, 1989.

Lynch DP: Oral candidiasis: History, classification and clinical presentation. Oral Surg Oral Med Oral Pathol 78:189, 1994.

MacPhail LA, Greenspan D, Feigal DW, Greenspan JS: Recurrent aphthous ulcers in association with HIV infection. Description of ulcer types and analysis of T-lymphocyte subsets. Oral Surg Oral Med Oral Pathol 71:678, 1991.

Manton SL, Scully C: Mucous membrane pemphigoid: An elusive diagnosis? Oral Surg Oral Med Oral Pathol 66:37, 1988.

McKenzie CD, Gobetti JP: Diagnosis and treatment of orofacial herpes zoster: Report of cases. J Am Dent Assoc 120:679, 1990.

Migliorati CA, Jones AC, Baughman PA: Use of exfoliative cytology in the diagnoses of oral hairy leukoplakia. Oral Surg Oral Med Oral Pathol 76:704, 1993.

Miller MF, Ship II, Ram C: A retrospective study of the prevalence and incidence of recurrent aphthous ulcers in a professional population, 1958–1971. Oral Surg Oral Med Oral Pathol 43:532, 1977.

Miller RL: The differential diagnosis of white lesions resembling oral hairy leukoplakia. J Tenn Dent Assoc 73:20, 1993.

Miller RL, Gould AR, Bernstein ML: Cinnamon induced stomatitis venenata. Oral Surg Oral Med Oral Pathol 73:708, 1992.

Morrow DJ, Sandhu HS, Daley TD: Focal epithelial hyperplasia (Heck's disease) with generalized lesions of the gingiva. A case report. J Periodontol 64:63, 1993.

Nossal GJV: The basic components of the immune system. N Engl J Med 316:1320, 1987.

Perna JJ, Eskinazi DP: Treatment of oro-facial herpes simplex infections with acyclovir: A review. Oral Surg Oral Med Oral Pathol 65:689, 1988.

Porter SR, Scully C, Standen GR: Autoimmune neutropenia manifesting as recurrent oral ulceration. Oral Surg Oral Med Oral Pathol 78:178, 1994.

Raghoebar GM, Brouwer TJ, Schoots CJ: Pemphigus vulgaris of the oral mucosa: Report of two cases. Quintessence International 22:199, 1991.

Rodu B, Mattingly G: Oral mucosal ulcers: Diagnosis and management. J Am Dent Assoc 123:83, 1992.

Ryan G, Majno G: Acute inflammation: A review. Am J Pathol 83:185, 1987.

Schofield JK, Tatnall FM, Leigh IM: Recurrent erythema multiforme: Clinical features and treatment in a large series of patients. Br J Dermatol 34:63, 1993.

Schonfeld S, Checchi L: Review of immunology for the periodontist. West Soc Periodontol 33:53, 1985 (abstract).

Sciubba JJ: Sjögren's syndrome: Pathology, oral presentation and dental management. Compend Contin Educ Dent 15:1084, 1994.

Scully C: Orofacial herpes simplex virus infections: Current concepts in the epidemiology, pathogenesis, and treatment, and disorders in which the virus may be implicated. Oral Surg Oral Med Oral Pathol 68:701, 1989.

Scully C, El-Kom M: Lichen planus: Review and update on pathogenesis. J Oral Pathol 14:431, 1985.

Sieggren M: Healing of physical wounds. Nurs Clin North Am 22:439, 1987.

Shaw L, Glenwright HD: Histiocytosis X: An oral diagnostic problem. J Clin Periodontol 15:312, 1988.

Turjanmaa K: Incidence of immediate allergy to latex gloves in hospital personnel. Contact Dermatitis 17:270, 1987.

Unanue E: Cooperation between mononuclear phagocytes and lymphocytes in immunity. N Engl J Med 303:997, 1980.

Vincent SD, Fotos PG, Baker KA, Williams TP: Oral lichen planus: The clinical, historical and therapeutic features of 100 cases. Oral Surg Oral Med Oral Pathol 70:165, 1990.

Vincent SD, Lilly GE, Baker KA: Clinical, historical and therapeutic features of cicatricial pemphigoid. A literature review and open therapeutic trial with corticosteroids. Oral Surg Oral Med Oral Pathol 76:453, 1993.

Williams BG: Oral drug reaction to methyldopa. Oral Surg Oral Med Oral Pathol 56:375, 1983.

Yazici H, Barnes CG: Practical treatment recommendations for pharmacotherapy of Behçet's syndrome. Drugs 42:796, 1991.

Zegarelli DJ: The treatment of oral lichen planus. Ann Dent 52:3, 1993.

Zhu WY, Leonardi C, Blauvelt A, et al: Human papillomavirus DNA in the dermis of condyloma acuminatum. J Cutan Pathol 20:447, 1993.

REVIEW QUESTIONS

1. The immune system defends the body against foreign substances that are called
   (A) Plasma cells
   (B) Antibodies
   (C) Antigens
   (D) Lymphocytes

2. Memory is an important function of the immune system because
    (A) It retains the memory of the antibody
    (B) It allows faster future immune responses
    (C) Like inflammation, it remembers the antigen
    (D) It weakens future immune responses

3. Immunization with a vaccine works by
    (A) Increasing the risk of an antigen-causing disease
    (B) Using antibodies produced by another person
    (C) Passing antibodies from the mother to the fetus
    (D) Producing active acquired immunity

4. A B lymphocyte is a cell in the immune system that is
    (A) Derived from a precursor stem cell
    (B) Matured and resides in the thymus
    (C) Produced from plasma cells
    (D) Active in foreign substance surveillance

5. A macrophage is a cell in the immune system that
    (A) Retains the memory of the encountered antigen
    (B) Serves as a link between the inflammatory and repair processes
    (C) Undergoes B-cell phagocytosis initially during inflammation
    (D) Can be activated by lymphokines

6. Which statement is TRUE of natural killer (NK) cells?
    (A) NK cells do not circulate
    (B) NK cells secrete antibodies
    (C) NK cells can recognize antigen
    (D) NK cells do not have memory

7. The cells of the body are no longer tolerated and the immune system treats them as antigens in which type of immunopathologic disease?
    (A) Hypersensitivity
    (B) Immunodeficiency
    (C) Hyperplasia
    (D) Autoimmune disease

8. During the anaphylactic type of hypersensitivity reaction, the plasma cells
    (A) Produce antibody called IgE
    (B) React with lymphocytes
    (C) Combine with antigen
    (D) Form immune complexes with antigen

9. Which type of hypersensitivity reaction involves activated complement?
    (A) Type I
    (B) Type II
    (C) Type III
    (D) Type IV

10. What type of lymphocyte matures in the thymus, produces lymphokines, and can increase or suppress the humoral immune response?
    (A) B cell
    (B) Plasma cell
    (C) T cell
    (D) Macrophage

11. In the immune system, antibodies are proteins that are
    (A) Also termed immunoglobulins
    (B) Directly produced from lymphocytes
    (C) Produced in response to other antibodies
    (D) Directly produced from mast cells

12. Which immunopathology involves a decreased number or activity of lymphoid cells?
    (A) Autoimmunity
    (B) Hypersensitivity
    (C) Immunodeficiency
    (D) Immunization

13. The humoral immune response involves the production of
    (A) Antigens
    (B) Antibodies
    (C) Autoimmune cells
    (D) Toxins

14. Measurement of a specific antibody level in the blood is called
    (A) Phagocytosis
    (B) Margination
    (C) Titer
    (D) Pavementing

15. Which type of immunity may be immediately provided to dental personnel following needle-stick accidents?
    (A) Natural passive immunity
    (B) Acquired passive immunity
    (C) Natural active immunity
    (D) Acquired active immunity

16. All of the following are examples of hypersensitivity reactions except
    (A) Lichen planus
    (B) Urticaria
    (C) Angioedema
    (D) Contact mucositis

17. Reiter's syndrome is
    (A) An infectious disorder
    (B) An autoimmune response
    (C) An immunologic disorder
    (D) More common in women than in men

18. The "target lesion" on the skin is associated with which disease?
    (A) Behçet's syndrome
    (B) Systemic lupus erythematosus
    (C) Lichen planus
    (D) Erythema multiforme

19. Tzanck cells are seen in which condition?
    (A) Pemphigus vulgaris
    (B) Erythema multiforme
    (C) Systemic lupus erythematosus
    (D) Behçet's syndrome

20. The oral lesions in Reiter's syndrome may resemble
    (A) Nicotine stomatitis
    (B) Lichen planus
    (C) Angioedema
    (D) Geographic tongue

21. Which systemic disease is NOT associated with aphthous ulcers?
    (A) Behçet's syndrome
    (B) Histiocytosis X
    (C) Ulcerative colitis
    (D) Crohn's disease

22. The two cells that histologically characterize the diseases categorized as histiocytosis X are
    (A) Lymphocytes and plasma cells
    (B) Fibroblasts and lymphocytes
    (C) Eosinophils and histiocytes (macrophages)
    (D) Neutrophils and lymphocytes

23. Which disease in the reticuloendothelial system is characterized by a triad of symptoms?
    (A) Letterer-Siwe disease
    (B) Hand-Schüller-Christian disease
    (C) Eosinophilic granuloma
    (D) Behçet's syndrome

24. The most benign type of histiocytosis X disease is
    (A) Hand-Schüller-Christian disease
    (B) Eosinophilic granuloma
    (C) Letterer-Siwe disease
    (D) Chronic disseminated reticulosis

25. The most significant oral manifestation of Sjögren's syndrome is
    (A) Leukoplakia
    (B) Geographic tongue
    (C) Erythema multiforme
    (D) Xerostomia

26. Which statement is FALSE?
    (A) The bullae of pemphigus vulgaris are more fragile than those of bullous pemphigoid
    (B) Acantholysis of the epithelium is seen in pemphigus vulgaris
    (C) In pemphigoid, the separation of the epithelium from the connective tissue occurs in the area of the basement membrane
    (D) Skin lesions are common in cicatricial pemphigoid

27. Which is the most distinct and definitive characteristic that distinguishes pemphigus from pemphigoid?
    (A) Size of the ulcerations
    (B) Age and sex of the patient
    (C) The histologic findings showing the location of the lesion being intraepithelial for pemphigus and subepithelial for pemphigoid
    (D) Amount of hyperkeratosis seen in both

28. Desquamative gingivitis may be seen in
    (A) Cicatricial pemphigoid
    (B) Pemphigus vulgaris
    (C) Lichen planus
    (D) All of the above

29. Which statement is FALSE?
    (A) The primary lesion of syphilis is called chancre
    (B) The secondary lesion of syphilis occurs at the site of inoculation with the organism
    (C) The tertiary lesion of syphilis is called a gumma
    (D) Syphilis is caused by the spirochete *Treponema pallidum*

30. Verruca vulgaris
    (A) Clinically resembles an irritative fibroma
    (B) Is caused by a human papillomavirus
    (C) Is most commonly seen on the buccal mucosa
    (D) All of the above

31. Which area, in a reaction to angioedema, could create very serious complications for the patient?
    (A) Lips
    (B) Mucosa
    (C) Eyelids
    (D) Epiglottis

32. Which form of lichen planus can simulate hyperkeratosis or leukoplakia?
    (A) Plaque-like
    (B) Erosive
    (C) Papular
    (D) Reticular

33. This pathologic condition occurs more frequently in females, and a blood test is of significant importance to the diagnosis. Oral lesions are ulcerated, and a characteristic butterfly-shaped lesion also appears on the skin. You suspect
    (A) Pemphigus
    (B) Erosive lichen planus
    (C) Desquamative gingivitis
    (D) Lupus erythematosus

34. Oral candidiasis is caused by a
    (A) Bacterium
    (B) Virus
    (C) Fungus
    (D) Protozoan

35. Which statement is FALSE?
    (A) Angular cheilitis may be caused by *Candida albicans*
    (B) White lesions resulting from candidiasis may not rub off
    (C) Erythematous candidiasis is usually completely asymptomatic
    (D) Denture stomatitis may be a form of oral candidiasis

36. Which type of infection is involved when normal oral flora can cause disease?
    (A) Chronic inflammatory
    (B) Opportunistic
    (C) Hyperplastic
    (D) Granulomatous

37. A characteristic clinical feature of herpes zoster is
    (A) Ulcer formation
    (B) Pain
    (C) Unilateral distribution of lesions
    (D) White lesions

38. A cytologic smear may be helpful in the diagnosis of
    (A) Coxsackievirus infection
    (B) Human papillomavirus infection
    (C) Tuberculosis
    (D) Candidiasis and herpes simplex infection

39. Which condition is not associated with the Epstein-Barr virus?
    (A) Hairy leukoplakia
    (B) Herpangina
    (C) Nasopharyngeal carcinoma
    (D) Infectious mononucleosis

4

Developmental Disorders

JOEN IANNUCCI HARING

•

OLGA A. C. IBSEN

•

Objectives

After studying this chapter, the student should be able to:

1. Define each of the words in the vocabulary list for this chapter.
2. Define inherited disorders.
3. Recognize developmental disorders of the dentition.
4. Describe the embryonic development of the face, oral cavity, and teeth.
5. Define, describe, and identify all the developmental anomalies discussed in this chapter.
6. Identify clinically, radiographically, or both, the developmental anomalies discussed in this chapter.
7. Distinguish between intraosseous cysts and extraosseous cysts.
8. Describe the differences between odontogenic and nonodontogenic cysts.
9. Name four odontogenic cysts that are intraosseous.
10. Name two odontogenic cysts that are extraosseous.
11. Name four nonodontogenic cysts that are intraosseous.
12. Name four nonodontogenic cysts that are extraosseous.
13. List and define three anomalies that affect the number of teeth.
14. List and define two anomalies that affect the size of the teeth.
15. List and define five anomalies that affect the shape of the teeth.
16. Identify anomalies affecting tooth eruption.
17. Identify the diagnostic process that contributes most significantly to the final diagnosis of each developmental anomaly discussed in this chapter.

Vocabulary

Ankyloglossia (ang″kĭ-lo-glos′e-ah)   Extensive adhesion of the tongue to the floor of the mouth or the lingual aspect of the anterior portion of the mandible.

Ankylosed teeth (ang′kĭ-lōsd tēth)   Teeth that are fused to the alveolar bone; a condition especially common with retained deciduous teeth

Anodontia (an″o-don′she-ah)   Congenital lack of teeth

Anomaly (ah-nom′ah-le)   Marked deviation from normal, especially as a result of congenital or hereditary defects

Commissure (kom′ĭ-shūr)   The site of union of corresponding parts, for example, the corners of the lips (labial commissure)

Concrescence (kon-kres′ens)   In dentistry, a condition in which two adjacent teeth become united by cementum

Congenital (kon-jen′ĭ-tal)   Present at and existing from the time of birth

Cyst (sist)   An abnormal sac or cavity lined by epithelium and enclosed in a connective tissue capsule

Dens in dente (dens in den′te)   "A tooth within a tooth"; a developmental anomaly

210

that results when the enamel organ invaginates into the crown of a tooth before mineralization

Dentinogenesis (den″tĭ-no-jen′ĕ-sis) The formation of dentin

Differentiation (dif′er-en″she-a′shun) The distinguishing of one thing from another

Dilaceration (di-las″er-a′shun) An abnormal bend or curve, as in the root of a tooth

Fusion (fu′zhun) The union of two adjacent tooth germs

Gemination (jem-ĭ-na′shun) "Twinning." A single tooth germ attempts to divide, resulting in the incomplete formation of two teeth; the tooth usually has a single root and root canal

Hypodontia (hi″po-don′she-ah) Partial anodontia; the lack of one or more teeth

Impacted teeth (im-pakt′ed tēth) Teeth that cannot erupt into the oral cavity because of a physical obstruction

Macrodontia (mak″ro-don′she-ah) Abnormally large teeth

Microdontia (mi″kro-don′she-ah) Abnormally small teeth

Multilocular (mul-tĭ-lok′ū-ler) A radiographic appearance in which there are many circular radiolucencies; these can appear "soap bubble–like" or "honeycomb-like."

Nodule (nod′ūl) A small solid mass that can be detected through touch

Predilection (prĕd-ĭ-lĕk′shun) A disposition in favor of something; preference

Proliferation (pro-lif″ĕ-ra′shun) The multiplication of cells

Stomodeum (sto″mo-de′um) The embryonic invagination that becomes the oral cavity

Supernumerary (soo″per-nu′mer-ar″e) In excess of the normal or regular number, as in teeth

The development of the human body is an extremely complex process that begins when an egg is fertilized by a sperm. It continues with a series of cell divisions, multiplications, and differentiation into various tissues and structures. A failure or disturbance that occurs during these processes may result in a lack, excess, or deformity of a body part. These disorders are called **developmental disorders**, or **developmental anomalies**.

Inherited disorders are different from developmental disorders in that they are caused by an abnormality in the genetic make-up (genes and chromosomes) of an individual and are transmitted from parent to offspring through the egg or sperm (see Chapter 6).

A **congenital disorder** is one that is present at birth. It can be either inherited or developmental; however, the cause of most congenital abnormalities is unknown.

The complex process of proliferation and differentiation that takes place in the human body provides numerous possibilities for errors or defects in development. The head and neck region is a common location for such errors because of its intricate sequence and pattern of development. This chapter includes descriptions of developmental disorders of the face, oral cavity, and teeth with which the dental hygienist should be familiar.

Some of the developmental disturbances discussed in this chapter can be identified clinically, whereas others are identified by radiographic examination, and still others require biopsy and histologic examinations. A thorough clinical examination, including extraoral as well as intraoral structures, is an essential component. Dental radiographs are an important part of the examination. Any developmental anomalies observed either clinically or radiographically are documented in the patient's record even if no treatment is indicated. The patient is informed of all dental anomalies, their possible implications, and the treatment necessary, if any. In some instances referral to a specialist is indicated. In order to better understand these developmental disorders, a brief review of the embryonic development of the face, oral cavity, and teeth is included in this chapter.

EMBRYONIC DEVELOPMENT OF THE FACE, ORAL CAVITY, AND TEETH

Face

Development of the face is a process of selective growth or proliferation and differentiation (Figs. 4–1 and 4–2). During the third week of embryonic life, an invagination or infolding of the ectoderm forms the primitive oral cavity, which is called the **stomodeum**. Just above the stomodeum is a process called the **frontal process**, and just below it is a structure called the first branchial arch. Additional branchial arches form below the first branchial arch. All of the face and most of the structures of the oral cavity develop from either the frontal process or the first branchial arch.

The first branchial arch divides into two **maxillary processes** and the **mandibular process**. The maxillary processes give rise to the upper part of the cheeks, the lateral portions of the upper lip, and part of the palate. The mandibular arch forms the lower part of the cheeks, the mandible, and part of the tongue.

As development continues, the future openings of the nose are marked by two pits called **olfactory pits** that develop on the surface of the frontal process. They divide the frontal process into three parts: one **median nasal process** and the right and left

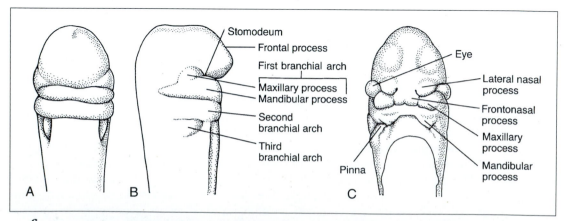

ƒ i g u r e 4–1   In the third week of embryonic life, an invagination or infolding of the ectoderm forms the primitive oral cavity called the stomodeum. *A* and *B,* As facial development continues, the first branchial arch divides into two maxillary processes. *C,* The fourth week of development.

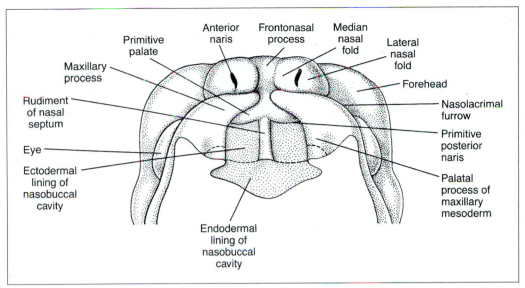

■ *figure* 4–2   The right and left palatine processes fuse to form the maxilla and premaxilla. A Y-shaped pattern results.

lateral nasal processes. The lateral nasal processes form the sides of the nose, whereas the median nasal process forms the center and tip of the nose. Later, the median nasal process grows downward between the maxillary processes to form a pair of bulges called the **globular process**. This continues to grow downward, forming the portion of the upper lip called the **philtrum**. Most of these developments are completed by the end of the eighth week of embryonic life.

Oral and Nasal Cavities

The area of the palate called the **premaxilla** develops from the globular process. The **lateral palatine processes** (left and right) are formed from the maxillary processes. These lateral palatine processes then fuse with the premaxilla. The fusion creates a Y-shaped pattern (see Fig. 4–2). The nasal septum arises from the median nasal process. The right and left maxillary processes fuse together with the nasal septum at the center of the palate.

The tongue develops from the first three branchial arches. The second and third branchial arches are located just below the first branchial arch (see Fig. 4–1B). The body of the tongue forms from the first branchial arch, and the base of the tongue forms from the second and third branchial arches.

Teeth

Tooth development, or **odontogenesis**, in the human embryo takes place at about the fifth week of embryonic life and involves both ectoderm and ectomesenchyme. The ectomesenchyme is derived from neural crest cells.

Odontogenesis begins with the formation of a band of ectoderm in each jaw called the **primary dental lamina**. Ten small knob-like proliferations of epithelial cells develop on the primary dental lamina in each jaw (Fig. 4–3A). Each of these proliferations extends into the underlying mesenchyme, becoming the early enamel organ for each of the primary teeth (Fig. 4–3B).

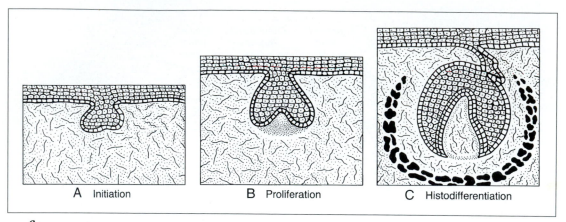

A   Initiation   B   Proliferation   C   Histodifferentiation

▪ *f* i g u r e 4–3   Development of a tooth germ showing initiation of dental lamina *(A)*, proliferation of dental lamina *(B)*, and differentiation of the components of the tooth germ *(C)*.

The tooth germ is composed of three parts: the enamel organ, the dental papilla, and the dental sac or follicle (Fig. 4–3*C*). The enamel organ develops from ectoderm, and the dental papilla and dental sac or follicle develop from mesenchyme. Cell differentiation in the enamel organ progresses to produce ameloblasts that form enamel. In the dental papilla, odontoblasts are produced to form dentin. The permanent or **succedaneous** enamel organs form at the same time.

Formation of dental hard tissues occurs during the fifth month of gestation (Fig. 4–4). **Dentinogenesis** is the formation of dentin. Dentin is the first mineralized tooth tissue to appear. When it begins to form, the mesenchymal tissue within the tooth germ is called the **dental papilla**. After dentin is produced, the dental papilla is called the dental pulp. Enamel is the product of the enamel organ. Enamel matrix begins to form shortly after dentin, and mineralization and maturation of enamel follow the formation of the matrix. **Amelogenesis** refers to the formation of enamel.

The dental sac or follicle that surrounds the developing tooth germ provides cells that form cementum, the periodontal ligament, and alveolar bone. **Cementogenesis** (the formation of cementum) occurs after crown formation is complete. An epithelial structure called **Hertwig's epithelial root sheath** proliferates to shape the root of the tooth and induces the formation of the root dentin. The cells of Hertwig's epithelial root sheath must break up and pull away from the root surface before cementum can be produced. Very little cementum is produced until the tooth has erupted and is in

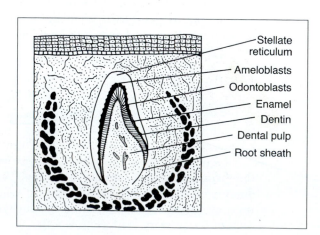

Stellate reticulum
Ameloblasts
Odontoblasts
Enamel
Dentin
Dental pulp
Root sheath

▪ *f* i g u r e 4-4
Deposition of enamel and dentin.

occlusion and functioning. Root length is not completed until 1 to 4 years after the tooth erupts into the oral cavity.

DEVELOPMENTAL SOFT TISSUE ABNORMALITIES

Ankyloglossia

Ankyloglossia is an extensive adhesion of the tongue to the floor of the mouth, which is often referred to as "tongue-tie." Ankyloglossia is derived from the Greek words "ankylos," meaning adhesion, and "glossa," meaning tongue. This adhesion results from the complete or partial fusion of the lingual frenum to the floor of the mouth. Total ankyloglossia is rare. Partial ankyloglossia appears clinically as a very short lingual frenum connecting the anteroventral portion of the tongue to the floor of the mouth (Fig. 4–5; Color Plate 34). Patients with a short lingual frenum may exhibit no adverse effects, but some may have problems with speech. Gingival recession and bone loss can occur if the frenum is attached high on the lingual alveolar ridge.

Treatment. Surgical removal of a portion of the lingual frenum, known as **frenectomy**, is the usual treatment for ankyloglossia.

Commissural Lip Pits

Commissural lip pits are epithelium-lined blind tracts located at the corners of the mouth (Fig. 4–6). These tracts may be shallow, or they may be several millimeters deep. They are a relatively common developmental anomaly. The cause of commissural lip pits is not clear; both the incomplete fusion of the maxillary and mandibular processes and the defective development of the horizontal facial cleft have been suggested. The commissural lip pit may be observed during examination.

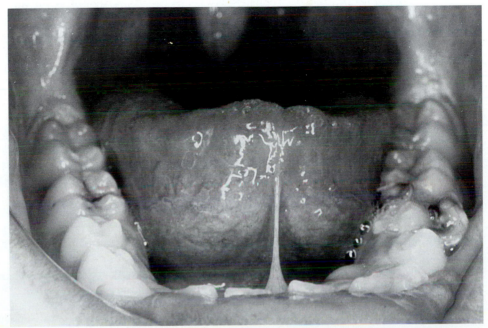

figure 4–5 Ankyloglossia. The short lingual frenum is attached near the tip of the tongue. (Courtesy of Dr. George Blozis.)

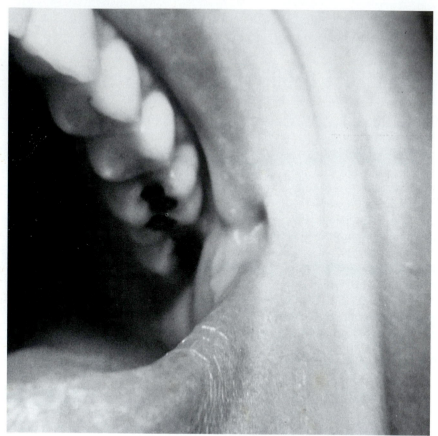

▪ *f* i g u r e 4–6   Commissural lip pit. A deep depression is seen at the labial commissure.

Another lip pit that occasionally may be seen is the **congenital lip pit**. It occurs
near the midline of the vermilion border of the lip and may appear as either a unilateral
or a bilateral depression.

Treatment. No treatment is indicated for lip pits.

Lingual Thyroid

Lingual thyroid, or **ectopic lingual thyroid nodule,** is a small mass of thyroid tissue
located on the tongue away from the normal anatomic location of the thyroid gland. It is
an uncommon developmental anomaly that results from the failure of the primitive thyroid
tissue to migrate from its developmental location in the area of the foramen caecum on
the posterior portion of the tongue to its normal position in the neck.

Clinically, the lingual thyroid nodule appears as a smooth nodular mass at the base
of the tongue posterior to the circumvallate papillae on or near the midline. It can be
asymptomatic or can cause a feeling of fullness in the throat or difficulty in swallowing.
Histologically, the lingual thyroid is composed of immature or mature thyroid tissue.

Treatment. On occasion, the size of the lingual thyroid necessitates its removal.
However, this nodule may be the patient's only functioning thyroid tissue. Therefore,
it is necessary to establish the presence of functioning thyroid tissue elsewhere before
any nodular lesion located in the posterior aspect of the tongue is removed. If a
normally located thyroid gland is lacking or nonfunctional, the lingual thyroid is not
removed.

DEVELOPMENTAL CYSTS

A **cyst** is an abnormal pathologic sac or cavity lined by epithelium and enclosed in a connective tissue capsule. Cysts occur throughout the body, including the oral region.

The cysts discussed in this chapter are all related to the development of the face, jaws, and teeth. Some have a distinctive histologic appearance, and a definitive diagnosis is based on microscopic examination of the tissue. Other cysts are lined by less distinctive epithelium. The diagnosis of these cysts is based on both the histologic appearance of the tissue and the location of the cyst.

The most common cyst observed in the oral cavity is caused by pulpal inflammation and is called the radicular cyst (see Chapter 2). The **residual cyst** is a radicular cyst that remains after extraction of the offending tooth.

Since cysts are commonly observed in the jaws and surrounding soft tissues, the dental hygienist should understand their diagnostic criteria, pathogenesis, and prognosis. The preliminary identification of a cystic lesion is within the scope of dental hygiene practice.

Developmental cysts are classified as **odontogenic** (related to tooth development) and **nonodontogenic** (not related to tooth development). Cysts are also classified according to location, cause, origin of the epithelial cells, and histologic appearance (Table 4–1). Developmental cysts can vary in size from small, asymptomatic lesions to large lesions that can cause expansion of bone. Very large and long-standing lesions can resorb tooth structure or move teeth.

Oral cysts that occur within bone are called **intraosseous cysts,** and cysts that occur in soft tissue are called **extraosseous cysts.**

Radiographically, cysts within bone generally appear as well-circumscribed radiolucencies. All cysts may appear **unilocular,** but some are more likely to appear as **multilocular** radiolucencies. When cysts are found within soft tissue, there is usually no radiographic change.

Odontogenic Cysts

Dentigerous Cyst

A **dentigerous cyst,** also called a **follicular cyst,** forms around the crown of an unerupted or developing tooth (Fig. 4–7). The epithelial lining originates from the reduced enamel epithelium after the crown has completely formed and calcified. Fluid accumulates between the crown and the reduced enamel epithelium. The reduced enamel epithelium results from remnants of the enamel organ. The most common location for the dentigerous cyst is around the crown of an unerupted or impacted

TABLE 4–1 Classification of Developmental Cysts			
Odontogenic		**Nonodontogenic**	
Intraosseous	*Extraosseous*	*Intraosseous*	*Extraosseous*
Dentigerous cyst	Eruption cyst	Nasopalatine duct cyst	Nasolabial cyst
Primordial cyst	Gingival cyst	(incisal canal cyst)	Epidermal cyst
Odontogenic keratocyst		Median palatal cyst	Dermoid cyst
Lateral periodontal cyst		Globulomaxillary cyst	Lymphoepithelial (branchial
		Median mandibular cyst	cleft) cyst
			Thyroglossal duct cyst

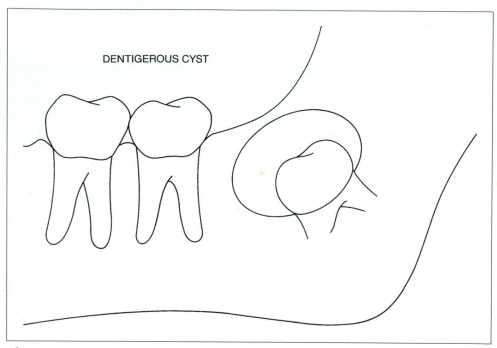

■ *figure 4-7*   Schematic of a dentigerous cyst located around the crown of an unerupted or impacted tooth.

third molar. However, a dentigerous cyst may form around the crowns of other unerupted or impacted teeth, such as the maxillary cuspid or a supernumerary tooth. This cyst is most often seen in young adults and can range from small and asymptomatic to very large. When large, it is capable of displacing teeth or causing a fracture of the mandible.

Radiographically, the dentigerous cyst appears as a well-defined, unilocular radiolucency around the crown of an unerupted or impacted tooth (Fig. 4–8A–C). Histologically, the lumen is most characteristically lined with cuboidal epithelium surrounded by a wall of connective tissue (Fig. 4–8D). It may also be lined with stratified squamous epithelium. The lumen may be filled with a watery or serous fluid.

Treatment. Treatment of a dentigerous cyst usually involves the complete removal of the cystic lesion and the tooth involved. If it is not removed, the cyst wall continues to enlarge. There is also a risk that a neoplasm (tumor) may develop.

Eruption Cyst

An **eruption cyst** is similar to a dentigerous cyst. It is found in the soft tissue around the crown of an erupting tooth.

Treatment. Since the tooth erupts through the cyst, this condition usually does not require treatment. Occasionally, the dome of the eruption cyst is removed to expose the crown. The tooth is allowed to erupt naturally.

Primordial Cyst

A **primordial cyst** develops in place of a tooth and is most commonly found in place of the third molar or posterior to an erupted third molar (Fig. 4–9). It originates from remnants and degeneration of the enamel organ. A history that the tooth was never present is an essential component of the diagnostic process.

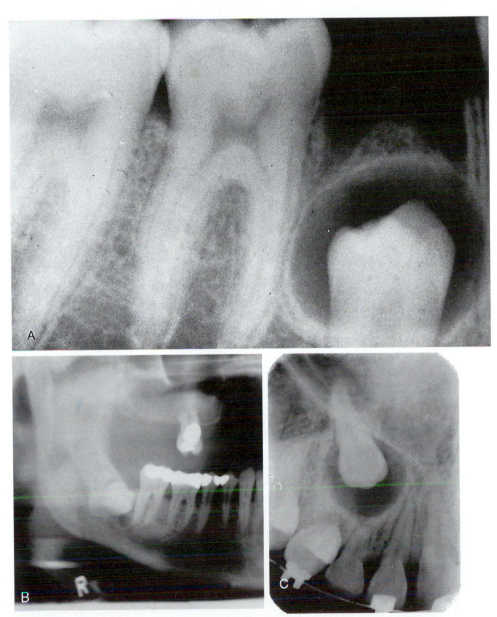

▪ *f i g u r e* **4–8**   Radiographs of dentigerous cysts around the crown of an unerupted bicuspid (*A*), an impacted third molar (*B*), and an unerupted maxillary cuspid (*C*).

Illustration continued on following page

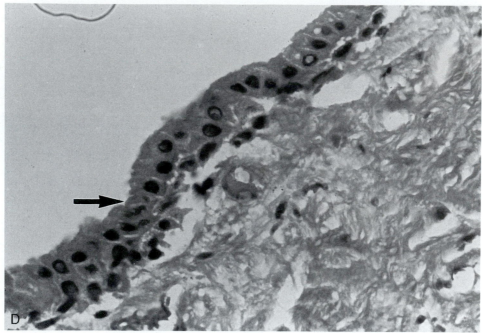

▪ *f* i g u r e **4–8**   *Continued (D),* Microscopic appearance of a dentigerous cyst. Arrow points to epithelial lining. *frequent reoccurence*

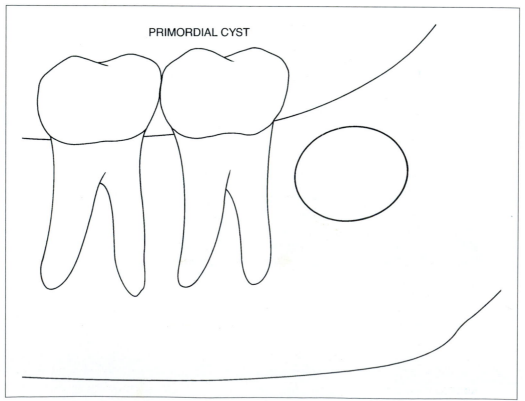

PRIMORDIAL CYST

▪ *f* i g u r e **4–9**   Schematic of a primordial cyst occurring in place of a tooth, the third molar.

Primordial cysts are most often seen in the young adult, and there is no reported sex predilection. Clinically, the cyst usually is asymptomatic and is discovered on radiographic examination. Radiographically, it is a well-defined, radiolucent lesion that can be either unilocular or multilocular. The histologic appearance and diagnosis of the primordial cyst may vary. Histologically, the lumen is lined by stratified squamous epithelium surrounded by parallel bundles of collagen fibers. The epithelium can be covered by a layer of orthokeratin or parakeratin. The term primordial cyst simply refers to its development in place of a tooth. For this reason biopsy and histologic examination of primordial cyst are essential. Histologically, a primordial cyst can be an odontogenic keratocyst or a lateral periodontal cyst.

Treatment. Treatment of a primordial cyst involves surgical removal of the entire lesion. The prognosis depends on the histology. The risk of recurrence depends on the histologic diagnosis. For example, if the cyst is histologically an odontogenic keratocyst, the risk of recurrence is greater than if the cyst is lined by nonkeratinized stratified squamous epithelium.

Odontogenic Keratocyst

An **odontogenic keratocyst** is an odontogenic cyst that is characterized by its unique histologic appearance and frequent recurrence. The lumen is lined by epithelium that is 8 to 10 cell layers thick and surfaced by parakeratin. The basal cell layer is palisaded and prominent. The interface between the epithelium and the connective tissue is flat (Fig. 4–10A,B).

These cysts are most often seen in the mandibular third molar region. Radiographically, the odontogenic keratocyst frequently appears as a well-defined, multilocular, radiolucent lesion (Fig. 4–10C). Unilocular lesions may also occur. The radiographic appearance of an odontogenic keratocyst can be identical to that of an odontogenic tumor. The odontogenic keratocyst is an expansive lesion that can move teeth and resorb tooth structure.

Treatment. Treatment of an odontogenic keratocyst is rather aggressive because of the high recurrence rate (Fig. 4–10D,E). The cyst generally extends beyond the borders that are seen on the radiograph because it extends between the trabeculae of bone. Therefore, thorough surgical excision and osseous curettage are recommended. Careful follow-up and evaluation are essential.

Lateral Periodontal Cyst and Gingival Cyst

The **lateral periodontal cyst** is named for its location. It is most often seen in the mandibular cuspid and premolar area. It presents as a unilocular or multilocular radiolucent lesion located on the lateral aspect of a tooth root (Fig. 4–11A). Histologically, the cyst is lined by a thin band of stratified squamous epithelium, which exhibits focal epithelial thickenings (Fig. 4–11C). The **gingival cyst** exhibits the same type of epithelial lining as the lateral periodontal cyst and is located in the soft tissue of the same area.

The lateral periodontal cyst is reported to be found most often in males. There is no reported sex predilection for gingival cysts. Clinically, the lateral periodontal cyst is asymptomatic. The gingival cyst appears as a small bulge or swelling of the attached gingiva or interdental papillae (Fig. 4–11B).

Treatment. Both the lateral periodontal cyst and the gingival cyst are treated by surgical excision. A few cases of recurrence of lateral periodontal cysts have been reported.

Text continued on page 226

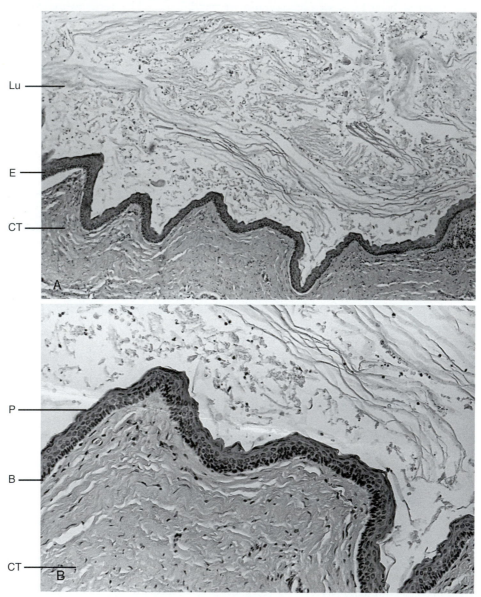

■ *f* i g u r e **4-10**   *A*, Microscopic appearance of an odontogenic keratocyst (OKC) showing
a thin uniform epithelial lining (low power). Lu = lumen; E = epithe-
lium; CT = connective tissue. *B*, Microscopic appearance of an OKC
showing a corrugated parakeratotic surface (P) and a prominent basal
cell layer (B) (high power).

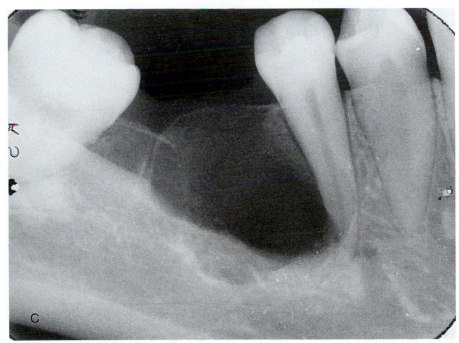

■ *f* i g u r e **4–10**   *Continued C,* Radiograph of an OKC showing a multilocular radiolucency.

Illustration continued on following page

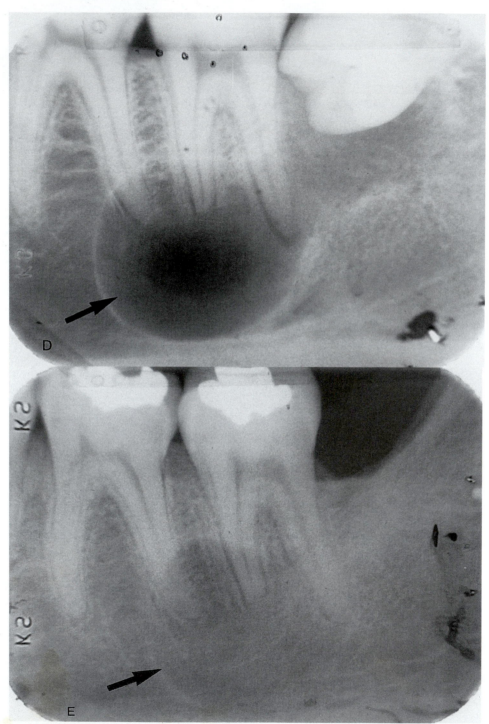

■ *f i g u r e* **4–10**   *Continued D*, Radiograph of an OKC extending to third molar. *E*, Patient in *D* 2 years later showing recurrence of OKC. Note third molar has been removed.

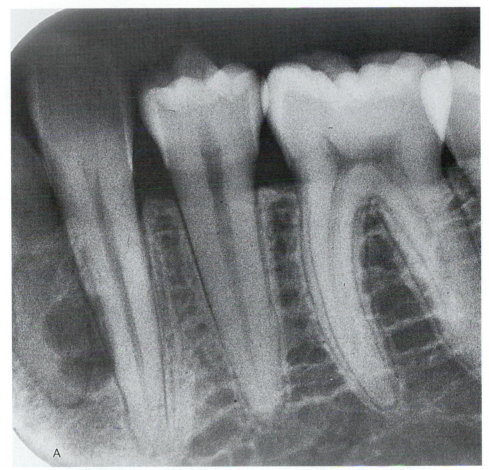

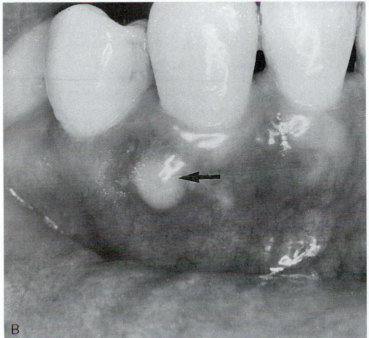

■ *f* i g u r e **4–11**   *A*, Radiograph of a lateral periodontal cyst. This biloculated, well-defined radiolucency is located lateral to the tooth root. *B*, Gingival cyst. (Courtesy of Drs. Paul Freedman and Stanley Kerpel.)

Illustration continued on following page

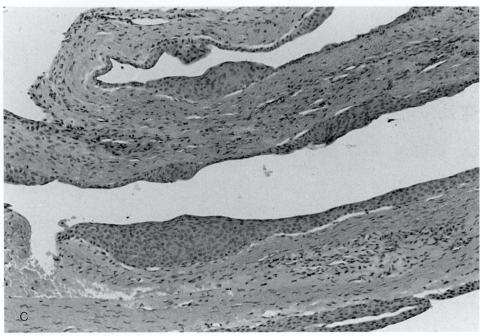

∎ f i g u r e 4–11   *Continued C*, Microscopic appearance of a lateral periodontal cyst showing a thin epithelial lining with focal epithelial thickenings.

Nonodontogenic Cysts

Nasopalatine Canal Cyst

A **nasopalatine canal cyst (incisive canal cyst)** is located within the nasopalatine canal or the incisive papilla. When found in the papilla, it is referred to as a cyst of the palatine papilla. This cyst arises from epithelial remnants of the embryonal nasopalatine ducts. The lesion is most commonly seen in adults between 40 and 60 years of age, and there is a strong predilection for males. The cyst is usually asymptomatic. There may be a small pink bulge near the apices and between the roots of the maxillary central incisors on the lingual surface. The adjacent teeth are usually vital. Radiographically, the nasopalatine canal cyst is a well-defined, radiolucent lesion that is often heart shaped (Fig. 4–12), resulting from the anatomic Y shape of the canal. When it is heart shaped, it is evenly distributed to the right and left of the midline.

Histologically, the cyst is lined by epithelium that varies from stratified squamous to pseudostratified ciliated columnar epithelium. The connective tissue wall contains nerves and blood vessels that are normally found in the area and may also contain inflammatory cells.

Treatment and Prognosis. Treatment of a nasopalatine canal cyst is surgical excision. It is especially important that surgery take place in the edentulous patient prior to the fabrication of a prosthesis. Recurrence is not expected.

Median Palatine Cyst

A **median palatine cyst** appears as a well-defined unilocular radiolucency and is located in the midline of the hard palate (Fig. 4–13). The cyst is now thought to be a more posterior form of a nasopalatine canal cyst. Histologically, the median palatine cyst is lined with stratified squamous epithelium that is surrounded by dense fibrous connective tissue.

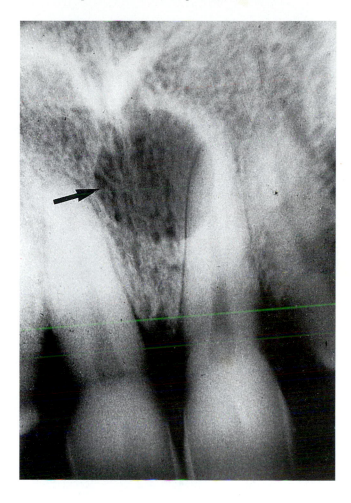

An incisive canal cyst may be located in
the anterior maxilla in either bone or
soft tissue, or both. This radiograph of
an incisive canal cyst shows a well-circumscribed radiolucency between the
maxillary central incisors.

Treatment and Prognosis. The median palatine cyst is treated by surgical enucleation. The prognosis is good, and recurrence is rare.

Globulomaxillary Cyst

Radiographically, a **globulomaxillary cyst** is a well-defined pear-shaped radiolucency found between the roots of the maxillary lateral incisor and cuspid (Fig. 4–14).
Although it was once thought to be a fissural cyst, it is now believed to be of
odontogenic epithelial origin. The size of the lesion can vary; however, when it is large
enough, a divergence of the roots can result. The adjacent teeth are usually vital.
Treatment and Prognosis. Surgical enucleation of the globulomaxillary cyst is
recommended. The prognosis is good, and recurrence is rare.

Median Mandibular Cyst

A **median mandibular cyst** is a rare lesion. It is located, as its name indicates, in
the midline of the mandible. The origin of the median mandibular cyst is also unclear.
Some believe it to be of odontogenic origin, possibly a primordial cyst. Since there is
no midline fusion between the bony processes, there can be no epithelial entrapment.
The cyst is lined with squamous epithelium, and the surrounding teeth are vital.
Radiographically, a well-defined radiolucency is seen below the apices of the mandibular incisors.

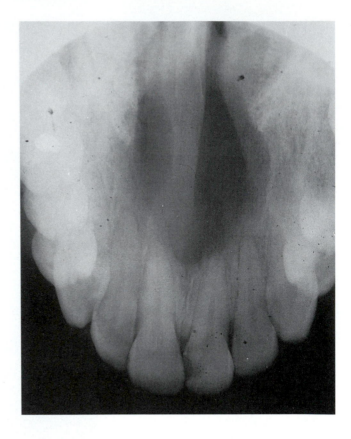

■ *figure* 4–13
Radiograph of a median palatine cyst showing a well-defined radiolucency located in the midline of the maxilla.

Treatment and Prognosis. A median mandibular cyst is treated by surgical removal, and prognosis is good. Recurrence is not expected.

Nasolabial Cyst

A **nasolabial cyst** is a soft tissue cyst with no alveolar bone involvement. The origin of this cyst is uncertain. At present it is thought to originate from the lower anterior portion of the nasolacrimal duct. The cyst is observed in adults 40 to 50 years of age, and there is a strong predilection (4:1) for females.

Clinically, there may be an expansion or swelling in the mucolabial fold in the area of the maxillary canine and the floor of the nose. There is usually no radiographic change associated with this cyst. However, when the lesion is large enough, expansive pressure can cause the resorption of bone (Fig. 4–15). Histologically, the cyst is lined with pseudostratified ciliated columnar epithelium and multiple goblet cells.

Treatment and Prognosis. Treatment of a nasolabial cyst is surgical excision, prognosis is good, and recurrence is rare.

Epidermal Cyst

An **epidermal cyst** presents as a raised nodule in the skin of the face or neck. Histologically, the cyst is lined by keratinizing epithelium that resembles the epithelium of skin (epidermis). The cyst lumen is usually filled with keratin scales. Most epidermal cysts are thought to originate from the epithelium of the hair follicle. Occasionally, when located in the skin of the cheek, the nodule may be noted from the buccal mucosal aspect as well as skin.

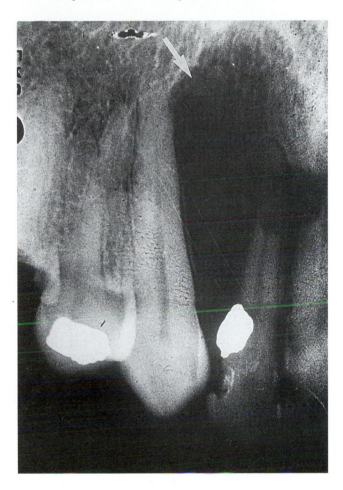

■ *f i g u r e* **4–14**
Radiograph of a globulomaxillary cyst showing a characteristic pear-shaped radiolucency between the maxillary lateral incisor and cuspid.

Treatment and Prognosis. An epidermoid cyst is treated by surgical excision, and prognosis is good.

Dermoid Cyst and Benign Cystic Teratoma

A **dermoid cyst** is a developmental cyst that is often present at birth or noted in young children. It is more common in other parts of the body than in the head and neck. When the dermoid cyst occurs in the oral cavity, it is usually found in the anterior floor of the mouth. The cyst may cause displacement of the tongue and may have a dough-like consistency when palpated.

Histologically, the dermoid cyst contains a stratified squamous epithelial lining surrounded by a connective tissue wall. Hair follicles, sebaceous glands, and sweat glands may be seen in the cyst wall. A **benign cystic teratoma** has a cystic component that resembles the dermoid cyst. In addition, teeth, bone, muscles, and nerve tissue may be found in the wall of this lesion. Teeth are usually not found in the malignant form of the teratoma.

Treatment and Prognosis. Treatment of the dermoid cyst is surgical excision, prognosis is good, and malignant transformation is rare.

Lymphoepithelial Cyst

A **lymphoepithelial cyst (branchial cleft cyst)** (Fig. 4–16) is most commonly found in the major salivary glands. It is composed of a stratified squamous epithelial

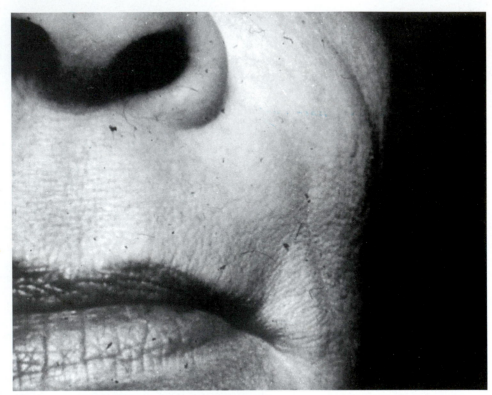

▪ *f* i g u r e **4–15**   Nasolabial cyst causing a swelling in the nasolabial fold area.

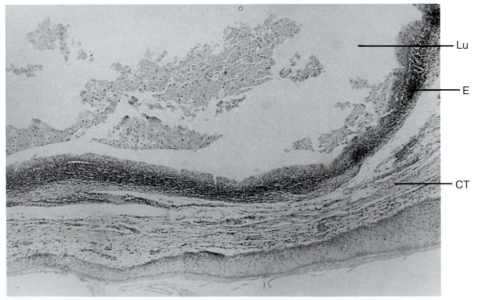

▪ *f* i g u r e **4–16**   Microscopic appearance of a lymphoepithelial cyst showing lumen (Lu), epithelial lining (E), surrounding lymphocytes, and connective tissue (CT) (low power).

lining surrounded by a well-circumscribed component of lymphoid tissue. It appears to arise from epithelium trapped in a lymph node during development. When found intraorally, the floor of the mouth and the lateral borders of the tongue are the most common locations. When occurring intraorally, the lymphoepithelial cyst appears as a pinkish-yellow, raised nodule.

Treatment and Prognosis. Treatment of a lymphoepithelial cyst consists of surgical excision, and prognosis is good.

Thyroglossal Tract Cyst

A **thyroglossal tract (duct) cyst** forms along the same tract that the thyroid gland follows in development, from the area of the foramen caecum to its permanent location in the neck (Fig. 4–17*A*,*B*). Most of these cysts occur below the hyoid bone. The epithelial lining varies from stratified squamous to ciliated columnar epithelium. Cysts above the hyoid bone are usually lined with squamous epithelium, and those below the hyoid bone with ciliated columnar epithelium. Thyroid tissue may also be found within the connective tissue wall.

The thyroglossal tract cyst is most often found in young individuals between 10 and 30 years of age, and there is a slight predilection for females. Clinically, if this cyst is located below the hyoid bone, it presents as a smooth bulge or swelling in the area of the midline of the neck. If located on the posterior aspect of the tongue, a smooth, rather firm mass of tissue is present, which can vary in size from a few millimeters to a centimeter. The patient may complain of dysphagia (difficulty in swallowing) or difficulty when extending the tongue.

Treatment and Prognosis. Treatment of a thyroglossal tract cyst consists of complete excision of the cyst and the tract, usually including a portion of the hyoid bone. Prognosis is generally good, but a few cases of malignant transformation have been reported.

Static Bone Cyst

A **static bone cyst (lingual mandibular bone concavity** or **Stafne's bone cyst)** is not a true cyst, since it is not a pathologic cavity and is not lined with epithelium. It is therefore often referred to as a pseudocyst. Radiographically, a well-defined cyst-like radiolucency is observed in the posterior region of the mandible inferior to the mandibular canal. The radiolucency is caused by a lingual depression in the mandible, which surrounds normal salivary gland tissue (Fig. 4–18). The salivary gland tissue may be an extension of the sublingual gland. The lesion is usually asymptomatic. Occasionally, the depression can be palpated.

Treatment. This variant of normal requires no treatment. If there is any question about the diagnosis, the patient is followed until it is determined that there is no enlargement of the radiolucency. If the radiolucency occurs above the mandibular canal, a biopsy may be indicated to establish the diagnosis and differentiate this variant of normal from cysts and tumors having a predilection for that location.

Simple Bone Cyst

A **simple bone cyst (traumatic bone cyst)** is a pathologic cavity in bone that is not lined with epithelium. The cause is uncertain, though an association with trauma has been suggested. The lesion is found most often in young individuals, and at one time it was reported to be more commonly found in males; more recently, an equal

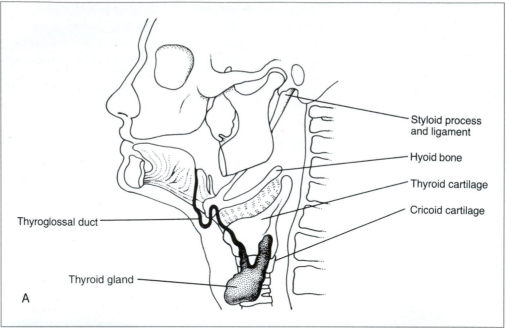

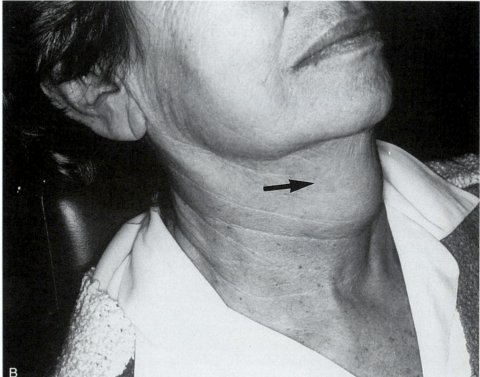

▪ *f* i g u r e **4–17**   *A,* The thyroglossal tract extends from the area of the foramen caecum lingual to the lower part of the neck. *B,* A thyroglossal tract cyst is the cause of this enlargement at the midline of the neck.

distribution among males and females has been reported. The lesion is observed radiographically as a well-defined unilocular or multilocular radiolucent lesion that characteristically shows scalloping around the roots of teeth (Fig. 4–19). The lesion is usually asymptomatic and is discovered on routine radiographs.

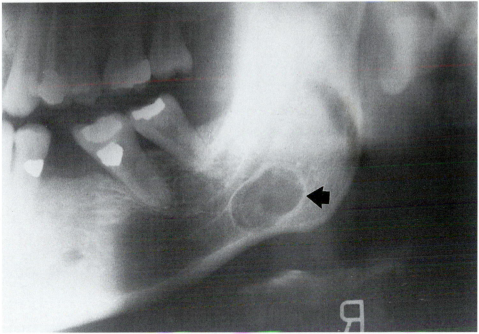

■ *f* i g u r e **4-18**   Panoramic radiograph of a lingual mandibular bone concavity (Stafne's bone cyst). Arrow points to a well-circumscribed radiolucency inferior to the mandibular canal.

Treatment and Prognosis. Surgical intervention reveals a void within the bone, which fills up with bone 6 months to 1 year after the surgical procedure. Prognosis is excellent, and recurrence is unusual.

Aneurysmal Bone Cyst

An **aneurysmal bone cyst** is a pseudocyst that consists of blood-filled spaces surrounded by multinucleated giant cells and fibrous connective tissue (similar to the giant cell granuloma). The radiolucent lesion has a multilocular appearance that is often described as a honeycomb or soap bubble. It is usually seen in individuals less than 30 years of age, and there is a slight predilection reported for females. The clinical presentation may be that of expansion of the involved bone.

A previous history of trauma to the area has been reported in some cases, but there is no direct correlation. Other reports have noted an association between the aneurysmal bone cyst and other bone lesions. It has frequently been associated with fibrous dysplasia.

Treatment. Surgical excision is the recommended treatment of an aneurysmal bone cyst and there may be excessive bleeding from the lesion during the procedure.

DEVELOPMENTAL ABNORMALITIES OF TEETH

Abnormalities in the Number of Teeth

Anodontia

Anodontia is the congenital lack of teeth. Total anodontia (lack of all teeth) is a rare condition that may affect either the deciduous or the permanent dentition. Since

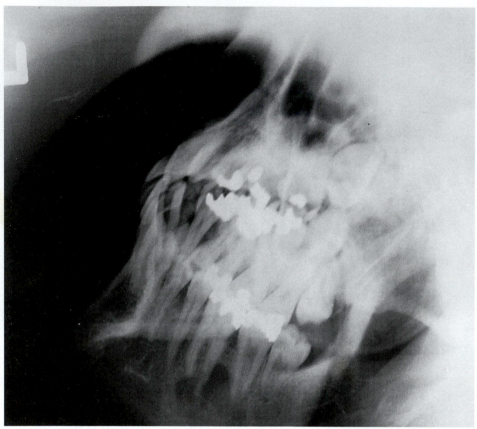

▪ *f i g u r e* **4–19**   Extraoral radiograph showing a simple (traumatic) bone cyst in the mandible with its unique radiolucent characteristic, scalloping around the roots. (Courtesy of Dr. Edward V. Zegarelli.)

development of both deciduous and permanent teeth begins before birth, their failure to develop is congenital. However, teeth may not be identified as missing until the time of normal eruption or initial radiographic examination. Total anodontia is often associated with the hereditary disturbance ectodermal dysplasia, which is described in Chapter 6.

Hypodontia

Hypodontia, also called **partial anodontia**, is the lack of one or more teeth. This developmental anomaly is rather common and may affect either deciduous or permanent teeth (Fig. 4–20*A*, *B*). Any tooth in either dentition may be missing. The permanent dentition is most commonly affected. The teeth most often missing are the maxillary and mandibular third molars, the maxillary lateral incisors, and the mandibular second premolars. Teeth are often missing bilaterally. The maxillary lateral incisor is the tooth most commonly missing in the deciduous dentition.

Teeth are identified as congenitally lacking by careful clinical and radiographic examination along with a thorough patient history.

There is a tendency for missing teeth to be **familial**, that is, affecting more members of a family than would be expected by chance. In addition, factors such as jaw lesions in infancy and radiation therapy during tooth formation may result in the destruction of tooth germs and the subsequent lack of affected teeth.

Treatment. Missing teeth may require prosthetic replacement. Their absence can

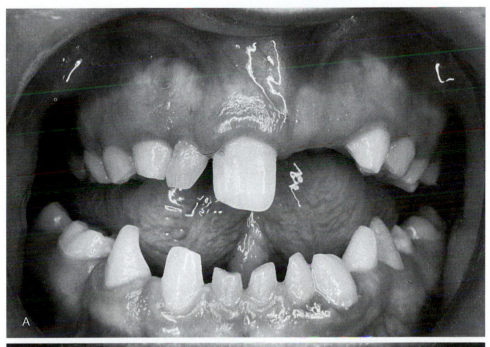

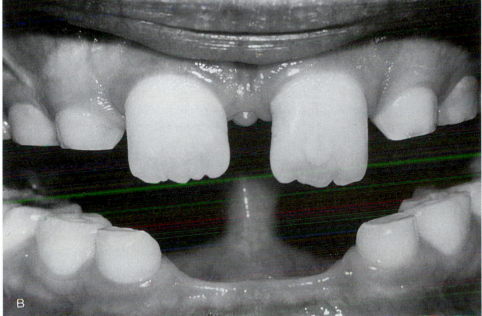

■ *f* i g u r e **4–20**   *A* and *B*, Hypodontia. Teeth missing have not been extracted; they never developed. (*A*, Courtesy of Dr. George Blozis; *B*, courtesy of Dr. Margot Van Dis.)

also result in problems in occlusion caused by drifting or tipping of teeth. Orthodontic evaluation and treatment may be necessary. In addition, congenitally missing teeth may be a component of a **syndrome**. A syndrome is a group of findings that occur together. Patients with congenitally missing teeth should be evaluated for other abnormalities.

Supernumerary Teeth

can be smaller -

Supernumerary teeth are extra teeth found in the dental arches (Fig. 4–21). **Supernumerary** means more than the normal or regular number. Supernumerary teeth result either from the formation of extra tooth buds in the dental lamina or from the cleavage of already existing tooth buds and may occur in either the deciduous or the permanent dentition. Extra teeth are most often seen in the maxilla and may occur singly or in multiples and unilaterally or bilaterally.

Typically, the supernumerary tooth is smaller than a normal-sized tooth and often does not erupt. Most are discovered on radiographs as incidental findings. A supernumerary tooth may or may not resemble a normal tooth in shape and position.

The most common supernumerary tooth is called the **mesiodens**, which is located between the maxillary central incisors at or near the midline. It is usually a small tooth with a conical crown and short roots (Fig. 4–22). It may occur singly or in pairs and may be inverted when seen on a radiograph. The mesiodens can erupt or remain embedded or impacted.

The second most common supernumerary tooth is the maxillary fourth molar, which is also called a **distomolar** because it is located distal to the third molar (Fig. 4–23). The distomolar can look like a miniature third molar or can be of normal third molar size and shape. It rarely erupts into the oral cavity and is usually discovered on a radiograph.

Other supernumerary teeth include mandibular and maxillary premolars, maxillary lateral incisors, and the maxillary paramolar, a small rudimentary tooth that occurs buccal to the third molar.

Treatment. Erupted supernumerary teeth can cause crowding, malpositioning of adjacent teeth, or noneruption of normal teeth; therefore, removal is often necessary. Nonerupted supernumerary teeth should be extracted because there is a risk of cyst development around the crown. Multiple supernumerary teeth may be a component of a syndrome such as cleidocranial dysplasia or Gardner's syndrome. These syndromes are described in Chapter 6.

Abnormalities in the Size of Teeth

Microdontia

Most common is peg shape laterals

Microdontia is a developmental anomaly in which one or more teeth in a dentition are smaller than normal. The term is derived from the Greek words "mikros," meaning small, and "odontos," meaning tooth. Microdontia is classified as true generalized microdontia, generalized relative microdontia, or microdontia involving a single tooth.

True generalized microdontia is seen in the pituitary dwarf and is extremely rare. All the teeth are smaller than normal. In **generalized relative microdontia**, normal-sized teeth appear small in large jaws. Heredity plays a role in generalized relative microdontia. For example, a child may inherit large jaws from one parent and normal-sized teeth from the other, resulting in the illusion of small teeth. **Microdontia involving a single tooth** is far more common than true generalized microdontia or generalized relative microdontia. The maxillary lateral incisor and the maxillary third molar are the teeth most often affected (Fig. 4–24). The maxillary lateral incisors often

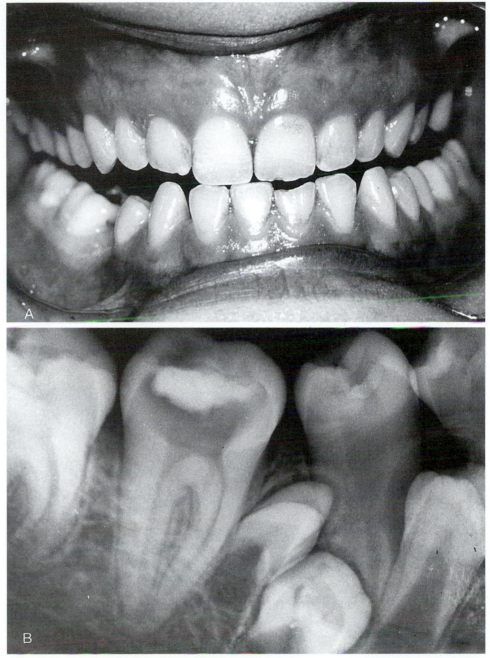

▪ *f i g u r e* 4–21   *A*, Supernumerary teeth. This patient has four maxillary lateral incisors. (Courtesy of Dr. Margot Van Dis.) *B*, Radiograph showing unerupted supernumerary teeth. (Courtesy of Dr. George Blozis.)

Illustration continued on following page

appear peg shaped, with the mesial and distal tooth surfaces converging toward the incisal edge. This "peg lateral" is smaller than normal, tends to occur bilaterally, has short roots, and is thought to be familial. The maxillary third molar microdont typically appears small but normally shaped. Microdonts are identified clinically if erupted or radiographically if unerupted.

Treatment. For cosmetic reasons, erupted microdonts may be restored to resem-

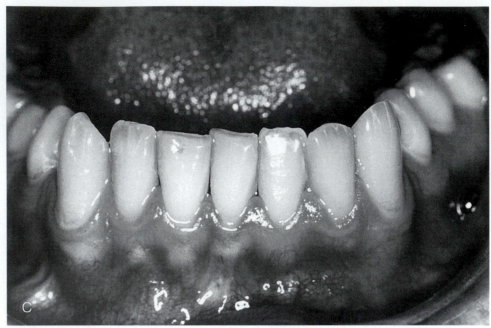

▪ *f i g u r e* **4–21**   *Continued C*, Supernumerary mandibular incisor.

ble teeth of normal size and shape. Impacted microdonts should be surgically removed to prevent cyst formation.

Macrodontia

Macrodontia is an uncommon developmental anomaly in which one or more teeth in a dentition are larger than normal. ("Makros" means large in Greek.) Macrodontia is classified in the same manner as microdontia: true generalized macrodontia, relative generalized macrodontia, and macrodontia involving a single tooth.

True generalized macrodontia is rare and is occasionally seen in cases of pituitary gigantism. **Relative generalized macrodontia** is seen in individuals with normal or slightly larger than normal teeth in small jaws and is generally caused by the patient's inheriting tooth size from one parent and jaw size from the other. **Macrodontia affecting a single tooth** is uncommon. Localized macrodontia affecting one side of the dental arches may be seen in a condition called **facial hemihypertrophy**, which involves the enlargement of half of the head with enlarged teeth on the involved side.

Treatment. No treatment is indicated for macrodontia.

Developmental Abnormalities in the Shape of Teeth

Gemination

Gemination is a developmental anomaly that occurs when a single tooth germ attempts to divide and results in the incomplete formation of two teeth. **Geminate** means paired or occurring in twos. The cause of this aborted twinning of a single tooth germ is unknown. Gemination is uncommon and is more frequently seen in the deciduous dentition, but occasionally it occurs in the permanent dentition. Gemination

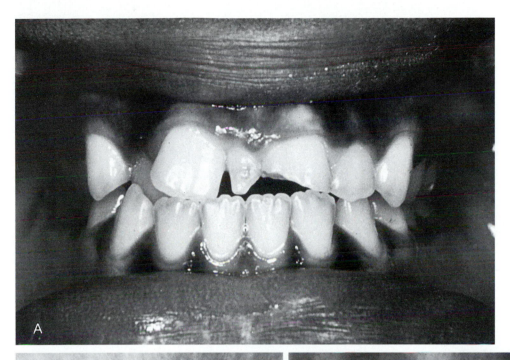

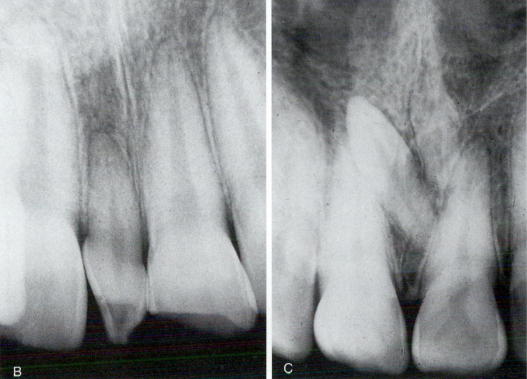

▪ *f i g u r e 4–22*   *A*, Mesiodens seen between the maxillary central incisors. *B*, Radiograph of a mesiodens. (*A* and *B*, Courtesy of Dr. George Blozis.) *C*, Radiograph showing a pair of inverted impacted mesiodens.

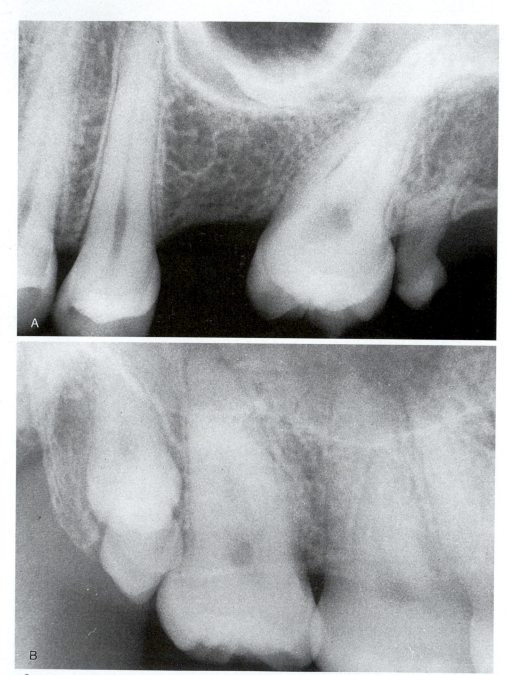

▪ *f* i g u r e 4–23   *A*, Small erupted microdont distal to the maxillary second molar. (Courtesy of Dr. Margot Van Dis.) *B*, Radiograph of a pair of distomolars, located distal to the second molar. (Courtesy of Dr. George Blozis.)

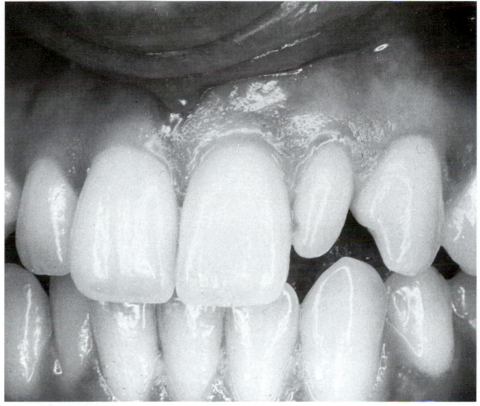

■ *f i g u r e* 4–24   Peg-shaped lateral incisor. (Courtesy of Dr. George Blozis.)

most often affects anterior teeth and is most often seen in the deciduous mandibular incisors and the permanent maxillary incisors.

Clinically, gemination appears as two crowns joined together by a notched incisal area (Fig. 4–25A,B). Radiographically, there is usually one single root and one common pulp canal (Fig. 4–25C). There is a full complement of teeth.

Treatment. A geminated tooth poses an aesthetic problem, particularly when it occurs in the maxillary anterior region. It also poses a prosthetic challenge. Treatment therefore usually involves alteration of the tooth so that it resembles a normal tooth in size and shape.

Fusion

Fusion results from the union of two normally separated adjacent tooth germs. The cause of fusion is uncertain—heredity, external pressure, and crowding have all been suggested. Fusion of adjacent teeth can be complete or incomplete, depending on the stage of tooth development at the time of contact. Early contact of developing tooth germs can result in a single, large tooth; later contact can result in the union of crowns only or the union of roots only. True fusion always involves confluence of dentin. Fusion tends to occur in the anterior region, and the incisors are the teeth most often affected. Fusion of deciduous teeth occurs more often than fusion of permanent teeth.

Clinically, fused teeth appear as a single large crown that occurs in place of two normal teeth and may exhibit an observable separation (Fig. 4–26). Radiographically, either separate or fused roots and root canals are seen. In order to differentiate fusion from gemination, the teeth must be counted. If the neighboring teeth of the tooth in

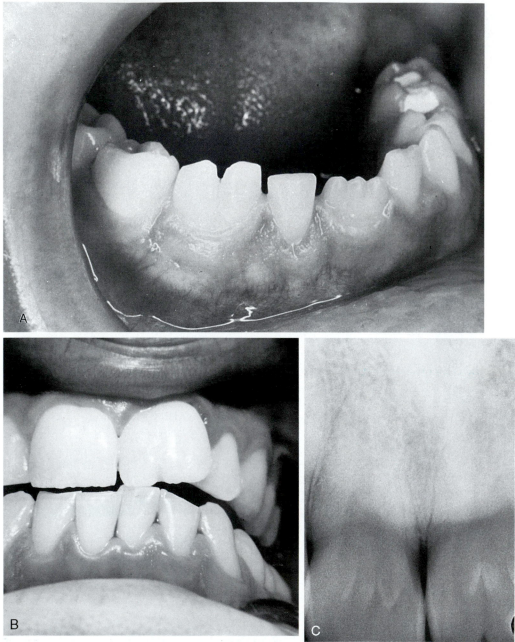

▪ *f* i g u r e 4–25   *A*, Clinical picture of gemination in a mandibular cuspid. (Courtesy of Dr. George Blozis.) *B*, Gemination seen in maxillary central. *C*, Radiograph of the same maxillary central incisor.

question are present, the tooth is geminated; if a neighboring tooth is lacking, the tooth in question is fused. Fusion can occur between two adjacent normal teeth or between a normal tooth and a supernumerary tooth. It may be difficult to distinguish between a geminated tooth and the fusion of a normal tooth to a supernumerary tooth.

Treatment. As with geminated teeth, fused teeth may present aesthetic and occlusal problems, and they also pose a restorative challenge. Treatment involves alteration of the size and shape of the tooth and may involve replacement of one of the fused teeth.

crown & bridge.

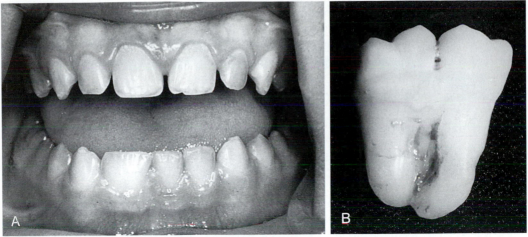

▪ *f i g u r e* **4–26**   *A,* Clinical picture of fusion involving a permanent mandibular lateral incisor. (Courtesy of Dr. George Blozis.) *B,* Fusion of mandibular molars. (Courtesy of Dr. Rudy Melfi.)

Concrescence

In dentistry, **concrescence** is a condition in which two adjacent teeth are united by cementum only. It is actually a form of fusion that takes place after tooth formation is complete and is usually discovered as an incidental radiographic finding (Fig. 4–27). The cause of concrescence is thought to be crowding or trauma that results in the close approximation of adjacent tooth roots. Subsequent cementum deposition acts to fuse the two adjacent roots. Concrescence is most often seen in adjacent maxillary

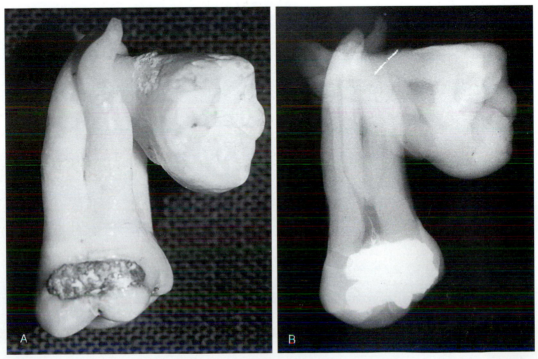

▪ *f i g u r e* **4–27**   Concrescence illustrated in a photograph *(A)* of extracted teeth and in a corresponding radiograph *(B).* (Courtesy of Dr. George Blozis.)

molars and adjacent supernumerary teeth and may involve erupted, unerupted, or impacted teeth.

Treatment. Concrescence generally does not require treatment. If one of the teeth joined by cementum requires extraction, extraction of the fused neighbor is inevitable. However, the extraction of involved teeth is difficult, and excessive fracture of the associated alveolar bone may result.

Dilaceration

In dentistry, **dilaceration** refers to an abnormal curve or angle in the root or crown of a tooth (Fig. 4–28). This dental anomaly is thought to be caused by trauma to the tooth germ during root development. The position of the calcified portion of the tooth is changed, and the remainder of the tooth forms at an angle. A dilaceration can appear anywhere along the root portion of a tooth and can occur in any tooth in either the deciduous or the permanent dentition. A root dilaceration is usually discovered as an incidental radiographic finding.

Treatment. Dilacerations do not require treatment. However, they may cause problems if extraction or endodontic therapy becomes necessary. The importance of a preoperative radiograph is obvious.

Enamel Pearl

An **enamel pearl**, or **enameloma**, is a small, spherical enamel projection located on a root surface (Fig. 4–29). This developmental anomaly is thought to occur as a result of the abnormal displacement of ameloblasts during tooth formation. The enamel pearl is usually found on maxillary molars. It is attached to cementum near the root bifurcation or trifurcation area. Occasionally, it is located near the cementoenamel junction. The enamel pearl may consist of enamel only or enamel, dentin, and pulp.

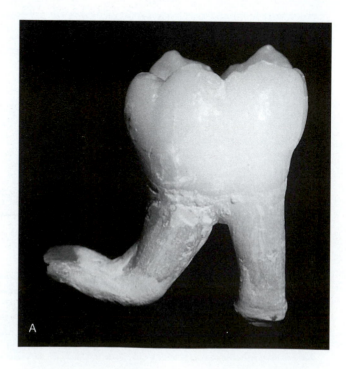

■ *f* i g u r e 4–28

A, Dilaceration on the distal root of an extracted tooth. (Courtesy of Dr. Rudy Melfi.)

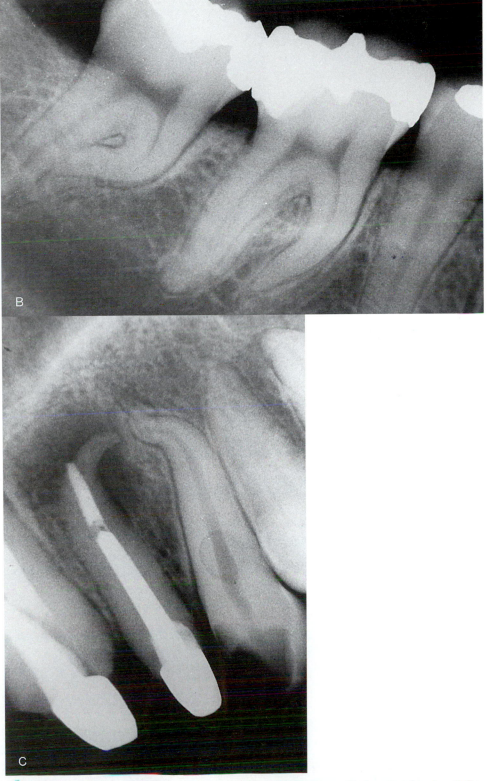

■ **figure 4-28**   *Continued B*, Mesial root dilaceration on a mandibular second molar. *C*, Radiograph of root dilaceration in maxillary lateral and cuspid.

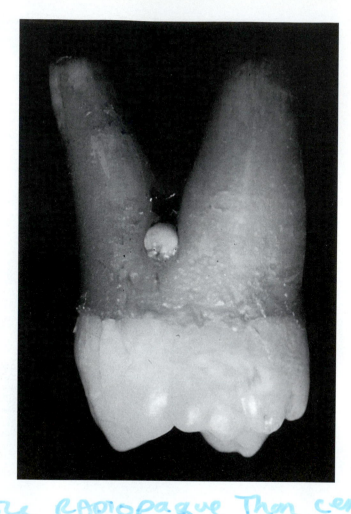

■ *f* i g u r e 4–29

Enamel pearl in the furcation area. (Courtesy of Dr. Rudy Melfi.)

[handwritten note: more RADIOPAQUE Than cementum]

The enamel pearl is an uncommon finding. It appears radiographically as a small, spherical radiopacity. Clinically, the enamel pearl may be mistaken for calculus.

Treatment. Generally, no treatment is necessary for this anomaly. Removal may be necessary if periodontal problems occur in the furcation area when an enamel pearl is present.

[handwritten note: Pulp stone NOT as radio paque]

Talon Cusp

A **talon cusp** is an accessory cusp located in the area of the cingulum of a maxillary or mandibular permanent incisor (Fig. 4–30). A talon is a claw of a predatory animal. The talon cusp is said to resemble an eagle's talon. The talon cusp often projects lingually to the height of the incisal edge of the involved tooth. The talon cusp is composed of normal enamel and dentin and contains a pulp horn. Frequently, a caries-susceptible fissure is present between the cusps.

Treatment. Removal of the talon cusp is often indicated because it interferes with occlusion. Because of the presence of the pulp horn, endodontic therapy is necessary.

Taurodontism

Taurodontism is a term used to describe a developmental dental anomaly in which the teeth exhibit elongated, large pulp chambers and short roots (Fig. 4–31). Taurodontism means "bull-like" teeth. The term was first used to describe teeth that

[handwritten notes: Board quest.; occlusion problem]

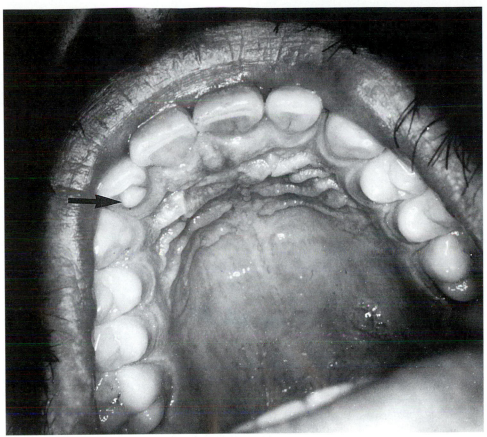

ƒ i g u r e 4–30 Talon cusp *(arrow)* on the lingual aspect of the maxillary right lateral permanent incisor.

resembled those of cud-chewing animals. Although the etiology of taurodontism is uncertain, a variety of causes have been suggested, ranging from a primitive pattern of tooth development to the developmental failure of Hertwig's epithelial root sheath to invaginate at the proper level.

Taurodontism is uncommon and is seen in both the deciduous and the permanent dentitions and usually affects a single molar tooth or several molars in the same quadrant. Taurodontism can occur unilaterally or bilaterally. The crown of the tooth appears clinically normal. A taurodont is identified by its characteristic radiographic appearance. The tooth tends to have a stretched appearance, and the pulp chamber is greatly enlarged and elongated without a constriction at the cementoenamel junction. The roots appear short, with the furcation located near the apices.   *lrg chamber*

Treatment. No treatment is indicated for taurodontism.

Dens in Dente   *tooth w/I a tooth.*

Dens in dente, also called **dens invaginatus,** is a developmental anomaly that results when the enamel organ invaginates into the crown of a tooth prior to mineralization (Fig. 4–32). **Invaginate** means that one portion infolds into another portion of a structure. Radiographically, a tooth-like structure appears within the involved tooth. An elongated bulb or pear-shaped mass of enamel is seen in dentin surrounding a radiolucent area—hence, the name dens in dente, or "tooth within a tooth." This defect is typically confined to the coronal third of the tooth, but in some cases it

more susept. to cavies cause enam is not as developed + STRONG.

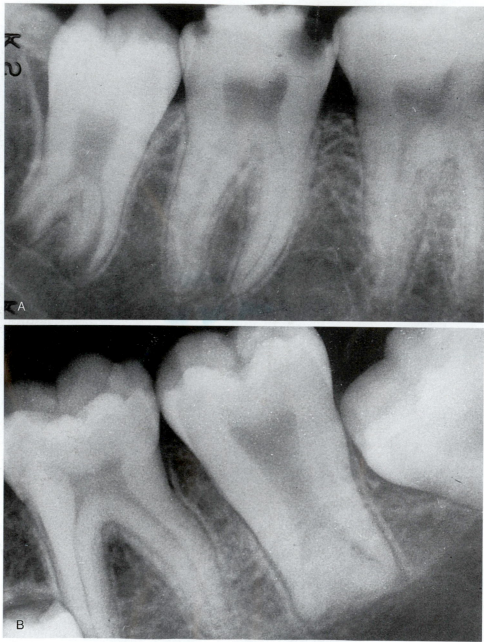

■ *f* i g u r e **4–31**   *A*, Taurodont in the mandibular third molar. (Courtesy of Dr. Margot Van Dis.) *B*, Taurodont in the mandibular second molar. (Courtesy of Dr. George Blozis.)

extends to include the entire root length. Clinically, the dens in dente may appear as either a normally shaped or malformed crown that exhibits a deep pit or crevice in the area of the cingulum. The invaginated tooth-like structure retains a communication with the outside of the tooth via the pit or crevice visible on the crown surface.

Dens in dente customarily affects a single tooth. Anterior teeth, particularly the maxillary and mandibular incisors, are more commonly affected than the posterior teeth. The maxillary lateral incisor is the most frequently affected tooth, and when affected it is often peg shaped.

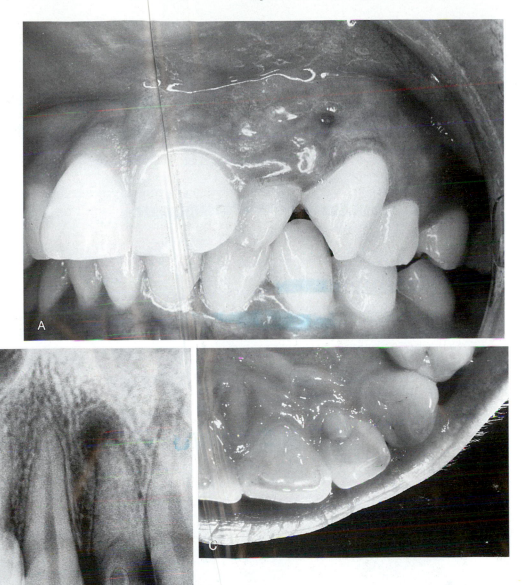

▪ *f* i g u r e 4–32   *A*, Clinical illustration of dens in dente in maxillary lateral incisor. (Courtesy of Dr. George Blozis.) *B*, Radiograph of dens in dente in maxillary lateral incisor. *C*, Dens in dente in maxillary lateral incisor. (Courtesy of Dr. Margot Van Dis.)

Treatment. The dens in dente is vulnerable to caries, pulpal infection, and necrosis as a result of the communication between the oral cavity and the invaginated area of the tooth. Consequently, the dens in dente is often nonvital and is seen in association with periapical pathosis. If the dens in dente is detected shortly after eruption, a prophylactic restoration can be placed in the deep pit or crevice to prevent caries and subsequent pulpal necrosis. A nonvital dens in dente may be treated endodontically. A malformed crown can be restored with composite materials or a full-coverage crown.

Dens Evaginatus

Dens evaginatus is an accessory enamel cusp found on the occlusal tooth surface (Fig. 4–33). This is a rare developmental anomaly that occurs most often on the mandibular premolars. When affected, they are called **tuberculated premolars**. Molars, cuspids, and incisors can also be affected. Dens evaginatus is thought to result from the proliferation and outpouching of enamel epithelium during tooth development.

Clinically, the dens evaginatus appears as a small, rounded nodule on the occlusal surface of a mandibular premolar between the buccal and lingual cusps. A pulp horn may extend into this extra cusp.

Treatment. The dens evaginatus may not require treatment. However, it can cause occlusal problems, and removal may be necessary. Occlusal wear or fracture of this accessory cusp may result in pulp exposure, and endodontic treatment may be necessary.

Supernumerary Roots

Supernumerary or extra roots can involve any tooth (Fig. 4–34). No cause for this developmental anomaly has been identified. External pressure, trauma, and metabolic dysfunction during root development have been suggested.

Supernumerary roots are not uncommon and tend to occur in teeth that exhibit root formation after birth. The multirooted teeth most often affected are the maxillary and mandibular third molars. The single-rooted teeth most often affected are the mandibular bicuspids and cuspids. Supernumerary roots may exhibit dilaceration and are diagnosed radiographically.

Treatment. Generally, no treatment is indicated for supernumerary roots. However, they become clinically significant if extraction of the involved tooth or endodontic therapy becomes necessary.

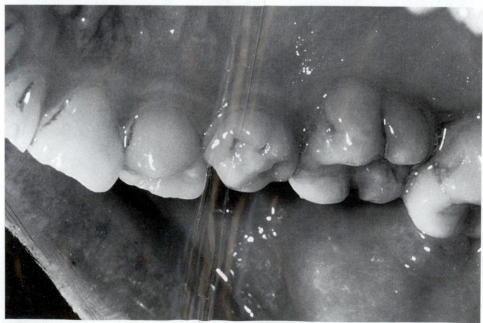

f i g u r e 4–33   Dens evaginatus of maxillary premolar. (Courtesy of Dr. Margot Van Dis.)

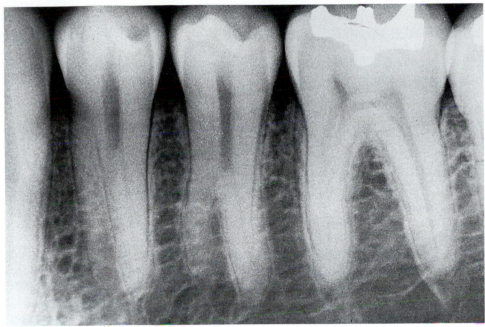

▪ *f* i g u r e **4–34**   Supernumerary roots in mandibular premolars.

Developmental Abnormalities of Tooth Structure

Enamel Hypoplasia

Enamel hypoplasia is the incomplete or defective formation of enamel, resulting in the alteration of tooth form or color. **Hypoplasia** is defined as the incomplete development of an organ or tissue. Enamel hypoplasia results from a disturbance of or damage to ameloblasts during enamel matrix formation. Enamel hypoplasia can affect either the deciduous or the permanent dentition.

Numerous factors can cause enamel hypoplasia (Color Plate 93):

- Amelogenesis imperfecta
- Febrile illness (measles, chickenpox, scarlet fever)
- Vitamin deficiency (vitamins A, C, D)
- Local infection of a deciduous tooth
- Ingestion of fluoride
- Congenital syphilis
- Birth injury, premature birth
- Idiopathic factors

Enamel hypoplasia that is inherited is called **amelogenesis imperfecta** (see Chapter 6). The factors that cause enamel hypoplasia by injuring the sensitive ameloblasts during enamel formation are discussed in this chapter.

Enamel Hypoplasia Caused by Febrile Illness or Vitamin Deficiency

Ameloblasts are one of the most sensitive cell groups in the body. It is believed that any serious systemic disease or severe nutritional deficiency is capable of producing enamel hypoplasia. Febrile illnesses (measles, chickenpox, and scarlet fever) and vitamin deficiencies (vitamins A, C, and D) that occur during the time of tooth formation can result in a type of enamel hypoplasia characterized by pitting of the enamel. Only the crowns of teeth that are developing at the time of the febrile illness or vitamin deficiency are affected. This type of hypoplasia usually involves the permanent central incisors, laterals, cuspids, and first molars, which are the teeth that form during the first year of life. One or more horizontal rows of tiny, deep pits are seen traversing the affected tooth surface. The number of pits and rows of pits may vary, depending on the extent and severity of injury to the ameloblasts. These enamel pits tend to stain and appear unsightly.

Treatment. Teeth affected with enamel hypoplasia of the pitting type may be restored with composites during childhood and later with porcelain veneers or full-crown coverage.

Enamel Hypoplasia Resulting from Local Infection or Trauma

Enamel hypoplasia of a permanent tooth may result from infection of a deciduous tooth. A single tooth is usually affected and is referred to as a **Turner's tooth**. A carious deciduous tooth with periapical involvement can disturb the ameloblasts of the underlying permanent tooth. The severity of the defect depends on the severity of the deciduous tooth infection, the degree of periapical tissue involvement, and the stage of development of the underlying permanent tooth.

The teeth most often affected are the permanent maxillary incisors and the permanent mandibular premolars. The clinical appearance of the affected tooth depends on the extent of the injury. The color of the enamel of these teeth may range from yellow to brown, or severe pitting and deformity may be involved. These enamel defects can frequently be identified radiographically before the eruption of the involved tooth.

Treatment. An anterior Turner's tooth may be restored to provide an improved aesthetic appearance; a posterior Turner's tooth may require a restoration to provide improved function.

Enamel Hypoplasia Resulting from Fluoride Ingestion

Enamel hypoplasia resulting from fluoride ingestion, or **dental fluorosis**, occurs as a result of the patient's ingesting high concentrations of fluoride during tooth formation, usually in drinking water. Affected teeth exhibit a mottled discoloration of enamel (Color Plate 94). **Mottling** refers to irregular areas of discoloration. The more fluoride ingested, the more severe the mottling. Minimal enamel changes are seen with fluoride levels of 0.9 to 1.0 part fluoride/million gallons of water. Ingestion of water with a fluoride concentration two to three times the recommended amount results in mild fluorosis that appears as white flecks and chalky opaque areas of enamel (Color Plate 94). Ingestion of water containing four times the recommended amount of fluoride causes brown or black staining and a pitted or overall corroded enamel appearance.

All permanent teeth are involved in this type of enamel hypoplasia. The teeth affected by fluorosis are generally decay resistant.

Treatment. In order to improve the aesthetic appearance of these teeth, bleaching, bonding, composites, porcelain veneers, or full-coverage crowns can be used.

Enamel Hypoplasia Resulting from Congenital Syphilis

Syphilis is a contagious venereal disease caused by the spirochete *Treponema pallidum*. It is described in detail in Chapter 2. Congenital syphilis is transmitted from an infected mother to her fetus via the placenta. Children with congenital syphilis have numerous developmental anomalies and may be blind, deaf, or paralyzed. In utero infection by *Treponema pallidum* results in enamel hypoplasia of the permanent incisors and first molars.

The affected incisors are shaped like screwdrivers—broad cervically and narrow incisally with a notched incisal edge (Fig. 4–35*A*). They are called **Hutchinson's incisors**. First molars appear as irregularly shaped crowns made up of multiple tiny globules of enamel instead of cusps (Fig. 4–35*B*). Because of their berry-like appearance, these molars are called **mulberry molars**. Not every case of congenital syphilis exhibits these dental findings, and similarly shaped teeth may be seen in individuals without congenital syphilis.

Treatment. Treatment to improve the aesthetic appearance of these teeth includes full-coverage crowns.

Enamel Hypoplasia Resulting from Birth Injury, Premature Birth, or Idiopathic Factors

Enamel hypoplasia can occur as a result of trauma or change of environment at the time of birth or in infants who were premature. Also, many cases of enamel hypoplasia do not have an identifiable cause despite careful and thorough history taking. The ameloblast is a sensitive cell that is easily damaged. For this reason, even a mild illness or systemic problem can result in enamel hypoplasia. Such illnesses may be so insignificant that they are not known to the patient or remembered by the patient's parents.

Treatment. To improve the aesthetic appearance of these teeth, composites, porcelain veneers, or full-coverage crowns can be used.

Enamel Hypocalcification

Enamel hypocalcification is a developmental anomaly that results in a disturbance of the maturation of the enamel matrix. It usually appears as a localized, chalky white spot on the middle third of smooth crowns. The underlying enamel may be soft and susceptible to caries. The cause of enamel hypocalcification is uncertain; however, trauma during the maturation of enamel matrix has been suggested.

Treatment. Bleaching, composites, porcelain veneers, or full-coverage crowns can be used to improve the aesthetic appearance of these teeth.

Endogenous Staining of Teeth

Endogenous or **intrinsic staining of teeth** occurs as a result of the deposition of substances circulating systemically during tooth development. For example, ingestion of tetracycline during tooth development causes a yellowish-green discoloration of dentin that is visible through the enamel. At the time of eruption, the teeth fluoresce under ultraviolet light. Later the tetracycline is oxidized, the color changes from yellowish to brown, and the teeth no longer fluoresce. Other conditions, such as Rh incompatibility (erythroblastosis fetalis), neonatal liver disease, and congenital porphyria, an inherited metabolic disease, also cause endogenous staining of teeth.

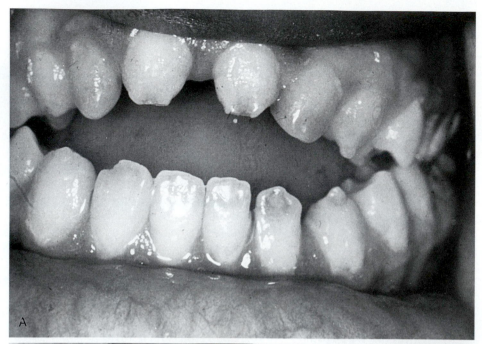

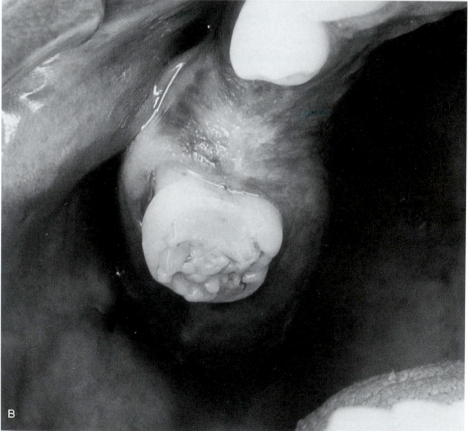

■ *f* i g u r e **4–35**   *A*, Hutchinson's incisors. *B*, Mulberry molars. (Courtesy of Dr. George Blozis.)

Regional Odontodysplasia

Regional odontodysplasia, or **ghost teeth,** is an unusual developmental problem in which one or several teeth in the same quadrant radiographically exhibit a marked reduction in radiodensity and a characteristic ghost-like appearance (Fig. 4–36). Very thin enamel and dentin are present. Occasionally, the enamel is not visible on the radiograph. The pulp chambers of these teeth are extremely large. Either the teeth do not erupt, or eruption is incomplete. If ghost teeth erupt into the oral cavity, they are typically nonfunctional and malformed.

Regional odontodysplasia can affect either the deciduous or the permanent dentition. The maxilla, especially the anterior maxilla, is more often involved than the mandible. The cause of regional odontodysplasia is unknown. A vascular phenomenon has been suggested.

Treatment. Extraction usually is the treatment of choice for ghost teeth.

Developmental Abnormalities of Tooth Eruption

Impacted and Embedded Teeth

Impacted teeth are teeth that cannot erupt because of a physical obstruction. **Embedded teeth** are those that do not erupt owing to a lack of eruptive force. An impacted tooth is one of the most common developmental defects occurring in humans. Any tooth can be impacted. The most commonly impacted teeth are the maxillary and mandibular third molars, the maxillary cuspids, the maxillary and mandibular premolars, and supernumerary teeth. Impacted teeth are identified radiographically (Fig. 4–37).

Third molar impactions are classified according to the position of the tooth: mesioangular, distoangular, vertical, and horizontal.

The most common position of an impacted third molar is mesioangular. The crown of the third molar points in a mesial direction and is in contact with the second

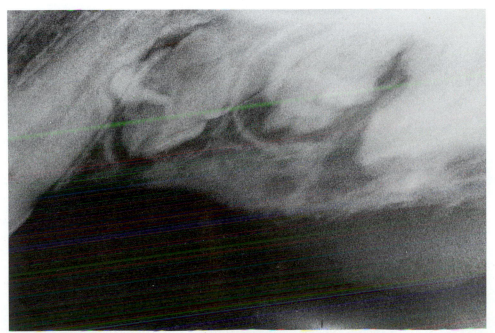

figure 4-36   Regional odontodysplasia.

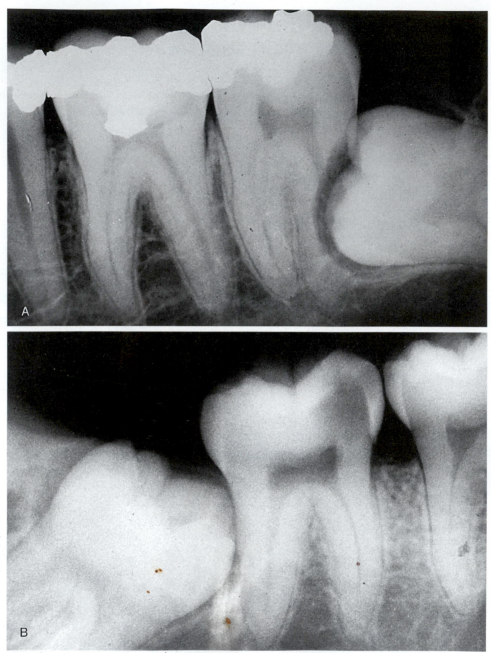

■ *f i g u r e 4–37*   *A,* Horizontal impaction of the third molar. *B,* Mesioangular impaction of the third molar.

1. Infects - can't keep clean.
2. dry socket causes - smoking - B.P's

molar, which is preventing its eruption. In a distoangular impaction, the crown of the third molar points in a distal direction toward the ramus, and the roots of the impacted tooth are adjacent to the distal root of the second molar. In a vertical impaction, the crown of the third molar is in a normal position for eruption, but eruption is prevented by the distal aspect of the second molar or by the anterior border of the ramus. In a horizontal impaction, the crown of the third molar is seen in a horizontal position relative to the inferior border of the mandible.

Teeth can be completely impacted in bone with no communication with the oral cavity, or they can be partially impacted. In a partial impaction, the tooth lies partly in soft tissue and partly in bone. Partially impacted teeth often have a communication with the oral cavity and are susceptible to infections (see pericoronitis, Chapter 3). For unknown reasons, some completely impacted teeth undergo resorption. This resorption usually begins in the crown portion of the tooth, and the tooth is slowly replaced by bone. Radiographically, this resorption should not be confused with caries. Caries of an impacted tooth is impossible unless there is communication with the oral cavity.

Treatment. Impacted teeth are surgically removed to prevent odontogenic cyst and tumor formation or damage (resorption) to adjacent teeth, and because in some cases the bone may be more susceptible to fracture. Partially impacted third molars are removed to prevent infections. Studies have shown that the optimal time to extract impacted third molars is between the ages of 12 and 24 years. With increased age, there is a greater incidence of nerve paresthesia.

Ankylosed Teeth

Ankylosed or **submerged teeth** are deciduous teeth in which bone has fused to cementum and dentin, preventing exfoliation of the deciduous tooth and eruption of the underlying permanent tooth (Fig. 4–38). Deciduous molars are most often affected by ankylosis. The cause is unknown. Trauma and infection of the periodontal ligament have been suggested.

Initially, the tooth erupts into the oral cavity into normal occlusion. The ankylosed tooth is not exfoliated. When the permanent teeth erupt, the permanent teeth adjacent to the ankylosed tooth have taller occlusocervical heights. Compared with the adjacent teeth, the ankylosed tooth appears submerged and has a different, more solid sound when percussed.

The presence of an ankylosed tooth is usually suspected on the basis of the clinical appearance and is confirmed radiographically. The periodontal ligament space is lacking or indistinct because of the union of bone and cementum, and the tooth usually exhibits root resorption. Ankylosis may be seen in permanent teeth that have been avulsed and reimplanted.

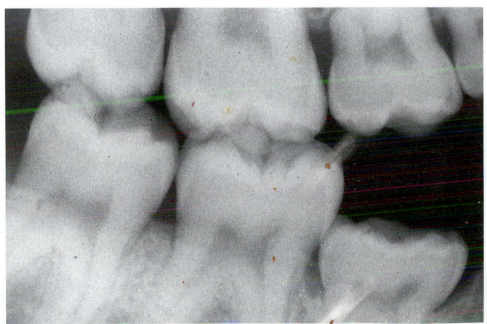

figure 4-38   Ankylosis of deciduous molar. (Courtesy of Dr. Margot Van Dis.)

Treatment. Extraction of ankylosed deciduous teeth is necessary to allow eruption of the underlying permanent tooth. Extraction of ankylosed permanent teeth is often necessary to prevent malocclusion, caries, and periodontal disease.

SELECTED REFERENCES

BOOKS

Eversole LR: Clinical Outline of Oral Pathology: Diagnosis and Treatment, 3rd ed. Philadelphia, Lea & Febiger, 1992.

Gibilisco JA (ed): Stafne's Oral Radiographic Diagnosis, 5th ed. Philadelphia, WB Saunders, 1985.

Gorlin RJ, Pindborg JJ, Cohen MM: Syndromes of the Head and Neck, 2nd ed. New York, McGraw-Hill, 1976.

Langlais RP, Bricker SL, Cottone JA, et al: Oral Diagnosis, Oral Medicine, and Treatment Planning. Philadelphia, WB Saunders, 1984.

Melfi RC: Permar's Oral Embryology and Microscopic Anatomy, 8th ed. Philadelphia, Lea & Febiger, 1988.

Miller BF: Encyclopedia and Dictionary of Medicine, Nursing, and Allied Health, 5th ed. Philadelphia, WB Saunders, 1992.

Neville BW, Damm DD, Allen CM, Bouquot JE: Oral and Maxillofacial Pathology. Philadelphia, WB Saunders, 1995.

Regezi JA, Sciubba JJ: Oral Pathology: Clinical-Pathologic Correlations, 2nd ed. Philadelphia, WB Saunders, 1993.

Shafer WG, Hine MK, Levy BM: A Textbook of Oral Pathology, 4th ed. Philadelphia, WB Saunders, 1983.

Sonis ST, Fazio RC, Fang L: Principles and Practice of Oral Medicine, 2nd ed. Philadelphia, WB Saunders, 1995.

Woelfel JB: Dental Anatomy: Its Correlation with Dental Health Service, 3rd ed. Philadelphia, Lea & Febiger, 1984.

Wood NK, Goaz PW: Differential Diagnosis of Oral Lesions, 4th ed. St. Louis, Mosby–Year Book, 1991.

JOURNAL ARTICLES

Alexander WN, Lilly GE, Irby WB: Odontodysplasia. Oral Surg 22:814, 1966.

Alfors E, Larson A, Sjögren S: The odontogenic keratocyst—a benign cystic tumor? J Oral Maxillofac Surg 42:10, 1984.

Al-Talabani NG, Smith CJ: Experimental dentigerous cysts and enamel hypoplasia: Their possible significance in explaining the pathogenesis of dentigerous cysts. J Oral Pathol 9:82, 1980.

Baker BR: Pits of the lip commissures in Caucasoid males. Oral Surg 21:56, 1966.

Barker GR: A radiolucency of the ascending ramus of the mandible associated with invested parotid salivary gland material and analogous with a Stafne bone cavity. Br J Oral Maxillofac Surg 26:81, 1988.

Baum BJ, Cohen MM: Patterns of size reduction in hypodontia. J Dent Res 50:779, 1971.

Black GV, McCay FA: Mottled teeth: An endemic developmental imperfection of the enamel of teeth heretofore unknown in the literature of dentistry. Dent Cosmos 58:129, 1916.

Bodin I, Julin P, Thomsson M: Hyperdontia III. Supernumerary anterior teeth. Dentomaxillofac Radiol 10:35, 1981.

Bodin I, Julin P, Thomsson M: Hyperdontia IV. Supernumerary premolars. Dentomaxillofac Radiol 19:99, 1981.

Brannon RB: The odontogenic keratocyst—a clinicopathologic study of 312 cases. Part I. Clinical features. Oral Surg 42:54, 1976.

Brannon RB: The odontogenic keratocyst—a clinicopathologic study of 312 cases. Part II. Histologic features. Oral Surg 43:233, 1977.

Buchner A, Hansen LS: Lymphoepithelial cysts of the oral cavity. A clinicopathologic study of 38 cases. Oral Surg 50:441, 1980.

Burton DJ, Saffos RO, Scheffer RB: Multiple bilateral dens in dente as a factor in the etiology of multiple periapical lesions. Oral Surg 49:496, 1980.

Cavanha AO: Enamel pearls. Oral Surg 19:373, 1965.

Christ TF: The globulomaxillary cyst—an embryologic misconception. Oral Surg 30:515, 1970.

Clayton JM: Congenital dental anomalies occurring in 3,557 children. J Dent Child 23:206, 1956.

Conklin WW: Bilateral dens invaginatus in the mandibular incisor region. Oral Surg 45:905, 1978.

Dachi SF, Howell FV: A survey of 3,874 routine full-mouth radiographs. II. A study of impacted teeth. Oral Surg 14:1165, 1961.

Darling AI, Levers BGH: Submerged human deciduous molars and ankylosis. Arch Oral Biol 18:1021, 1973.

Dean HT, Arnold FA: Endemic dental fluorosis or mottled teeth. J Am Dent Assoc 30:1278, 1943.

Dehlers FAC, Lee KW, Lee EC: Dens evaginatus (evaginated odontome). Dent Pract 17:239, 1967.

Delany GM, Goldblatt LI: Fused teeth: A multidisciplinary approach to treatment. J Am Dent Assoc 103:732, 1981.

DiFiore PM, Hartwell GR: Median mandibular lateral periodontal cysts. Oral Surg Oral Med Oral Pathol 63:545, 1987.

Dolder E: Deficient dentition. Dent Res 56:142, 1937.

Eisenbud LE, Attie JN, Gaslick J, et al: Aneurysmal bone cyst of the mandible. Oral Surg Oral Med Oral Pathol 64:202, 1987.

el-Mofty SK, Shannon MT, Mustoe TA: Lymph node metastasis in spindle cell carcinoma arising in an odontogenic cyst. Oral Surg Oral Med Oral Pathol 71:209, 1991.

Everett FG, Wescott WB: Commissural lip pits. Oral Surg 14:202, 1961.

Fantasia JE: Lateral periodontal cyst. An analysis of 46 cases. Oral Surg 48:237, 1979.

Freedman PD, Lumerman H, Gee JK: Calcifying odontogenic cyst. Oral Surg 40:93, 1975.

Gardner DG: An evaluation of reported cases of median mandibular cysts. Oral Surg Oral Med Oral Pathol 65:208, 1988.

Gardner DG: The dentinal changes in regional odontodysplasia. Oral Surg 38:887, 1974.

Gardner DG, Girgis SS: Taurodontism, shovel-shaped incisors and the Klinefelter syndrome. J Can Dent Assoc 8:372, 1978.

Gardner DG, Sapp JP: Regional odontodysplasia. Oral Surg 35:351, 1973.

Graber LW: Congenital absence of teeth: A review with emphasis on inheritance patterns. J Am Dent Assoc 96:266, 1978.

Grahnen H, Granath LE: Numerical variations in primary dentition. Odontol Rev 12:342, 1961.

Grahnen H, Larsson PG: Enamel defects in deciduous dentition of prematurely born children. Odontol Rev 9:143, 1958.

Hamner JE III, Witko CJ, Metro PS: Taurodontism. Report of a case. Oral Surg 18:409, 1964.

Henderson HZ: Ankylosis of primary molars: A clinical, radiographic, and histologic study. J Dent Child 46:117, 1979.

Hernandez GA, Castro A, Castro G, Amador E: Aneurysmal bone cyst versus hemangioma of the mandible. Oral Surg Oral Med Oral Pathol 76:790, 1993.

Holt RD, Brook AH: Taurodontism: A criterion for diagnosis and its prevalence in mandibular first molars in a sample of 1,115 British school children. J Int Assoc Dent Child 10:41, 1979.

Howell RE, Handlers JP, Aberle AM, et al: CEA immunoreactivity in odontogenic tumors and keratocysts. Oral Surg Oral Med Oral Pathol 66:576, 1988.

Hutchinson ACW: A case of total anodontia of the permanent dentition. Br Dent J 94:16, 1953.

Keith A: Problems relating to the teeth of the earlier forms of prehistoric man. Proc R Soc Med 6 (Part 3):103, 1913.

Kelly JR: Gemination, fusion, or both? Oral Surg 45:326, 1978.

King RC, Smith BR, Burk JL: Dermoid cyst in the floor of the mouth. Oral Surg Oral Med Oral Pathol 78:567, 1994.

Kitchin PC: Dens in dente. J Dent Res 15:1176, 1935.

Krolls SO, Donalhue AH: Double-rooted maxillary primary canines. Oral Surg 49:379, 1980.

Levitas TC: Gemination, fusion, twinning, and concrescence. J Dent Child 32:93, 1965.

Ligh RA: Coronal dilaceration. Oral Surg 51:567, 1981.

Mader CL: Fusion of teeth. J Am Dent Assoc 98:62, 1979.

Mangion JJ: Two cases of taurodontism in modern human jaws. Br Dent J 113:309, 1962.

Mathewson RJ, Siegel MJ, McCanna DL: Ankyloglossia: A review of the literature and a case report. J Dent Child 33:238, 1966.

Mellor JK, Ripa LW: Talon cusp: A clinically significant anomaly. Oral Surg 29:224, 1970.

Merrill RG: Occlusal anomalous tubercles on premolars of Alaskan Eskimos and Indians. Oral Surg 17:484, 1964.

Milazzo A, Alexander SA: Fusion, gemination, oligodontia and taurodontism. J Pedodontics 6:194, 1982.

Mlynarczyk G: Enamel pitting: A common symptom of tuberous sclerosis. Oral Surg Oral Med Oral Pathol 71:63, 1991.

Morningstar CH: Effect of infection of deciduous molar on the permanent tooth germ. J Am Dent Assoc 24:786, 1937.

Oehlers FA: Dens invaginatus (dilated composite odontome). I. Variations of the invagination process on associated anterior crown forms. Oral Surg 10:1204, 1957.

Partridge M, Towers JF: The primordial cyst (odontogenic keratocyst): Its tumor-like characteristics and behavior. Br J Oral Maxillofac Surg 25:271, 1987.

Pendrys DG: Dental fluorosis in perspective. J Am Dent Assoc 122:63, 1991.

Ray GE: Congenital absence of permanent teeth. Br Dent J 90:213, 1951

Reaume CE, Sofie VL: Lingual thyroid: Review of the literature and a report of a case. Oral Surg 45:841, 1978.
Redman RS: Respiratory epithelium in an apical periodontal cyst of the mandible. Oral Surg Oral Med Oral Pathol 67:77, 1989.
Rushton MA: Hereditary enamel defects. Proc R Soc Med 57:53, 1964.
Rushton MA: Invaginated teeth (dens in dente): Contents of the invagination. Oral Surg 11:1378, 1958.
Rushton MA: Odontodysplasia: "Ghost teeth." Br Dent J 119:109, 1965.
Sapp PJ, Stark M: Self-healing traumatic bone cysts. Oral Surg Oral Med Oral Pathol 69:597, 1990.
Sauk JJ Jr: Ectopic lingual thyroid. J Pathol 102:239, 1970.
Shafer WG: Dens in dente. NY Dent J 19:220, 1953.
Suchina JA, Ludington JR Jr, Madden RM: Dens invaginatus of a maxillary lateral incisor: Endodontic treatment. Oral Surg Oral Med Oral Pathol 68:467, 1989.
Swallow JN: Complete anodontia of the permanent dentition. A case report. Br Dent J 107:143, 1959.
van Gool AV: Injury to the permanent tooth germ after trauma to the deciduous predecessor. Oral Surg 35:2, 1973.
Vorheis JM, Gregory GT, McDonald RE: Ankylosed deciduous molars. J Am Dent Assoc 44:68, 1952.
Weinmann JP, Svoboda JF, Woods RW: Hereditary disturbances of enamel formation and calcification. J Am Dent Assoc 32:397, 1945.
Yip WK: The prevalence of dens evaginatus. Oral Surg 38:80, 1974.
Yoshikazu S, Tanimoto K, Wada T: Simple bone cyst: Evaluation of contents with conventional radiography and computed tomography. Oral Surg Oral Med Oral Pathol 77:296, 1994.
Zegarelli DJ, Zegarelli EV: Radiolucent lesions in the globulomaxillary region. J Oral Surg 31:767, 1973.

REVIEW QUESTIONS

1. Which term refers to a defect present at birth?
   (A) Anomaly
   (B) Inherited defect
   (C) Congenital defect
   (D) Developmental defect

2. Which term refers to the origin and tissue formation of teeth?
   (A) Odontogenesis
   (B) Dentinogenesis
   (C) Amelogenesis
   (D) Cementogenesis

3. Which term refers to the joining of teeth by cementum *only*?
   (A) Fusion
   (B) Gemination
   (C) Twinning
   (D) Concrescence

4. Which teeth are most often missing?
   (A) Canines
   (B) Third molars
   (C) Lateral incisors
   (D) Premolars

5. Which tooth is the most common supernumerary tooth?
   (A) Mesiodens
   (B) Distomolar
   (C) Paramolar
   (D) Hutchinson's incisor

6. Which teeth most often appear smaller than normal?
   (A) Mandibular premolars and maxillary third molars
   (B) Maxillary premolars and mandibular third molars
   (C) Mandibular lateral incisors and mandibular third molars
   (D) Maxillary lateral incisors and maxillary third molars

7. Which term refers to the developmental anomaly that arises when a single tooth germ attempts to divide and results in the incomplete formation of two teeth?
   (A) Fusion
   (B) Gemination
   (C) Concrescence
   (D) Dilaceration

8. Which term refers to the developmental anomaly that arises from the union of two normally separated adjacent tooth germs?
   (A) Fusion
   (B) Gemination
   (C) Concrescence
   (D) Dilaceration

9. Which term refers to an abnormal angulation or curve in the root or crown of a tooth?
   (A) Fusion
   (B) Gemination
   (C) Concrescence
   (D) Dilaceration

10. Which term refers to a developmental anomaly in which teeth exhibit elongated, large pulp chambers and short roots?
    (A) Dens in dente
    (B) Dens evaginatus
    (C) Taurodontism
    (D) Dilaceration

11. Which developmental anomaly is often associated with a nonvital tooth and periapical lesions?
    (A) Dens in dente
    (B) Dens evaginatus
    (C) Taurodontism
    (D) Talon cusp

12. Which of the following teeth most often exhibit supernumerary roots?
    (A) Maxillary premolars
    (B) Maxillary third molars
    (C) Mandibular first molars
    (D) Maxillary first molars

13. Which one of the following describes the appearance of enamel hypoplasia resulting from a febrile illness or vitamin deficiency?
    (A) Pitting defects
    (B) Yellowish-brown discoloration
    (C) Blackish-brown staining
    (D) Chalky white spots

14. Which one of the following is associated with enamel hypoplasia resulting from congenital syphilis?
    (A) Turner's tooth
    (B) Hutchinson's incisors
    (C) Taurodont
    (D) Dens evaginatus

15. Which one of the following describes the appearance of enamel hypocalcification?
    (A) Pitting defects
    (B) Yellowish-brown discoloration
    (C) Blackish-brown stains
    (D) Chalky white spots

16. Which term describes a tooth that has not erupted because of the lack of eruptive force?
    (A) Ankylosed
    (B) Impacted
    (C) Embedded
    (D) Fused

17. Which teeth are most often impacted?
    (A) Maxillary and mandibular third molars
    (B) Maxillary and mandibular first molars
    (C) Mandibular cuspids
    (D) Mandibular bicuspids

18. Which term describes a tooth in which bone has fused to cementum and dentin and prevents the eruption of an underlying permanent tooth?
    (A) Ankylosed
    (B) Embedded
    (C) Impacted
    (D) Fused

19. Which cyst is not an odontogenic cyst?
    (A) Dentigerous cyst
    (B) Primordial cyst
    (C) Median palatal cyst
    (D) Lateral periodontal cyst

20. The most common cause of the radicular cyst is
    (A) Caries
    (B) Trauma
    (C) Malignant infiltration
    (D) Food impaction

21. Which cyst is an odontogenic intraosseous cyst that forms around the crown of a developing tooth?
    (A) Coronal cyst
    (B) Dentigerous cyst
    (C) Lateral periodontal cyst
    (D) Eruption cyst

22. Which cyst develops in place of a tooth?
    (A) Dentigerous cyst
    (B) Primordial cyst
    (C) Follicular cyst
    (D) Odontogenic keratocyst

23. Which cyst is characterized by its unique histologic appearance and frequent recurrence?
    (A) Residual cyst
    (B) Stafne's bone cyst
    (C) Odontogenic keratocyst
    (D) Eruption cyst

24. The lateral periodontal cyst is defined by its location. In which area is the lateral periodontal cyst most commonly found?
    (A) Mandibular third molar area
    (B) Maxillary tuberosity area
    (C) Between the maxillary premolars
    (D) Between the mandibular cuspid and first premolar

25. The teeth are vital with all of the following cysts except
    (A) Nasopalatine canal cyst
    (B) Cyst of the palatine papilla
    (C) Radicular cyst
    (D) Median mandibular cyst

26. Which cyst is characteristically pear shaped?
    (A) Globulomaxillary cyst
    (B) Median palatal cyst
    (C) Incisal canal cyst
    (D) Median mandibular cyst

27. Which cyst was probably a radicular cyst left behind after the extraction of the offending tooth?
    (A) Periodontal cyst
    (B) Gingival cyst
    (C) Odontogenic cyst
    (D) Residual cyst

28. With which cyst may the patient complain of dysphagia?
    (A) Thyroglossal tract cyst
    (B) Median palatal cyst
    (C) Static bone cyst
    (D) Traumatic bone cyst

29. Which cyst is considered a pseudocyst?
    (A) Traumatic bone cyst
    (B) Dentigerous cyst
    (C) Lymphoepithelial cyst
    (D) Primordial cyst

30. In addition to the odontogenic keratocyst, which lesion would you suspect if a radiograph revealed a multilocular radiolucency?
    (A) Globulomaxillary cyst
    (B) Aneurysmal bone cyst
    (C) Stafne's bone cyst
    (D) Radicular cyst

31. Which term refers to the adhesion of the tongue to the floor of the mouth?
    (A) Ankylosis
    (B) Ankyloglossia
    (C) Anodontia
    (D) Amelogenesis

32. Which location is the most common for lip pits?
    (A) Commissure
    (B) Philtrum
    (C) Nasolabial groove
    (D) Labiomental groove

33. Which term refers to an ectopic mass of thyroid tissue located on the dorsal tongue?
    (A) Thyroid cyst
    (B) Thyroid tumor
    (C) Lingual tonsil
    (D) Lingual thyroid

34. Which term refers to the total absence of all teeth?
    (A) Anodontia
    (B) Hypodontia
    (C) Hyperdontia
    (D) Microdontia

35. Which term refers to the lack of one or more teeth?
    (A) Anodontia
    (B) Hypodontia
    (C) Hyperdontia
    (D) Microdontia

36. Which tooth is the second most common supernumerary tooth?
    (A) Taurodont
    (B) Mesiodens
    (C) Paramolar
    (D) Distomolar

37. Which term refers to abnormally small teeth?
    (A) Taurodontia
    (B) Macrodontia
    (C) Microdontia
    (D) Hypodontia

38. Which term refers to abnormally large teeth?
    (A) Taurodontia
    (B) Macrodontia
    (C) Microdontia
    (D) Hypodontia

39. Which location is the most likely for an enamel pearl?
    (A) Maxillary molars
    (B) Maxillary premolars
    (C) Mandibular premolars
    (D) Mandibular molars

40. Which location is the most likely for a talon cusp?
    (A) Canines
    (B) Incisors
    (C) Molars
    (D) Premolars

41. Which term refers to an accessory cusp located on the occlusal surface of a tooth?
    (A) Mulberry cusp
    (B) Talon cusp
    (C) Dens invaginatus
    (D) Dens evaginatus

42. Which term refers to the enamel hypoplasia of a permanent tooth that results from infection of a deciduous tooth?
    (A) Hutchinson's tooth
    (B) Talon's tooth
    (C) Turner's tooth
    (D) Gorlin's tooth

43. Which term refers to the irregular areas of discoloration that result from fluoride ingestion?
    (A) Pitting defects
    (B) Mottling defects
    (C) Endogenous staining
    (D) Extrinsic staining

44. Which term refers to teeth that appear ghost-like on a dental radiograph?
    (A) Taurodontism
    (B) Enamel hypocalcification
    (C) Regional odontodysplasia
    (D) Enamel hypoplasia

45. Which term refers to teeth that cannot erupt because of physical obstruction?
    (A) Fused
    (B) Ankylosed
    (C) Embedded
    (D) Impacted

5

Neoplasia

PAUL D. FREEDMAN

·

ANNE CALE JONES

·

JOAN A. PHELAN

·

Objectives

After studying this chapter, the student should be able to:

1. Define each of the words in the vocabulary list for this chapter.
2. Explain the difference between a benign tumor and a malignant tumor.
3. Define leukoplakia and erythroplakia.
4. Define the neoplasms listed below.
5. Describe the clinical features of each neoplasm listed below.
6. Explain the usual treatment for each neoplasm listed below.

Papilloma	Lipoma
Squamous cell carcinoma	Neurofibroma and schwannoma
Verrucous carcinoma	Granular cell tumor
Basal cell carcinoma	(granular cell myoblastoma)
Pleomorphic adenoma	Congenital epulis
(benign mixed tumor)	Rhabdomyosarcoma
Monomorphic adenoma	Hemangioma
Papillary cystadenoma	Lymphangioma
lymphomatosum	Melanocytic nevi
Adenoid cystic carcinoma	Melanoma
Mucoepidermoid carcinoma	Osteoma
Ameloblastoma	Ossifying fibroma
Calcifying epithelial odontogenic	Osteogenic sarcoma
tumor (Pindborg tumor)	Chondrosarcoma
Calcifying odontogenic cyst	Leukemia
Adenomatoid odontogenic tumor	Lymphoma
Myxoma	Multiple myeloma
Cementifying fibroma	Metastatic jaw tumors
Cementoblastoma	
Ameloblastic fibroma	
Odontoma	

7. Describe the clinical and histologic features of the calcifying odontogenic cyst, and explain why it is sometimes considered a neoplasm.
8. Describe the clinical features, radiographic appearance, and management of periapical cemental dysplasia and florid osseous dysplasia.

Vocabulary

(handwritten, top margin): anaplastic -Characterized by a loss of differentiation of cells and their orientation to one another; a charc. of malignant tumors

(handwritten, right margin): undifferentiated – absence of normal differentiation; a characteristic of tumor tissue

Benign (be-nīn′)   Not malignant; favorable for recovery

Carcinoma (kar″si-no′mah)   A malignant tumor of epithelium

Central (sen′tral)   Occurring within bone

Dysplasia (dis-pla′ze-ah)   Disordered growth

Encapsulated (en-kap′su-lāt-ed)   Surrounded by a capsule of fibrous connective tissue

Hyperchromatic (hi″per-kro-mat′ik)   Staining more intensely than normal

Hyperplasia (hi″per-pla′zĕ-ah)   An abnormal increase in the number of normal cells in normal arrangement in a tissue

Invasion (in-va′zhun)   The infiltration and active destruction of surrounding tissues

Leukoplakia (loo-kō-plā′kē-ah)   A clinical term used to identify a white, plaque-like lesion of the oral mucosa that cannot be wiped off and cannot be diagnosed as any other disease

Malignant (mah-lig′nant)   Likely to cause the death of the host

Malignant tumor (mah-lig′nant too′mor)   Cancer; a tumor that is resistant to treatment and frequently causes death; a tumor that has the potential for uncontrolled growth and dissemination or recurrence, or both

(handwritten, left margin): In situ - Confined to origin w/out invasion of other tissue.

Metastasis (mĕ-tas′tah-sis) (plural, metastases; mĕ-tas′tah-sēz)   The transport of neoplastic cells to parts of the body remote from the primary tumor and the establishment of new tumors in those sites

Metastatic tumor (met″ah-stat′ik too′mor)   Tumor formed by cells that have been transported from the primary tumor to sites not connected to the original tumor

Mitotic figure (mi-tot′ik fig′ur); mitosis (mi-to′sis)   Dividing cells caught in the process of mitosis

Neoplasia (ne″o-pla′ze-ah)   The formation of tumors by the uncontrolled proliferation of cells

Neoplasm (ne′o-plazm)   Tumor; a new growth of tissue in which growth is uncontrolled and progressive

(handwritten, left margin): Neoplastic - pertains to formation of tumors by uncontrolled proliferation of cells.

Nevus (ne′vus) (plural, nevi; ne′vi)   A benign, localized overgrowth of melanocytes; also, a birthmark *(handwritten:* pigmented not a*)*

Odontogenic (o-don″to-jen′ik)   Tooth forming

Oncology (ong-kol′o-je)   The study of tumors or neoplasms

Peripheral (pĕ-rif′er-al)   Occurring outside of bone

Pleomorphic (ple″o-mor′fik)   Occurring in various forms

Primary tumor (pri′mer-e too′mor)   The original tumor; the source of metastasis

Sarcoma (sar-ko′mah)   A malignant tumor of connective tissue

Tumor (too′mor)   A neoplasm; also, a swelling or enlargement

(handwritten, bottom margin): Pedunculated & Sessile other vocab

DESCRIPTION

Neoplasia means new growth. It is a process in which cells exhibit uncontrolled proliferation. A **neoplasm** is a mass of such cells. Although the word **tumor** means swelling, it is commonly used as a synonym for neoplasm. The study of tumors is called **oncology.** "Onco," from Greek, means swelling or mass.

In order for neoplasia to occur, an irreversible change must take place in the cells, and this change must be passed on to new cells, resulting in uncontrollable cell multiplication. For most neoplasms, the initial stimulus that triggers the process of cell change is not known. The size of normal tissues is maintained by regulatory processes. A neoplasm is not controlled by the regulatory processes that maintain the size of normal tissues, and it exhibits unlimited and unregulated growth.

Like hyperplasia, which is described in Chapter 2, neoplasia is an abnormal process. With hyperplasia, normal cells proliferate in a normal arrangement in response to tissue damage, and the proliferation stops when the stimulus is removed. Although the size of the tissue may be greater than normal, the growth of the tissue is still under control. Reactive lesions, such as the irritation fibroma, denture-related hyperplasia (epulis fissuratum), and the pyogenic granuloma, described in Chapter 2, are examples of hyperplasia. Neoplasia, in contrast, is a completely abnormal process—the cells are abnormal, and the proliferation of those cells is uncontrolled and unlimited.

CAUSES OF NEOPLASIA

Many agents—principally chemicals, viruses, and radiation—have been shown to cause neoplastic transformation of cells in the laboratory. Hundreds of chemicals have been shown to cause cancer in animals. In addition, certain chemicals, viruses, and radiation have been shown to cause some cancers in humans. Neoplastic transformation can also occur spontaneously secondary to a genetic mutation. Viruses that cause tumors are called **oncogenic viruses.** Radiation from sunlight, x-rays, nuclear fission, or other sources is well established as a cancer-producing agent in humans.

CLASSIFICATION OF TUMORS

Tumors are divided into two categories: benign and malignant. A **benign tumor** or **neoplasm** remains localized. It may be **encapsulated,** which means that it is walled off by surrounding fibrous connective tissue. Sometimes a benign tumor can invade adjacent structures, but it does not have the ability to spread to distant sites. A **malignant tumor,** in contrast, both invades and destroys surrounding tissue and also has the ability to spread throughout the body. **Cancer** is synonymous with malignancy.

Benign and Malignant Tumors

Benign tumors almost always resemble normal cells, whereas malignant tumors vary in their histologic appearance. Malignant tumors in which the cells though abnormal still resemble normal cells are called well-differentiated tumors. Malignant tumors may also be poorly differentiated. The cells of these tumors have only some of the characteristics of the tissue from which they are derived. Still other malignant tumors may be undifferentiated or anaplastic and do not resemble the tissue from which they are derived at all. Malignant tumors are often composed of cells that vary in size and shape **(pleomorphic)** (Fig. 5–1). The nuclei of the cells look darker than

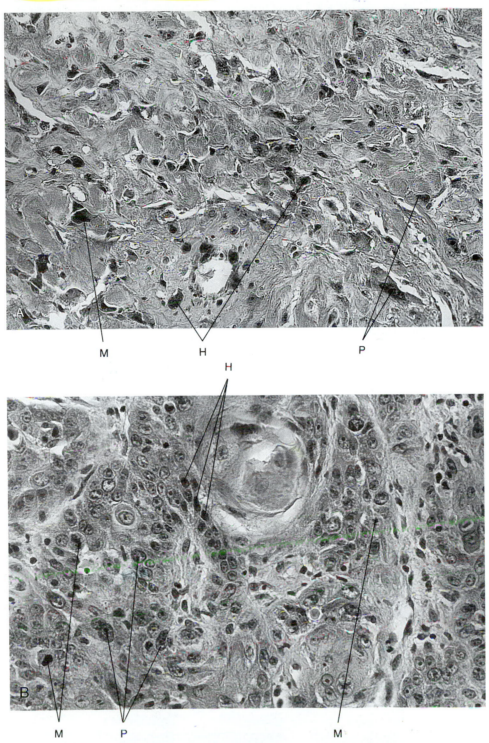

■ *f i g u r e* 5–1   Photomicrographs of malignant tumors showing pleomorphic (P) and hyperchromatic (H) nuclei and mitotic figures (M). *A,* Osteogenic sarcoma. *B,* Squamous cell carcinoma.

TABLE 5–1 Comparison of Benign and Malignant Tumors

Benign	Malignant
Usually well differentiated	Well differentiated to anaplastic
Usually slow growing	Slow to rapid growth
Mitotic figures rare	Mitotic figures may be numerous
Usually encapsulated	Invasive and unencapsulated
No metastasis	Metastasis likely

nota classification

those of normal cells **(hyperchromatic)**, are larger, and may also be pleomorphic (see Fig. 5–1). **Mitotic figures** are seen microscopically in cells in which the nucleus is caught in the process of dividing. Normal and abnormal mitotic figures are seen in many malignant tumors (see Fig. 5–1). Abnormal mitotic figures are those that are not dividing normally and, therefore, the shape of the dividing nucleus does not follow the shape of a normal mitotic figure. Table 5–1 compares benign and malignant tumors.

NAMES OF TUMORS

The prefix of the name of a tumor is determined by the tissue or cell of origin. The suffix "oma" is used to indicate a tumor. For example, a benign tumor of fat is called a **lipoma,** and a benign tumor of bone is called an **osteoma.** Malignant tumors are named in a similar fashion. Malignant tumors of epithelium are called **carcinomas,** and malignant tumors of connective tissue are called **sarcomas.** The prefix of the name of a malignant tumor is also determined by the tissue or cell of origin. Therefore, a malignant tumor of squamous epithelium is called **squamous cell carcinoma,** and a malignant tumor of bone is called an **osteosarcoma.** Carcinomas are about 10 times more common than sarcomas. Table 5–2 lists tumors according to their tissue of origin.

TABLE 5–2 Names of Tumors

Tissue of Origin	Benign Tumor	Malignant Tumor
Epithelium		
Squamous cells	Papilloma	Squamous cell or epidermoid carcinoma
Basal cells		Basal cell carcinoma
Glands or ducts	Adenoma	Adenocarcinoma
Neuroectoderm		
Melanocytes	Nevus	Melanoma
Connective Tissue		
Fibrous	Fibroma	Fibrosarcoma
Cartilage	Chondroma	Chondrosarcoma
Bone	Osteoma	Osteosarcoma
Fat	Lipoma	Liposarcoma
Endothelium		
Blood vessels	Hemangioma	Angiosarcoma
Lymphatic vessels	Lymphangioma	Lymphangiosarcoma
Muscle		
Smooth muscle	Leiomyoma	Leiomyosarcoma
Striated muscle	Rhabdomyoma	Rhabdomyosarcoma

TREATMENT OF TUMORS

Benign tumors are generally treated by surgical excision, which can be accomplished through wide local excision or enucleation. Malignant tumors can be treated by surgery, chemotherapy, or radiation therapy; a combination is often used.

Since many different types of tissues are present in the oral cavity, many different types of tumors can arise in this location. These neoplasms can be either benign or malignant. In this chapter, the neoplasms are classified according to their tissue of origin. Benign tumors are described first, followed by their malignant counterparts.

EPITHELIAL TUMORS

Three different types of epithelial tumors occur in the oral cavity: Tumors derived from squamous epithelium, tumors derived from salivary gland epithelium, and tumors derived from odontogenic epithelium. A few of the lesions included in this section are not true tumors. The reasons for their inclusion are explained in their descriptions.

Tumors of Squamous Epithelium

Papilloma

The **papilloma** is a benign tumor of squamous epithelium that appears clinically as a relatively small exophytic pedunculated or sessile growth. These tumors are composed of numerous projections that may be either white or the color of normal mucosa (Fig. 5–2). They are often described as cauliflower-like in appearance. Histologically, the papilloma consists of numerous finger-like or papillary projections surfaced by normal stratified squamous epithelium. Each papillary projection is supported by a central core of fibrous connective tissue. The color of the lesion depends on the amount of surface keratin. The more keratin, the whiter the surface (Color Plate 70).

Other oral lesions that may look like a papilloma clinically are verruca vulgaris (common wart) and condyloma acuminatum (venereal wart). These two lesions are caused by papillomaviruses and are described in Chapter 3. They are differentiated from the papilloma by microscopic examination. Special staining procedures can be used to identify viral particles in these lesions.

A papilloma can occur at any age. Although the most common location is the soft palate, it can occur anywhere on the oral mucosa.

Treatment and Prognosis. The papilloma is treated by surgical excision, which must include the base of the growth. With adequate excision, the papilloma usually does not recur.

Premalignant Lesions

Leukoplakia

It is important to define the term **leukoplakia** in any discussion of premalignant lesions of the oral mucosa because in the past this term was used to refer to a microscopically premalignant oral mucosal lesion. However, this is no longer the way this term is used. Leukoplakia is a clinical term and does not refer to a specific histologic appearance. Leukoplakia is defined as a white plaque-like lesion of the oral

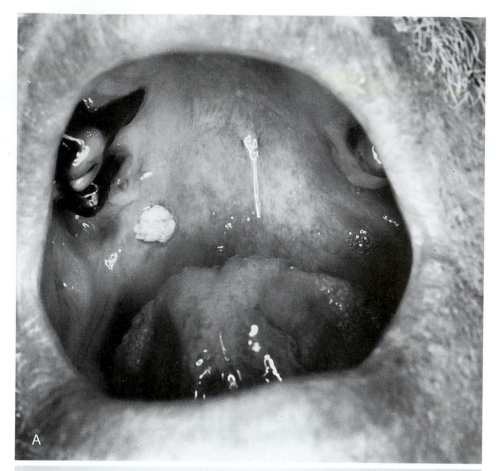

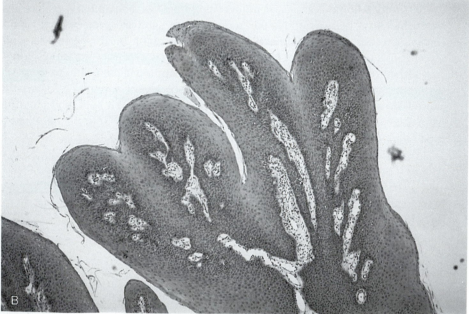

■ *f* i g u r e 5–2   *A,* Clinical appearance of a papilloma of the oral mucosa showing cauliflower-like appearance and rough surface resulting from finger-like
projections. *B,* Microscopic appearance of a papilloma showing finger-like
projections surfaced by squamous epithelium and supported by thin cores
of fibrous connective tissue.

mucosa that cannot be rubbed off and cannot be diagnosed as a specific disease (Fig. 5–3; Color Plates 49, 56, and 71). Leukoplakia is sometimes referred to as **idiopathic leukoplakia** to emphasize that the specific cause of the lesion is not known. The white lesion illustrated in Figure 5–4 and Color Plate 20 is more accurately called a tobacco chewer's white lesion than a leukoplakia because the direct cause of the lesion is known.

The histologic appearance of lesions that appear clinically as leukoplakia varies, and therefore a biopsy is essential to establish the diagnosis. Most leukoplakias are due to hyperkeratosis (thickening of the keratin layer) or a combination of epithelial hyperplasia (thickening of the prickle cell or spinous layer) and hyperkeratosis. When examined histologically, a leukoplakia may also show epithelial dysplasia, a premalignant condition, or even squamous cell carcinoma, a malignant tumor of squamous epithelium. In one study, approximately 16% of leukoplakias examined microscopically showed epithelial dysplasia. Studies have also revealed that leukoplakia found on the floor of the mouth and on the lateral and ventral tongue are more likely to be epithelial dysplasia or squamous cell carcinoma than leukoplakias occurring in other areas of the oral cavity.

When a white lesion is identified in the oral cavity, the first goal is to find the cause. Any associated irritation should be removed. If the lesion does not resolve, a biopsy and histologic examination must be performed. Any white lesion that is diagnosed as epithelial dysplasia or that cannot be diagnosed as a specific disease should be completely removed. When leukoplakia is found on the floor of the mouth or the lateral or ventral tongue, the lesion is often removed even if the histologic appearance is that of hyperkeratosis or epithelial hyperplasia because of the increased risk of squamous cell carcinoma in these areas.

The treatment of leukoplakia is dependent on histologic diagnosis.

The treatment of epithelial dysplasia and squamous cell carcinoma is discussed in the sections that follow.

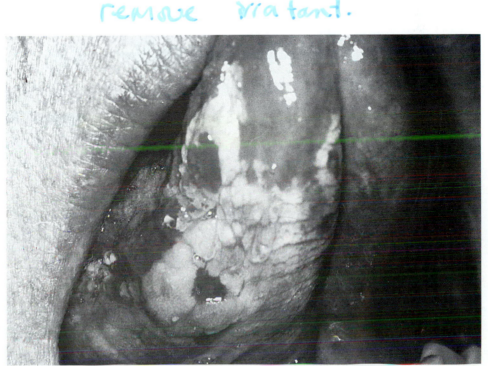

f i g u r e **5–3**   Clinical appearance of leukoplakia on the right ventral aspect of the tongue in a 48-year-old woman. The cause of the lesion could not be identified.

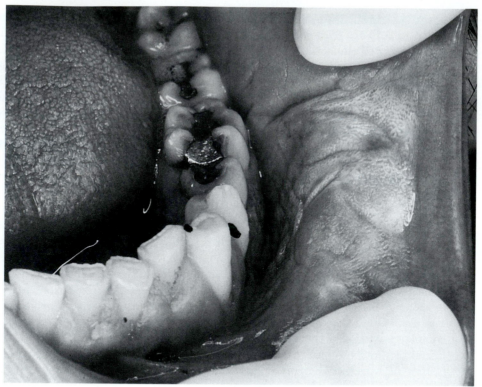

■ *f i g u r e* 5–4   Clinical appearance of a white lesion that was associated with tobacco chewing. This lesion developed at the site at which the tobacco was held.

Erythroplakia *worse than white*

Erythroplakia is a clinical term that is used to describe an oral mucosal lesion that may appear as a smooth red patch or a granular red and velvety patch. A lesion that shows a mixture of red and white areas is generally called **speckled leukoplakia** rather than erythroplakia. Erythroplakia is much less common than leukoplakia. In one study, 60 cases of leukoplakia were seen for every 1 case of erythroplakia. When examined microscopically, erythroplakia more frequently shows epithelial dysplasia or squamous cell carcinoma than does leukoplakia.   *dysplasia — biopsy.*

Treatment of erythroplakia depends on the histologic diagnosis.

Epithelial Dysplasia

Epithelial dysplasia is a histologic diagnosis. It is considered a premalignant condition. Lesions histologically exhibiting epithelial dysplasia frequently precede squamous cell carcinoma. Unlike those of squamous cell carcinoma, the cellular changes in epithelial dysplasia may revert to normal if the stimulus, such as tobacco smoking, is removed. Epithelial dysplasia may present clinically as an erythematous lesion (erythroplakia), as a white lesion (leukoplakia), or as a mixed erythematous and white lesion (speckled leukoplakia). **Dysplasia** means disordered growth. The term dysplasia is used to describe lesions of other tissues as well. Dysplasias of other tissues (e.g., bone) may not be considered premalignant lesions.

Histologically, epithelial dysplasia shows abnormal maturation of epithelial cells, hyperplasia of the basal cells, disorganization of the epithelial layers, cells with enlarged and hyperchromatic nuclei, abnormal keratinization, and increased numbers of both normal and abnormal mitotic figures (Fig. 5–5). Histologically, epithelial dysplasia differs from squamous cell carcinoma in that there is no invasion of the abnormal epithelial cells through the basement membrane into the underlying tissue as there is in squamous cell carcinoma. Severe dysplasia is sometimes called **carcinoma in situ.**

Squamous Cell Carcinoma

Squamous cell carcinoma, or **epidermoid carcinoma,** is a malignant tumor of squamous epithelium. It is the most common primary malignancy of the oral cavity and, like other malignant tumors, can infiltrate adjacent tissues and metastasize to distant sites. Squamous cell carcinomas usually metastasize first to lymph nodes of the neck and then to more distant sites such as the lungs and liver. Clinically, squamous cell carcinoma is usually an exophytic ulcerative mass (Fig. 5–6; Color Plates 50, 51, 57, 58, 72), but early tumors may be erythematous and plaque-like (erythroplakia), white and plaque-like (leukoplakia), or a mixture of erythematous and white areas (speckled leukoplakia).

The essential feature of squamous cell carcinoma is the invasion of tumor cells through the epithelial basement membrane into the underlying connective tissue (Fig. 5–7A), which is seen on microscopic examination of the tissue. Histologically, the tumor is characterized by invasive sheets and nests of neoplastic squamous cells. Although squamous cell carcinoma is a malignant tumor, it exhibits features that allow the cells to be recognized as squamous epithelial cells. In well-differentiated tumors, these features are easily recognized; however, in a poorly differentiated squamous cell carcinoma, they may not be. Since keratin is a product of squamous epithelium, well-differentiated tumors show keratin formation. In addition to normal surface keratin, the keratin may be seen in individual cells within the tumor and as structures called

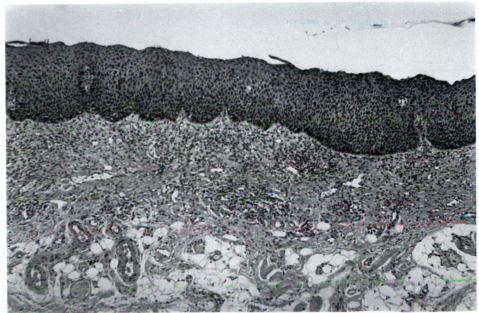

f i g u r e 5–5   Microscopic appearance of epithelial dysplasia. There is loss of the normal stratification of the epithelium, hyperplasia of the basal cells, and enlarged and hyperchromatic nuclei.

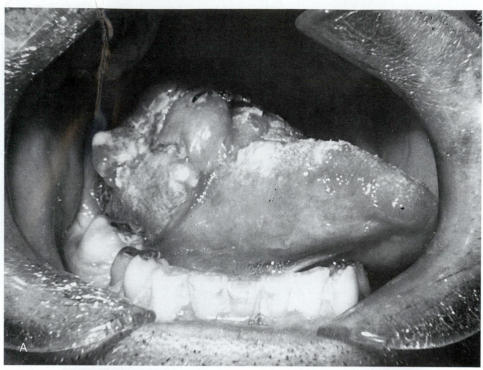

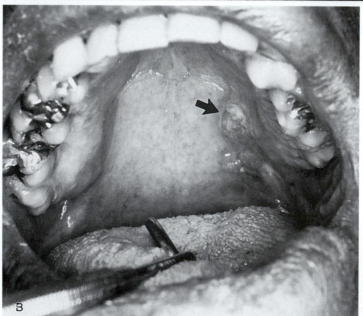

■ *f* i g u r e 5–6   *A*, Clinical appearance of a squamous cell carcinoma of the posterolateral tongue showing an exophytic, ulcerated mass. *B*, Clinical appearance of a squamous cell carcinoma of the left side of the soft palate and fauces.

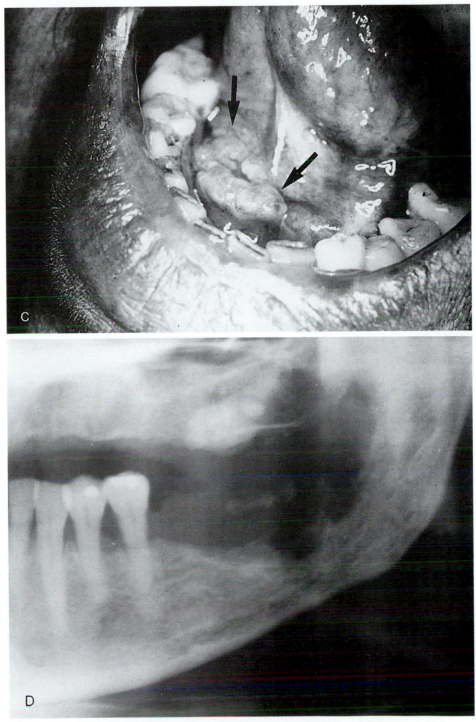

■ f i g u r e 5-6   *Continued C*, Clinical appearance of a squamous cell carcinoma on the floor of the mouth. *D*, Left side of a panoramic radiograph showing destruction of the mandible by squamous cell carcinoma.

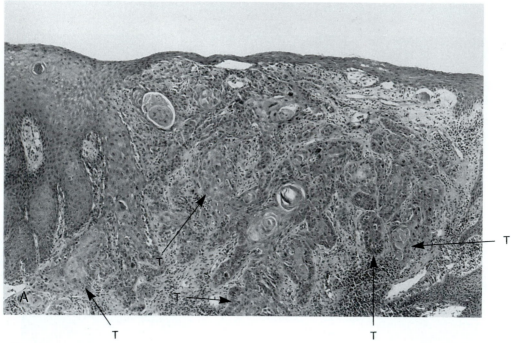

f i g u r e 5–7   *A,* Microscopic appearance (low power) of a squamous cell carcinoma showing infiltration of the tumor (T) into the connective tissue.

keratin pearls (Fig. 5–7*B*). The neoplastic cells are not normal cells. They contain large hyperchromatic nuclei and numerous mitotic figures. Some of the mitotic figures appear normal, whereas others are bizarre (Fig. 5–7*B*).

Intraoral squamous cell carcinomas can occur anywhere in the oral cavity, but most tumors occur on the floor of the mouth, ventrolateral tongue, soft palate, tonsillar pillar, and retromolar areas. The clinical appearance of squamous cell carcinoma occurring in several different locations is seen in Figure 5–6.

Squamous cell carcinomas can occur on the vermilion border of the lips and skin of the face (Fig. 5–8; Color Plate 7). In this location, it is associated with sun exposure and tends to be more common in individuals with fair skin. The prognosis for squamous cell carcinoma of the lips and skin is much better than that for squamous cell carcinoma of the oral mucosa. Sun exposure causes recognizable changes of the vermilion border of the lips. The color changes from dark pink and uniform to mottled grayish pink. The interface of the vermilion border and the skin becomes blurred, and linear fissures are seen at right angles to the line of the interface. Histologically, damage from sun exposure is seen as changes that range from degeneration of the collagen under the epithelium to a condition called **solar cheilitis,** in which there is mild to severe epithelial dysplasia. Fair-skinned individuals are prone to the development of squamous cell carcinoma of the lips and skin resulting from sun exposure and therefore should be advised either to avoid the sun or to use sun block.

The majority of squamous cell carcinomas occur in patients older than 40 years of age. In the past, men have outnumbered women; however, in the last 30 years, there has been an increased incidence of squamous cell carcinoma in women. This most likely results from an increase in the number of women who smoke and the fact that women outnumber men in older age groups.

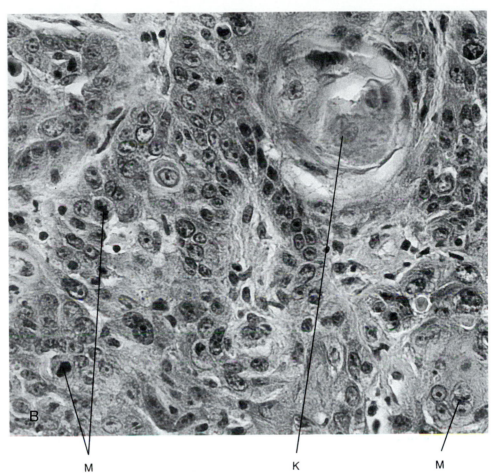

B

M   K   M

■ *f* **i g u r e 5–7**   *Continued B,* High-power photomicrograph showing atypical mitotic figures (M) and abnormal keratinization (K).

Risk Factors. Several risk factors have been associated with the development of squamous cell carcinoma. The most significant is tobacco—including cigar, pipe, and cigarette smoking, snuff dipping, and tobacco chewing. Alcohol consumption appears to add to the risk of oral squamous cell carcinoma. It has been suggested that chronic irritation is related to the development of oral cancer. However, there is no evidence that it is an initiating factor.

Treatment and Prognosis. Squamous cell carcinoma is generally treated by surgical excision. Radiation therapy or chemotherapy may be used in combination with surgery, depending on the location, size of the tumor, and presence of metastases. Occasionally, radiation therapy is used alone. The prognosis is related to the size and location of the tumor and the presence or absence of metastases. The smaller the tumor at the time of treatment, the better the prognosis (Color Plate 50). Therefore, it is important to identify early lesions while they are small and to remove potentially premalignant lesions.

Patients who have undergone irradiation for malignant tumors of the head and neck can experience severe xerostomia (dry mouth) from the destruction of salivary gland tissue by radiation. These patients require preventive dental care, including nutritional counseling, topical fluoride application, and meticulous home care.

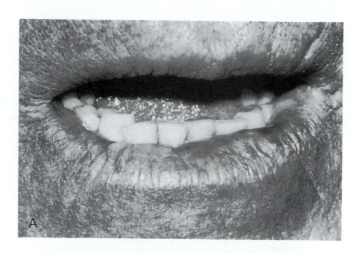

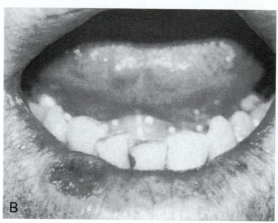

■ *f* i g u r e 5–8

A, Clinical appearance of solar cheilitis. *B,* Clinical appearance of squamous
cell carcinoma of the lower lip. (From
Regezi JA, Sciubba JJ: Oral Pathology:
Clinical-Pathologic Correlations. Philadelphia, WB Saunders, 1989, pp 73
and 94.)

Verrucous Carcinoma

Verrucous carcinoma is a form of squamous cell carcinoma that is separated
from other squamous cell carcinomas because it has a much better prognosis (Color
Plate 8). Clinically, it appears as a slow-growing exophytic tumor with a pebbly white
and red surface (Fig. 5–9). Histologically, the tumor shows many papillary epithelial
proliferations. The spaces between these papillary projections are filled with keratin.
The epithelium is well differentiated, does not contain atypical cells, and exhibits
broad-based rete pegs that penetrate deeply into the connective tissue. The epithelial
basement membrane is intact, and the tumor does not show invasion of tumor cells
through the basement membrane, as is seen in squamous cell carcinomas.

Treatment. Verrucous carcinoma is treated by surgical excision. Although it is a
carcinoma, it usually does not metastasize, and therefore the prognosis is better for
verrucous carcinoma than for squamous cell carcinoma. If it is not treated, it can cause
extensive local damage. Close long-term follow-up is necessary for patients with this
condition.

Basal Cell Carcinoma

Basal cell carcinoma is a malignant skin tumor composed of basal cells derived
from squamous epithelium. The development of basal cell carcinoma is associated with
sun exposure. Since it occurs frequently on the skin of the face, it is important that the
dental hygienist be familiar with this lesion. The basal cell carcinoma appears clinically

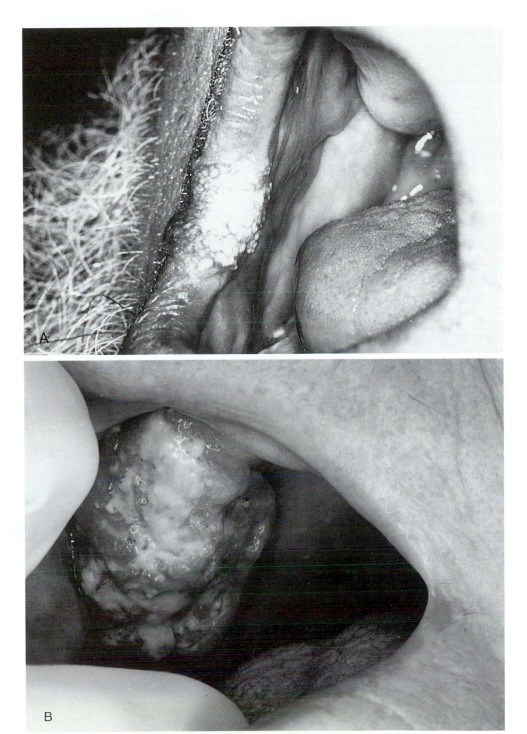

■ *f* i g u r e 5–9   *A,* Clinical appearance of a verrucous carcinoma occurring on the commissure and anterior buccal mucosa. *B,* Maxillary alveolar ridge.

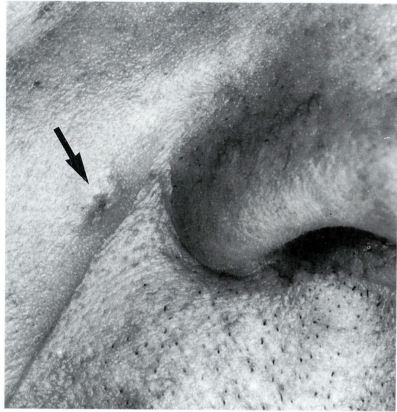

■ *figure 5-10*   Clinical appearance of a basal cell carcinoma illustrating the characteristic "rolled" borders.

as a nonhealing ulcer of the skin with characteristic rolled borders (Fig. 5-10). Basal cell carcinoma does not occur in the oral cavity. Histologically, there is a proliferation of basal epithelial cells. Broad rete pegs penetrate deeply into the connective tissue. The basal cell carcinoma is generally a locally invasive tumor that can become large and disfiguring if not removed. Only rarely does the basal cell carcinoma metastasize. Patients often believe that the ulcer is healing because of the rolled borders. They should be referred to a dermatologist, or a biopsy should be considered for any ulcer of the skin or lips that does not heal within 10 days.

SALIVARY GLAND TUMORS

Benign and malignant tumors of both the major and minor salivary glands occur in the oral region. Tumors can occur within the parotid, submandibular, or sublingual glands, or they can involve any of the minor salivary glands located in the oral cavity. Intraorally, minor salivary gland tumors are most commonly located at the junction of the hard and soft palates. They can also occur on the labial and buccal mucosa, the retromolar area, the floor of the mouth, and, rarely, the tongue (Fig. 5-11). Tumors of minor salivary glands are much more common in the upper lip than in the lower lip.
Since the source of these tumors is glandular epithelium, benign tumors of salivary gland origin are called **adenomas.** Although some of the malignant tumors of salivary gland epithelium are called **adenocarcinomas,** most have more specific names such as **adenoid cystic carcinoma** and **mucoepidermoid carcinoma.** All salivary gland tumors

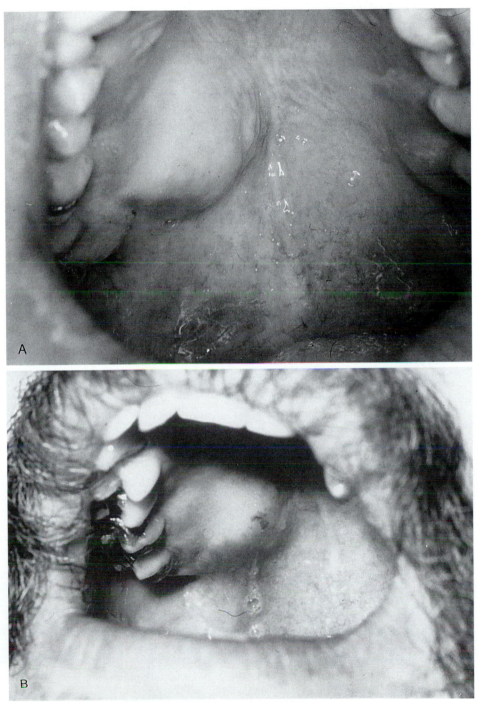

f i g u r e 5–11   *A,* Benign salivary gland tumor of the palate (pleomorphic adenoma). *B,*
Malignant salivary gland tumor of the palate (adenoid cystic carcinoma).
Illustration continued on following page

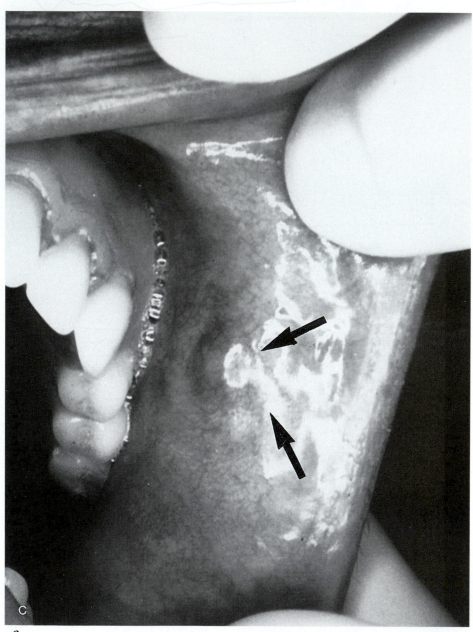

■ *f i g u r e* **5–11**   *Continued C*, Benign salivary gland tumor of the upper lip (monomorphic adenoma).

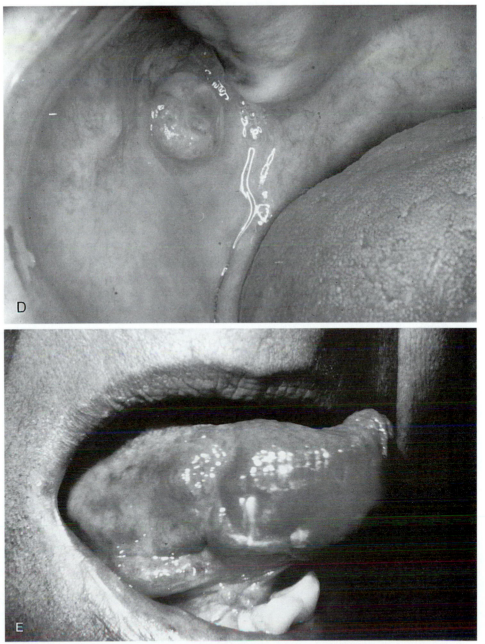

■ *f i g u r e* 5–11   *Continued D,* Malignant salivary gland tumor of the buccal mucosa (mucoepidermoid carcinoma). *E,* Malignant salivary gland tumor of the
tongue (adenoid cystic carcinoma).

are diagnosed on the basis of their histologic appearance, and therefore biopsy and histologic examinations of the tissue are required. Benign tumors tend to grow more slowly than malignant ones.

Pleomorphic Adenoma (Benign Mixed Tumor)

The **pleomorphic adenoma** is a benign salivary gland tumor. It is the most common salivary gland neoplasm and accounts for about 90% of all benign salivary gland tumors. Histologically, it is an encapsulated tumor composed of tissue that appears to be a mixture of both epithelium and connective tissue (Fig. 5–12). For this reason, the tumor is often called the **benign mixed tumor.** The connective tissue–like part can vary from loose and dense fibrous connective tissue to cartilage. The tissue that looks like connective tissue is derived from a salivary gland cell called the **myoepithelial cell.**

The most common extraoral location for the pleomorphic adenoma is the parotid gland. The most common intraoral site is the palate. However, these tumors can occur wherever salivary gland tissue is present. Clinically, the pleomorphic adenoma appears as a slowly enlarging, nonulcerated, painless, dome-shaped mass (see Fig. 5–11A,B; Color Plates 16 and 69). The surface can be ulcerated if traumatized. Its size can range from a few millimeters to several centimeters. Most individuals in whom pleomorphic adenomas develop are older than 40 years of age, but these tumors have also been reported in children.

Treatment and Prognosis. The pleomorphic adenoma is treated by surgical removal. The extent of the surgery depends on the location of the tumor. Parotid gland tumors are treated by removing the part of the parotid gland containing the tumor (partial parotidectomy), whereas minor salivary gland tumors are treated by more conservative surgical excision. The pleomorphic adenoma grows by extension of projections of tumor into the surrounding tissue, and therefore some tumors are difficult to remove completely. Recurrence rates vary and are related to the adequacy of the initial surgical removal. Pleomorphic adenomas have been known to undergo malignant transformation, and this occurrence is called **carcinoma arising in pleomorphic adenoma.**

Monomorphic Adenoma

Monomorphic adenomas are benign encapsulated salivary gland tumors that are much rarer than pleomorphic adenomas. They are composed of a uniform pattern of epithelial cells (Fig. 5–13). These tumors do not have the connective tissue–like component seen in pleomorphic adenomas. They occur most commonly in adults in the upper lip, though they can occur wherever salivary gland tissue is found (see Fig. 5–11C).

Treatment. Monomorphic adenomas are treated by surgical excision. Recurrence is rare.

Papillary Cystadenoma Lymphomatosum (Warthin's Tumor, Adenolymphoma)

The **papillary cystadenoma lymphomatosum** is a unique type of monomorphic adenoma. It is also called **Warthin's tumor.** Histologically, it is an encapsulated tumor in which two types of tissue are seen: epithelial and lymphoid (Fig. 5–14). The epithelial component is the neoplastic component. The epithelial component lines cystic structures. The epithelial-lined cystic structures are surrounded by sheets of lymphocytes.

f i g u r e 5–12   Microscopic appearance of a pleomorphic adenoma. *A*, Low power photo-micrograph shows capsule. *B*, High-power photomicrograph shows mixture of epithelium (E) and connective tissue (CT).

CAPSULE

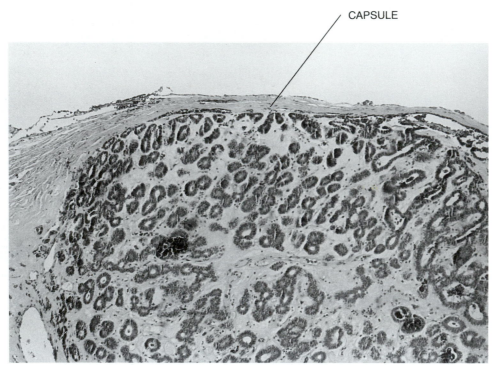

▪ *f i g u r e* **5-13**   Microscopic appearance (low power) of a monomorphic adenoma showing capsule and uniform pattern of epithelial cells.

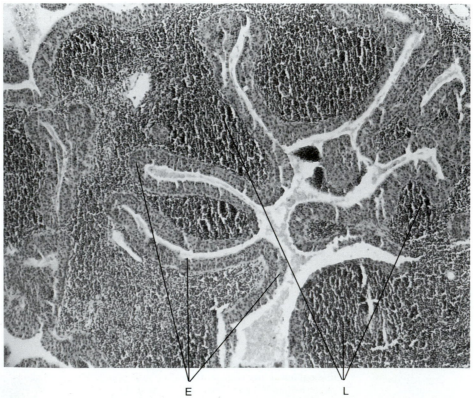

E   L

▪ *f i g u r e* **5-14**   Microscopic appearance of a papillary cystadenoma lymphomatosum (Warthin's tumor) showing space lined by epithelium (E) surrounded by lymphocytes (L).

The lymphoid component is usually derived from pre-existing lymph nodes in which the epithelial component has proliferated. The tumor presents as a painless, soft, compressible or fluctuant mass, usually in the parotid gland and very rarely in the oral cavity. It often develops bilaterally and occurs predominantly in adult men.

This tumor has also been called an **adenolymphoma**. This name is confusing because it is a benign tumor and is in no way related to the malignant tumor of lymphoid tissue—the lymphoma.

Treatment and Prognosis. This tumor is treated by surgical excision and generally does not recur.

Adenoid Cystic Carcinoma (Cylindroma)

Adenoid cystic carcinoma is a malignant tumor of salivary gland origin that can originate from either major or minor salivary gland tissue. It is unencapsulated and infiltrates surrounding tissue. This tumor is composed of small, deeply staining, uniform epithelial cells arranged in perforated round to oval islands. The microscopic appearance of adenoid cystic carcinoma has been likened to that of Swiss cheese (Fig. 5–15). These round and oval islands represent cylinders of tumor, and therefore this tumor has also been called a **cylindroma**. Although it is malignant, pleomorphic cells and mitotic figures are rarely seen. Malignancy is recognized on the basis of the unique histologic features. The adenoid cystic carcinoma is a slow-growing malignant tumor. It may be many years before metastasis occurs.

The most common extraoral site for these tumors is the parotid gland. The most common intraoral site is the palate. Most tumors appear as slowly growing masses that can exhibit surface ulceration (see Fig. 5–11B,E). Pain is often present because of the tendency of these tumors to surround nerves. Adenoid cystic carcinoma is more

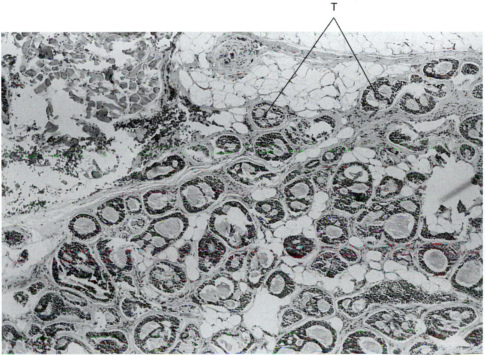

■ *figure* **5–15**   Microscopic appearance of an adenoid cystic carcinoma showing perforated islands of uniform cells. Tumor (T) is seen infiltrating adjacent adipose tissue.

common in women than in men and is a tumor of adults, the majority occurring in the fifth and sixth decades of life.

Treatment and Prognosis. The treatment of choice for adenoid cystic carcinoma is complete surgical excision. Radiation treatment has been attempted and has been shown to be of benefit in some cases. However, recurrence and persistent local invasion are common. About 30% of patients experience cervical lymph node involvement. Distant metastases, most often involving the lungs, can occur after many years. In these cases the prognosis is poor.

Mucoepidermoid Carcinoma

Mucoepidermoid carcinoma is a malignant salivary gland tumor. It is an unencapsulated infiltrating tumor composed of a combination of mucous cells and squamous-like epithelial cells called **epidermoid cells** (Fig. 5–16).

The parotid gland is the most likely site for mucoepidermoid carcinomas of the major glands, whereas minor gland tumors are most common on the palate. They appear clinically as slowly enlarging masses (see Fig. 5–11D). Occasionally, mucoepidermoid tumors occur centrally within bone, usually in the mandibular premolar and molar region. They appear either as unilocular or multilocular radiolucencies on x-ray film (Fig. 5–16B). Central mucoepidermoid carcinomas are probably derived either from salivary gland tissue trapped within bone or from the transformed epithelial lining of a dentigerous cyst (a developmental odontogenic cyst that forms around the crown of an unerupted or impacted tooth; see Chapter 4).

Mucoepidermoid carcinoma affects a wide age range of individuals. Although it usually occurs in adults after middle age, this tumor is the most common malignant salivary gland tumor in children.

Treatment and Prognosis. Treatment of the mucoepidermoid carcinoma consists of complete surgical excision, with close long-term follow-up for signs of recurrence and metastasis. The behavior of any one tumor is difficult to predict and is related to the histologic appearance of the tumor. For low-grade tumors, 92% of patients survive

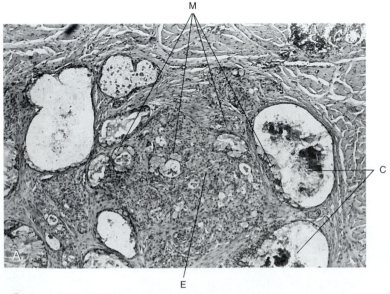

f i g u r e 5–16   *A*, Microscopic appearance (low power) of a mucoepidermoid carcinoma showing cystic structures (C), mucous cells (M), and epidermoid cells (E).
Illustration continued on opposite page

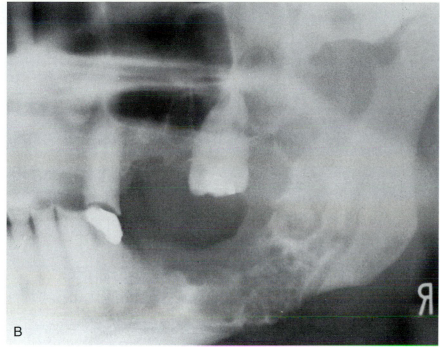

B

f i g u r e **5-16**   *B,* Radiograph of a central mucoepidermoid carcinoma showing a multilocular radiolucency.

5 years after the initial treatment. For high-grade (more malignant) tumors, only 49% survive 5 years after the initial treatment.

Other Malignant Salivary Gland Tumors

In addition to the adenoid cystic carcinoma and the mucoepidermoid carcinoma, there are several other malignant salivary gland tumors, including polymorphous low-grade adenocarinoma (lobular carcinoma, terminal duct carcinoma), acinic cell adeno-carcinoma, and other adenocarcinomas.

ODONTOGENIC TUMORS

Odontogenic tumors are derived from tooth-forming tissues. Tooth formation results from an interaction between odontogenic epithelium and mesenchymal tissue. Some odontogenic tumors are composed of epithelium only, some are composed of mesenchymal tissue only, and others are a mixture of both elements. Most odontogenic tumors are benign. Malignant odontogenic tumors occur but are rare. Table 5–3 presents a classification of odontogenic tumors according to the type of tissue they contain.

In addition to the odontogenic tumors described in this text, there are other, rarer odontogenic tumors such as the squamous odontogenic tumor and the central odontogenic fibroma. (See the references at the end of this chapter for more detailed information on these tumors.)

TABLE 5–3 Classification of Odontogenic Tumors

Epithelial Odontogenic Tumors	Mesenchymal Odontogenic Tumors	Mixed Odontogenic Tumors
Ameloblastoma	Myxoma	Ameloblastic fibroma
Calcifying epithelial odontogenic tumor (CEOT)	Cementifying fibroma	Adenomatoid odontogenic tumor (AOT or OAT)
Squamous odontogenic tumor*	Odontogenic fibroma*	Odontoma
Clear cell odontogenic tumor*	Peripheral odontogenic (ossifying) fibroma	
	Cementoblastoma	

Description not included in this text.

Epithelial Odontogenic Tumors

Ameloblastoma

The **ameloblastoma** is a benign, slow-growing but locally aggressive epithelial odontogenic tumor that occurs in both the maxilla and the mandible. It is an unencapsulated tumor that infiltrates into surrounding tissue and can cause extensive destruction. When it occurs in the maxilla, death can result from direct extension into vital structures. It is composed of ameloblast-like epithelial cells that surround areas resembling stellate reticulum. These cells are arranged in either dental follicle–like islands or interconnecting strands (Fig. 5–17). An ameloblastoma can also exhibit other, less common histologic patterns.

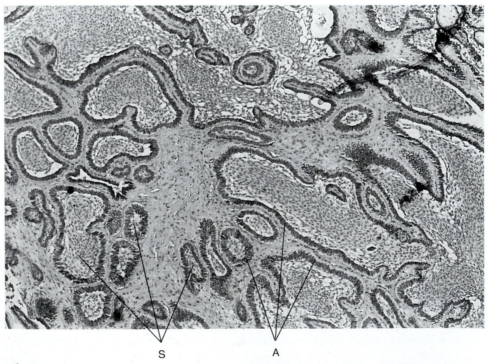

▪ *figure 5–17*   Microscopic appearance (low power) of a follicular ameloblastoma showing dental follicle-like islands composed of epithelial cells consisting of peripheral ameloblast-like cells (A) and stellate reticulum-like areas (S).

The classic radiographic appearance of an ameloblastoma is a multilocular soap-bubble–like or honeycombed radiolucency (Fig. 5–18). In smaller tumors, the radiolucency may be unilocular. An ameloblastoma can arise anywhere in the jaws and can occur in association with a dentigerous cyst (Fig. 5–19). However, 80% of ameloblastomas arise in the mandible, and most mandibular ameloblastomas occur in the molar-ramus area. The molar area is the most common location when they occur in the

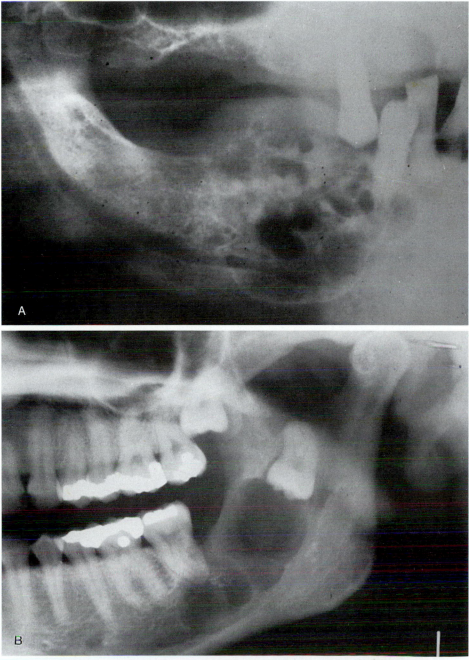

figure 5–18 *A*, Radiograph of ameloblastoma showing multilocular radiolucencies in the molar area of the mandible. *B*, Radiograph of ameloblastoma showing multilocular radiolucencies in the molar area of the mandible.

Illustration continued on following page

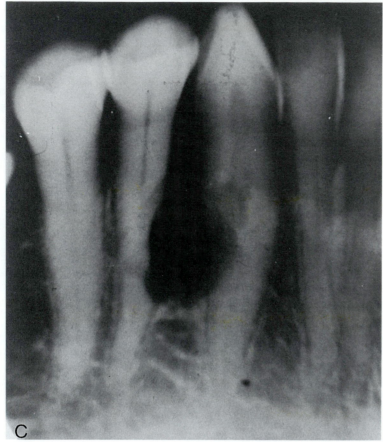

▪ *f* **i g u r e 5–18**   *Continued C*, Radiograph of an ameloblastoma showing a small but multilocular radiolucency in the man-
dibular cuspid-bicuspid region.

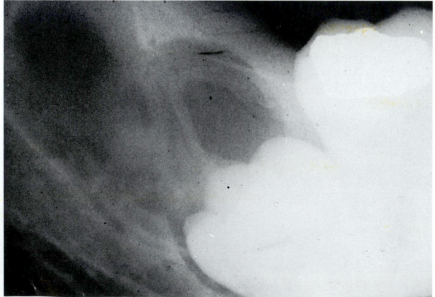

▪ *f* **i g u r e 5–19**   Radiograph of an ameloblastoma that formed in association with
an impacted tooth and dentigerous cyst.

maxilla as well. The tumor may cause expansion of bone. The usual initial presentation is a slowly developing, asymptomatic swelling of the affected bone. The age range of individuals affected is broad, but most ameloblastomas occur in adults.

Treatment and Prognosis. Ameloblastomas are treated by complete surgical removal. Recurrence is common. Occasionally, these tumors occur in the gingiva and do not involve bone, in which case they are called **peripheral ameloblastomas.** These are also treated by surgical excision and differ from the central ameloblastomas in that they generally do not recur.

Calcifying Epithelial Odontogenic Tumor

The **calcifying epithelial odontogenic tumor (CEOT),** also known as a **Pindborg tumor,** is a benign epithelial odontogenic tumor that occurs much less frequently than the ameloblastoma (Fig. 5–20). It is a unique odontogenic tumor because the proliferating cells do not resemble odontogenic epithelium. The tumor is composed of islands and sheets of polyhedral (multisided) epithelial cells. Deposits that look like amyloid are seen in the tumor, and calcifications are seen within these deposits. The amyloid-like material is thought to be a form of abnormal enamel protein. Radiographically, the CEOT is a unilocular or multilocular radiolucency. Calcifications that form within the tumor appear as radiopacities within the radiolucency (Fig. 5–20B).

The majority of patients affected with this tumor are adults. However, the CEOT affects a broad age range, which extends from young adults to elderly individuals. Reports of this tumor occurring in the mandible are twice as common as reports of those occurring in the maxilla, and though it can occur anywhere in the maxilla or mandible, the bicuspid-molar area is the most common location. Many CEOTs are associated with impacted teeth.

Treatment and Prognosis. Treatment of the CEOT depends on the size and location of the tumor and involves complete surgical excision. Recurrence has been reported, but the recurrence rate is lower than that for ameloblastoma.

Mesenchymal Odontogenic Tumors

Odontogenic Myxoma

The **odontogenic myxoma** is a benign nonencapsulated infiltrating tumor composed of a pale-staining mucopolysaccharide substance that contains dispersed cells that have long processes (Fig. 5–21A). This tissue closely resembles tissue seen in the dental papilla, the mesenchymal component of tooth-forming tissue.

The odontogenic myxoma most often occurs in young people between 10 and 29 years of age.

The classic radiographic appearance of a myxoma is a multilocular, honeycombed radiolucency with poorly defined margins (Fig. 5–21B). The tumor may be extensive and can cause tooth displacement. It can occur anywhere in the maxilla or mandible.

Treatment and Prognosis. Myxomas are treated by complete removal of the tumor. The extent of the surgery depends on the size of the tumor. The recurrence rate is 25%. When they recur, most myxomas recur within the first 2 years after treatment.

Cementifying and Ossifying Fibromas

The **cementifying fibroma** is a benign well-circumscribed tumor composed of fibrous connective tissue and rounded or globular calcifications resembling cementum

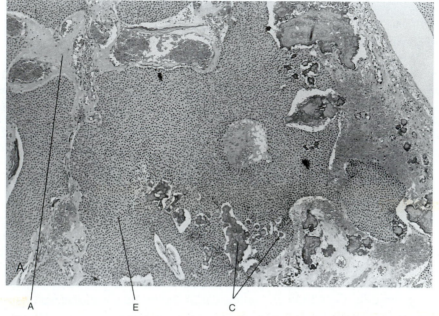

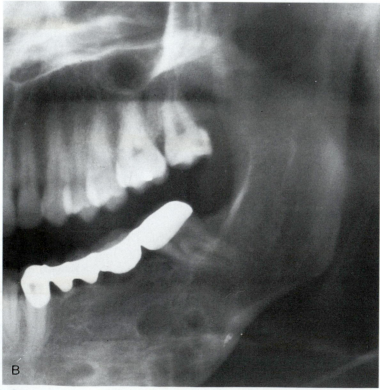

ƒigure 5–20   Calcifying epithelial odontogenic tumor. *A*, Microscopic appearance (low power) of a calcifying epithelial odontogenic tumor showing sheets of epithelial cells (E), amorphous material (A), and calcifications (C).

ƒigure 5–20   *Continued B*, Radiograph of a calcifying epithelial odontogenic tumor showing a multilocular radiolucency.

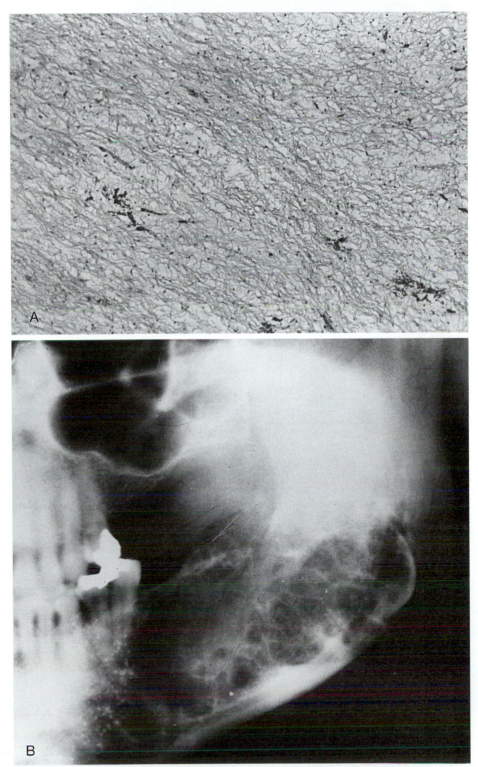

■ *f i g u r e* **5–21** *A,* Photomicrograph of a myxoma showing background substance containing widely dispersed cells with long processes. *B,* Radiograph of a myxoma showing a multilocular, honeycombed radiolucency.

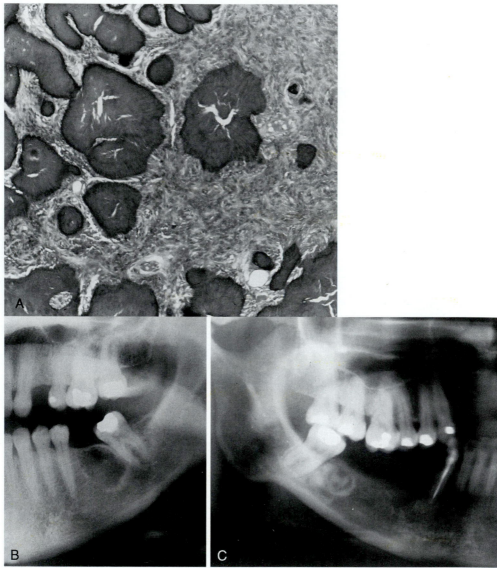

■ *f* i g u r e 5-22   *A,* Photomicrograph of a cementifying fibroma showing rounded, globular calcifications and cellular fibrous connective tissue. *B,* Radiograph of a cementifying fibroma showing a well-circumscribed radiolucent lesions. *C,* Radiograph
of a cementifying fibroma showing a radiolucent-radiopaque lesion.

(Fig. 5–22*A*). Because histologically it is composed of fibrous connective tissue and
calcifications, it is one of the lesions classified as a fibro-osseous lesion. The cementifying fibroma and ossifying fibroma are variants of the same tumor. In the **ossifying
fibroma,** the calcifications more closely resemble bone trabeculae. Some tumors have
both globular calcifications resembling cementum and bone trabeculae. These are
called **cemento-ossifying fibromas.** The variation in the appearance of these tumors
results from the potential of periodontal ligament cells to produce either cementum or
bone. The tumor usually occurs in adults. Radiographically, it is well defined and varies
from radiolucent to radiopaque, depending on the amount of calcified tissue present
(Fig. 5–22*B,C*).

Other fibro-osseous lesions, such as periapical cemental dysplasia (discussed later in this chapter) and fibrous dysplasia (discussed in Chapter 7), may be histologically identical to the cementifying and ossifying fibroma. The radiographic appearance of these lesions is important in distinguishing them from each other.

Treatment and Prognosis. Cementifying and ossifying fibromas surgical excision. They separate easily from the surrounding bone. They generally do not recur.

Benign Cementoblastoma

The benign cementoblastoma is a cementum-producing lesion that is fused to the root of the tooth. The radiographic appearance of this lesion is distinctive (Fig. 5–23). It consists of a well-defined radiopaque mass that is in continuity with the root or roots of the affected tooth and obliterates the apex of the tooth. The mass is surrounded by a radiolucent halo.

The tumor usually occurs in young adults. It is commonly associated with a mandibular molar or premolar. Unlike in other odontogenic tumors, pain is a frequent symptom of the cementoblastoma.

Treatment and Prognosis. Treatment of the cementoblastoma consists of enucleation of the tumor and removal of the involved tooth. It does not recur.

Periapical Cemental Dysplasia

Periapical cemental dysplasia is a relatively common condition of unknown cause that affects periapical bone (Fig. 5–24). The term cementoma is often used for this condition. However, it is not a neoplasm. It is included in this section to differentiate it clearly from the cementoblastoma, a true odontogenic tumor. In this lesion, the term dysplasia refers to the disordered production of cementum and bone, and unlike epithelial dysplasia, it is not a premalignant condition. The diagnosis of periapical cemental dysplasia is usually made on the basis of the characteristic radiographic and clinical features. The lesion is asymptomatic and is discovered on routine radiographic examination. It occurs most commonly in the anterior mandible of patients older than 30 years of age. It is more common in women than in men, and many studies have shown a predominance in black women. Early lesions are well circumscribed and radiolucent and can mimic periapical disease. The teeth in the area are vital unless they have been affected coincidentally by caries or trauma. The lesions become increasingly calcified with time, and therefore older lesions become increasingly radiopaque. Histologically, periapical cemental dysplasia is a fibro-osseous lesion. Like other fibro-osseous lesions, it is composed of both fibrous tissue and calcifications. The calcifications in this lesion may resemble bone, cementum, or both. Early lesions consist of mostly fibrous tissue, whereas the tissue of older lesions is mostly calcified.

Treatment. Once the condition is recognized, no treatment is necessary. The lesion remains asymptomatic and localized. A biopsy may be necessary for lesions that do not present with the characteristic radiographic features. Follow-up of patients with early lesions may be necessary to ensure that the diagnosis is correct.

Florid Osseous Dysplasia

Florid osseous dysplasia, another fibro-osseous lesion, is also a condition of disordered cementum and bone development. The condition usually involves multiple quadrants. Dense, sclerotic masses of bone or cementum, or both, appear as large

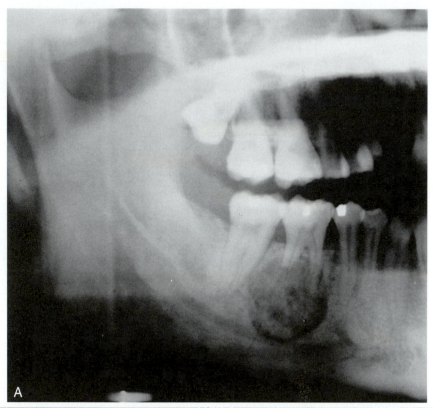

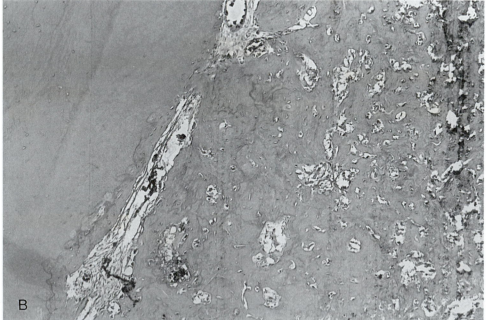

▪ *f* i g u r e 5–23   *A*, Radiograph of a benign cementoblastoma showing a well-circumscribed radiopaque mass surrounded by a radiolucent halo and attached to the roots of a mandibular first molar. *B*, Microscopic appearance (high power) of a cementoblastoma showing the tumor attached to a tooth root.

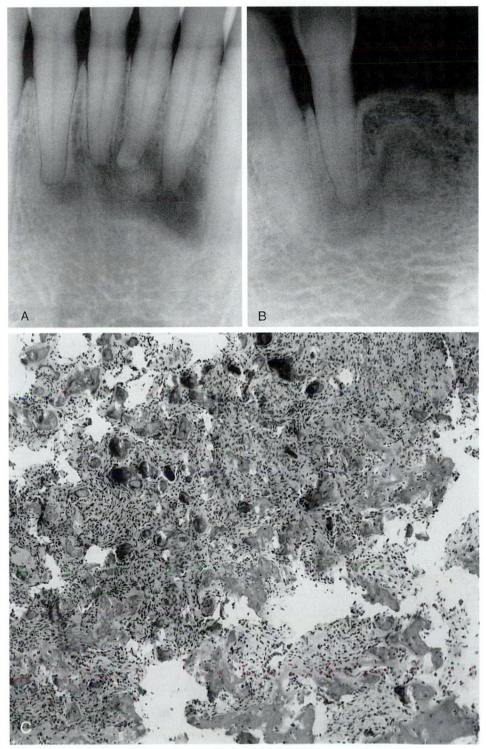

f i g u r e 5–24   *A* and *B*, Radiographs of periapical cemental dysplasia, *C*, Microscopic appearance of periapical cemental dysplasia showing a combination of cellular fibrous tissue and calcified tissue.

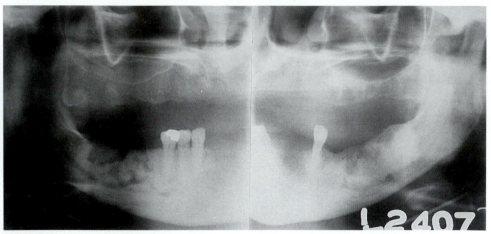

■ *f i g u r e* **5–25**   Florid osseous dysplasia. Irregular radiopaque masses are seen in both the left and the right mandible.

radiopaque areas (Fig. 5–25). Radiographically, it differs from periapical cemental dysplasia in the extent of the involvement of the maxilla and mandible. In addition, the early radiolucent phase, which precedes the radiopacities in periapical cemental dysplasia, is generally not identified. Florid osseous dysplasia occurs most often in black women older than 40 years of age. Its cause is not known.

The diagnosis of florid osseous dysplasia can usually be made on the basis of the characteristic radiographic appearance.

Treatment. No treatment is indicated. The most common complication of florid osseous dysplasia is the development of osteomyelitis in patients who wear full or partial dentures. The dense sclerotic bone resorbs unevenly and often perforates the mucosa, allowing saliva and bacteria to enter the bone.

*potential fa
Then might have
TO Treat.*

Mixed Odontogenic Tumors

Ameloblastic Fibroma

mesenchymal + epith.

The ameloblastic fibroma is a benign, nonencapsulated odontogenic tumor composed of both strands and small islands of odontogenic epithelium and tissue that resembles the dental papilla (Fig. 5–26). The ameloblastic fibroma occurs in young children as well as in adults. However, most occur in individuals less than 20 years of age. The most common location is the mandibular bicuspid-molar region.

Radiographically, the ameloblastic fibroma appears as either a well-defined or a poorly defined unilocular or multilocular radiolucency.

Treatment and Prognosis. Ameloblastic fibroma is treated by surgical removal of the tumor. The recurrence rate is low.

Adenomatoid Odontogenic Tumor

The **adenomatoid odontogenic tumor (AOT)**, also known as **odontogenic adenomatoid tumor (OAT)**, is an encapsulated, benign epithelial odontogenic tumor that has a distinctive age, sex, and site distribution. It also differs from other epithelial odontogenic tumors in that it does not recur. The tumor is surrounded by a dense, fibrous connective tissue capsule and consists of duct-like structures, whorls, and large

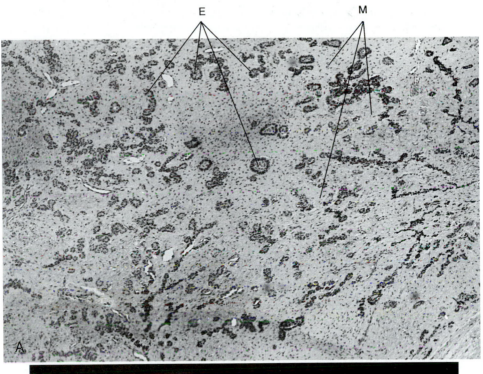

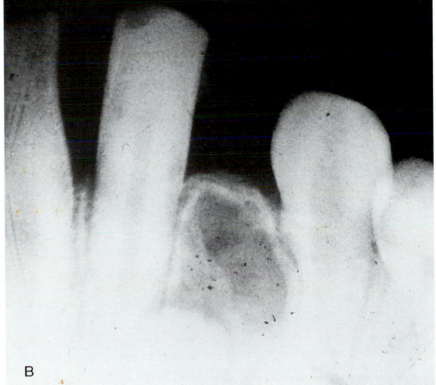

■ *f* i g u r e 5–26   *A,* Microscopic appearance of an ameloblastic fibroma showing a combination of odontogenic epithelium (E) and mesenchymal tissue (M). *B,* Radiograph of an ameloblastic fibroma showing a poorly defined multilocular radiolucency.

masses of cuboidal and spindle-shaped epithelial cells (Fig. 5–27A). The duct-like structures are one of the distinctive features of this tumor and are the reason for the name **adenomatoid,** or gland-like. These structures are not ducts but actually ameloblast-like cells that resemble ducts because of their circular arrangement. Eosinophilic

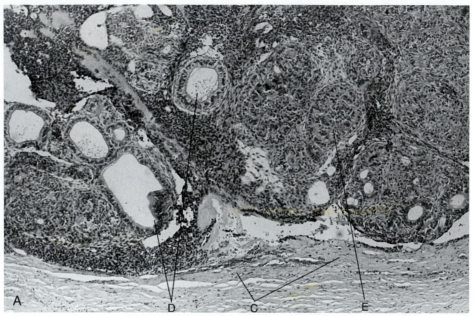

■ *f* i g u r e 5–27   Adenomatoid odontogenic tumor. *A,* Microscopic appearance of an adenomatoid odontogenic tumor showing the capsule (C), epithelial cells (E), and duct-like structures (D).

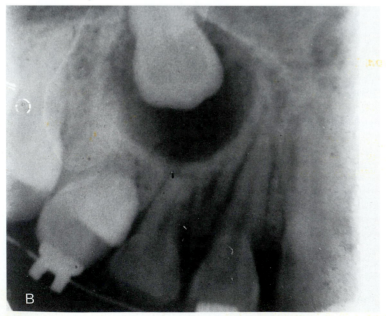

■ *f* i g u r e 5–27   *Continued B,* Radiograph of an adenomatoid odontogenic tumor showing unilocular radiolucency surrounding the crown of an unerupted maxillary cuspid.

material is seen in the centers of these structures, and calcifications also form in this tumor.

Approximately 70% of AOTs occur in females less than 20 years of age, and 70% involve the anterior part of the jaws. The maxilla is more commonly involved than the mandible. Many AOTs are associated with impacted teeth. There may be a swelling in the area of the tumor. Most AOTs are asymptomatic and are discovered on routine radiographic examination.

Radiographically, the AOT appears as a well-circumscribed radiolucency (Fig. 5–27*B*). Because of the frequent association with an impacted tooth, an AOT often simulates a dentigerous cyst. However, unlike the dentigerous cyst (see Chapter 4), the AOT extends beyond the cementoenamel junction and can involve 50% to 60% of the root. As calcifications form within the tumor, radiopaque areas of varying size are visible on the radiograph.

Treatment and Prognosis. The AOT can be treated very conservatively by a process called enucleation, in which the tumor is removed in its entirety. The tumor is easily separated from the surrounding bone, and recurrence is rare.

and tooth + replace w/ prost.

Calcifying Odontogenic Cyst

The **calcifying odontogenic cyst** is usually a nonaggressive cystic lesion lined by odontogenic epithelium with associated ghost cell keratinization. The epithelium resembles that seen in an ameloblastoma, consisting of ameloblast-like cells and stellate reticulum–like areas. Ghost cells are round structures with clear centers (Fig 5–28*A*). The calcifying odontogenic cyst is usually a radiographically well-defined lesion that can present as either a unilocular or a multilocular radiolucency (Fig 5–28*B*). Calcifications can occur and are seen as radiopaque areas. The calcifying odontogenic cyst affects a broad range of ages and is most commonly seen in individuals younger than 40 years of age. It is treated by conservative surgical enucleation and generally does not recur. Occasionally, this lesion exhibits aggressive behavior, and a solid variant has been reported. It has been suggested that it is a neoplasm rather than a cyst.

Odontoma

Board —

The odontoma is an odontogenic tumor composed of mature enamel, dentin, cementum, and dental pulp. The odontoma is the most common of the odontogenic tumors. There are two types of odontomas: compound and complex. A compound odontoma consists of a collection of numerous small teeth (Fig. 5–29). A complex odontoma consists of a mass of enamel, dentin, cementum, and pulp that does not resemble a normal tooth (Fig. 5–30).

Most odontomas are detected in adolescents and young adults. The compound odontoma is usually located in the anterior maxilla, and the complex odontoma most commonly occurs in the posterior mandible. The most common clinical manifestation of an odontoma is the failure of a permanent tooth to erupt. Most odontomas are small, but large lesions can cause swelling and displacement of erupted teeth. Odontomas can be associated with impacted or unerupted teeth as well as with odontogenic cysts and tumors.

Radiographically, compound odontomas appear as a cluster of numerous miniature teeth surrounded by a radiolucent halo (see Fig. 5–29). A complex odontoma appears as a radiopaque mass surrounded by a thin radiolucent halo (see Fig. 5–30).

Treatment and Prognosis. Treatment of an odontoma consists of surgical excision. Odontomas generally do not recur.

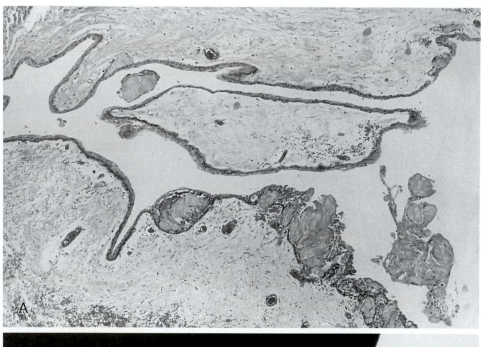

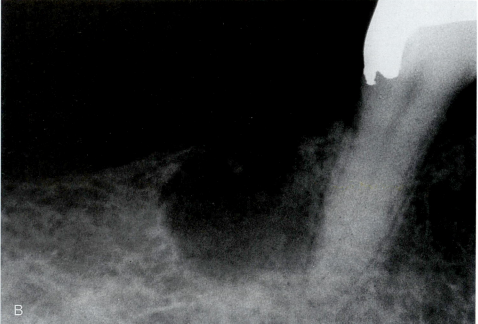

■ *f i g u r e 5-28*   Calcifying odontogenic cyst. *A*, Microscopic appearance of a calcifying odontogenic cyst showing a cystic structure lined by odontogenic epithelium with associated ghost cells. *B*, Radiograph of a calcifying odontogenic cyst showing a unilocular radiolucency of the mandible.

Peripheral Odontogenic Tumors

Peripheral Ossifying Fibroma

The **peripheral ossifying fibroma** is an exophytic lesion that occurs only on the gingiva and is most likely derived from cells of the periodontal ligament (Fig. 5–31*A*).

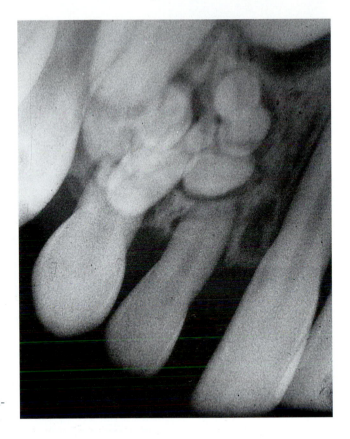

▪ *f* **i g u r e** 5–29

Radiograph of a compound odontoma showing a collection of numerous, small, tooth-like radiopacities surrounded by a radiolucent halo.

It is composed of cellular connective tissue interspersed with scattered bone or cementum-like calcifications (Fig. 5–31*B*). The cementifying fibroma and ossifying fibroma that occur within bone are histologically similar to the peripheral ossifying fibroma.

The peripheral ossifying fibroma usually presents as a well-demarcated sessile or pedunculated lesion that appears to originate from the gingival interdental papilla. It

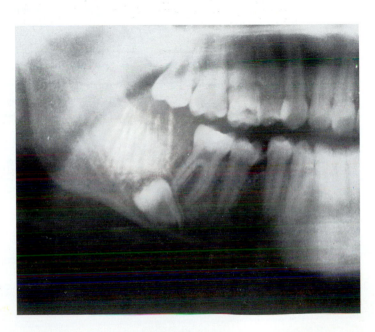

▪ *f* **i g u r e** 5–30

Radiograph of a complex odontoma showing a radiopaque mass surrounded by a radiolucent halo.

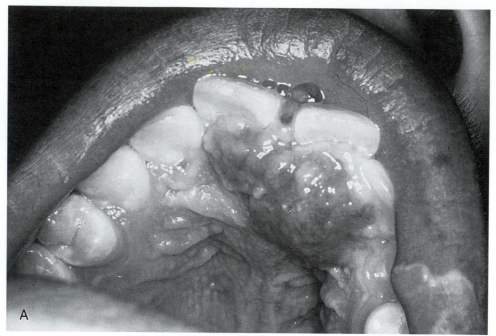

A

■ ƒ i g u r e 5–31   *A*, Clinical appearance of a peripheral odontogenic fibroma showing an exophytic lesion involving the palatal gingiva of the maxillary anterior teeth.

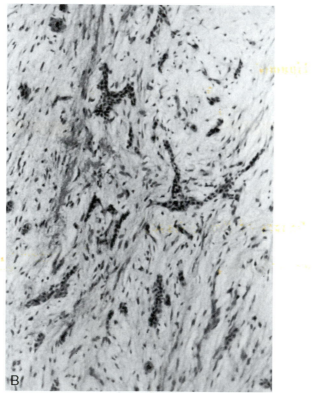

B

■ ƒ i g u r e 5–31   *Continued B*, Photomicrograph of a peripheral odontogenic fibroma. (*B*, From Regezi, JA, Sciubba JJ: Oral Pathology: Clinical-Pathologic Correlations. Philadelphia, WB Saunders, 1989, p 187.)

has been more commonly reported in females than in males and often occurs in young individuals. It has been reported in children as well as in adults.

Treatment and Prognosis. Treatment of the peripheral ossifying fibroma consists of surgical excision with thorough scaling of the adjacent teeth to remove any irritants that can induce regrowth of the lesion. The recurrence rate for peripheral ossifying fibromas is about 16%.

Other Peripheral Odontogenic Tumors

Several other odontogenic tumors have been reported to occur in the gingiva without underlying bone involvement. Although rare, these lesions are of importance to the dental hygienist because of their gingival location. The peripheral ossifying fibroma is the most common of these tumors. The peripheral ameloblastoma has also been mentioned. The calcifying epithelial odontogenic tumor (CEOT) has been reported to occur in the gingiva, as has the peripheral odontogenic fibroma, which is composed of fibrous connective tissue with a proliferation of odontogenic epithelium with or without calcifications.

Treatment and Prognosis. The treatment of each of these tumors is surgical excision. The peripheral ossifying fibroma often recurs. However, the other peripheral odontogenic tumors rarely recur following complete excision.

TUMORS OF SOFT TISSUE

Tumors of soft tissue include benign and malignant tumors of adipose tissue (fat), nerve, muscle, blood, and lymphatic vessels.

Ex Liposarcoma –

Lipoma

The **lipoma** is a benign tumor of mature fat cells (Fig. 5–32). Clinically, it appears as a yellowish mass that is surfaced with thin overlying epithelium. Because of this thin epithelium, a delicate pattern of blood vessels is usually seen on its surface. Histologically, the lipoma is a well-delineated tumor composed of lobules of mature fat cells that are uniform in size and shape.

Treatment and Prognosis. The lipoma is treated by surgical excision and generally does not recur.

Tumors of Nerve Tissue

The **neurofibroma** (Fig. 5–33) and the **schwannoma** are benign tumors derived from nerve tissue. The schwannoma is also called a **neurilemmoma.** Both of these tumors are derived from Schwann cells, which are a component of the connective tissue surrounding a nerve. Although the neurofibroma and schwannoma are histologically distinct tumors, they are quite similar in their clinical presentation and behavior and are therefore discussed together. The tongue is the most common intraoral site for these tumors, which can occur at any age. Whereas microscopic examination of a neurofibroma reveals a fairly well delineated diffuse proliferation of spindle-shaped Schwann cells (Fig. 5–33A), in a schwannoma the spindle-shaped Schwann cells are arranged in palisaded whorls around a central pink zone. The schwannoma is surrounded by a connective tissue capsule.

Treatment and Prognosis. The treatment for benign tumors of nerve is surgical excision. They generally do not recur. Malignant tumors of nerve tissue occur but are extremely rare.

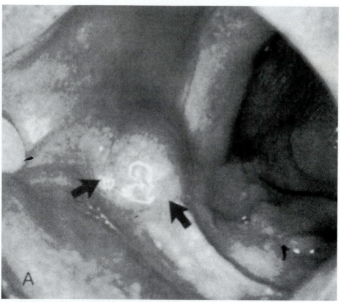

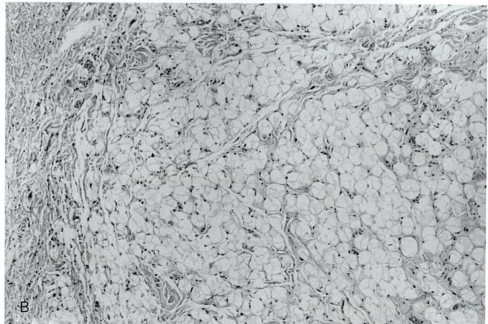

▪ *f i g u r e* 5–32   *A*, Clinical appearance of a lipoma. *B*, Photomicrograph of a lipoma showing mature fat cells. (*B*, From Regezi JA, Sciubba JJ: Oral Pathology: Clinical-Pathologic Correlations. Philadelphia, WB Saunders, 1989, p 222.)

Neurofibromas occur in the **multiple neurofibromatosis syndrome,** also called
von Recklinghausen's disease. Patients with this syndrome have numerous neurofibromas on the skin and other sites in addition to other abnormalities. This syndrome
is genetically inherited and is described in detail in Chapter 6.

Granular Cell Tumor

The **granular cell tumor,** or **granular cell myoblastoma,** is a benign tumor
composed of large cells with granular cytoplasm. It most likely arises from neural or

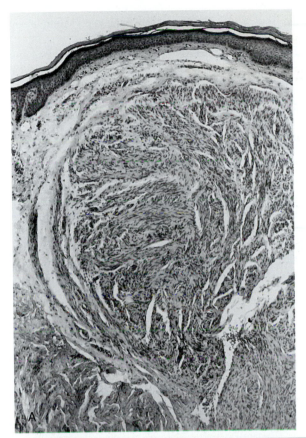

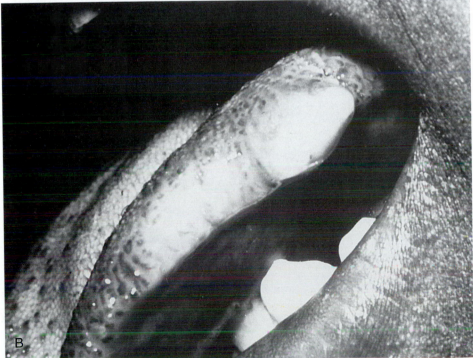

■ *figure* 5–33   *A,* Photomicrograph of a neurofibroma. *B,* Clinical appearance of a neurofibroma showing a nonulcerated mass on the lateral border of the tongue.

primitive mesenchymal cells. The name **myoblastoma** was used when it was thought that these tumors were of muscle origin.

The intraoral granular cell tumor almost always occurs on the tongue and clinically appears as a painless, nonulcerated nodule (Fig. 5–34*A*). Microscopic examination reveals large oval-shaped cells with granular cytoplasm. The granular cells are found in the connective tissue (Fig. 5–34*B*). The overlying surface epithelium exhibits pseudo-

[handwritten margin notes: "— like a nerve", "firm + embedded in tongue"]

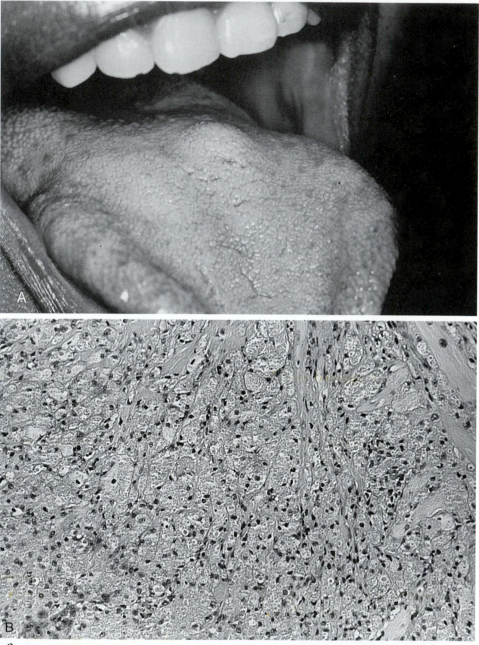

▪ *f i g u r e* **5–34**   *A*, Clinical appearance of a granular cell tumor of the tongue showing a nonulcerated mass. (Courtesy of Dr. Sidney Eisig.) *B*, Cells with granular cytoplasm.

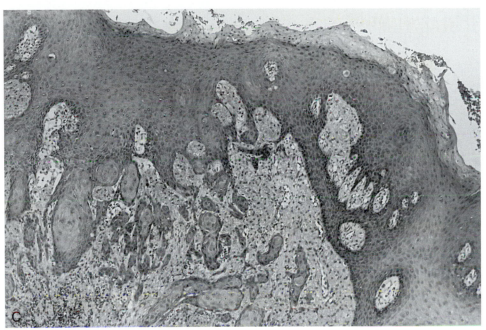

■ *f i g u r e* **5–34**   *Continued C,* Microscopic appearance of a granular cell tumor showing overlying pseudoepitheliomatous hyperplasia.

epitheliomatous hyperplasia, which is a benign proliferation of epithelium into the
connective tissue (Fig. 5–34*C*).

Treatment and Prognosis. This tumor is treated by surgical excision and does
not recur.

Congenital Epulis

The **congenital epulis,** or **gingival granular cell tumor of the newborn,** is
composed of cells that closely resemble those of the granular cell tumor. The cell of
origin is not certain, but it is probably different from that of the granular cell tumor
of adults despite the similarity of the histologic appearance of the granular cells. This
tumor is present at birth as a sessile or pedunculated mass on the gingiva. It usually
occurs on the anterior maxillary gingiva and almost always occurs in girls.

Treatment and Prognosis. The congenital epulis is treated by surgical excision
and does not recur.

TUMORS OF MUSCLE

Tumors of muscle are extremely rare in the oral cavity. The **rhabdomyoma,** a
benign tumor of striated muscle, has been reported to occur on the tongue. Tumors of
smooth muscle, leiomyomas, are even more rare, except for those that occur in
association with blood vessels. These tumors are called vascular leiomyomas and
occasionally occur in the oral cavity. The **rhabdomyosarcoma,** a malignant tumor of
striated muscle, is the most common malignant soft tissue tumor of the head and neck
in children. It presents as a rapidly growing, destructive tumor.

Treatment and Prognosis. The rhabdomyosarcoma is an aggressive, malignant
tumor that is best treated by a combination of multidrug chemotherapy and surgery.
The prognosis, despite treatment, is poor.

VASCULAR TUMORS

Hemangioma

The **hemangioma** is a benign proliferation of capillaries (Fig. 5–35; Color Plates 5 and 26). It is a common vascular lesion considered by many to be a developmental lesion rather than a tumor because hemangiomas do not generally exhibit unlimited growth potential. Some contain numerous small capillaries and are called **capillary hemangiomas.** Others contain larger blood vessels and are called **cavernous hemangiomas.**

Most are present at birth or arise shortly thereafter. More than half the hemangiomas that occur in the body occur in the head and neck area. The tongue is the most common intraoral location for hemangiomas. When they occur in this location, enlargement of the tongue (macroglossia) can result. They are more common in girls than in boys. Hemangiomas also occur in adults and may be caused by an abnormal proliferation of blood vessels during the healing process. They appear as variably sized deep red or blue lesions that frequently blanch when pressure is applied.

Treatment. Many hemangiomas undergo spontaneous remission. Others can enlarge rapidly because of hemorrhage, thrombosis, or inflammation. Treatment is variable and includes surgery or the injection of a sclerosing solution into the lesion, which causes it to resolve.

Lymphangioma

The **lymphangioma** is a benign tumor composed of lymphatic vessels. It is less common than the hemangioma. Most lymphangiomas are present at birth, and half are in the head and neck area. The most common intraoral location is the tongue. These tumors can cause macroglossia. A cystic lymphangioma in the neck is called a **cystic hygroma.** It is usually present at birth or develops shortly thereafter.

Treatment and Prognosis. Lymphangiomas are generally treated by surgical excision and tend to recur.

Malignant Vascular Tumors

Several different types of malignant vascular tumors can occur in the oral cavity, but they are quite rare. **Kaposi's sarcoma** (Color Plates 90 and 91) is a malignant vascular tumor. It usually occurs in multiple sites and is composed of spindle-shaped cells mixed with slit-like spaces containing red blood cells. Classic Kaposi's sarcoma presents as multiple purplish tumors of the lower extremities in elderly men. The condition in these patients progresses slowly, usually resolves with low doses of radiation, and rarely causes death. With the advent of the human immunodeficiency virus (HIV) epidemic in the 1980s, Kaposi's sarcoma has appeared in a much more aggressive form. In HIV-positive patients, these lesions are often seen in the oral cavity. The hard palate and gingiva are the most common intraoral sites. Kaposi's sarcoma also occurs in other patients with immunodeficiency, such as patients receiving drugs to suppress the immune system. Kaposi's sarcoma associated with HIV infection is also described in Chapter 7.

The cause of Kaposi's sarcoma is unknown, but infectious agents have been proposed because of the epidemiology and behavior of the lesions.

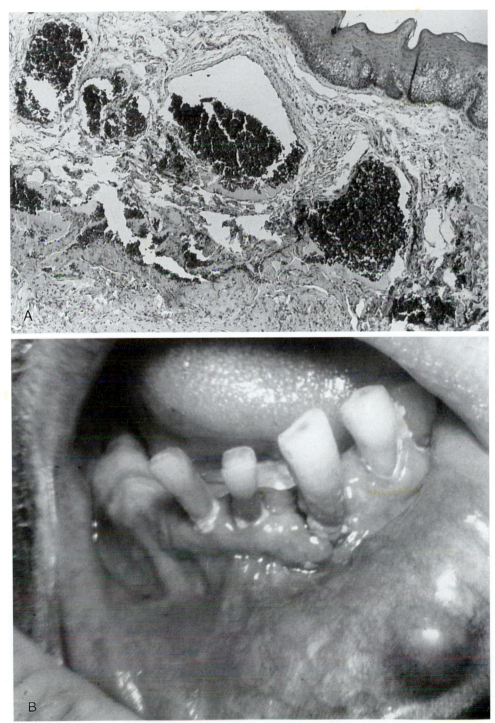

■ *f* **i g u r e 5–35**   *A,* Photomicrograph of a hemangioma showing numerous capillaries. *B,* Clinical appearance of a hemangioma of the lower lip.

TUMORS OF MELANIN-PRODUCING CELLS

Melanocytic Nevi

The word **nevus** (plural, nevi) has two meanings. Here the word is used to mean a tumor of melanocytes (melanin-producing cells), which are called **nevus cells.** Nevus also refers to a pigmented congenital lesion (a lesion present at birth). A hemangioma present at birth is an example of this type of nevus.

Melanocytic nevi can arise on the skin or the oral mucosa. Intraoral tumors consist of tan to brown macules or papules that are most commonly located on the hard palate. The buccal mucosa is the second most common location (Fig. 5–36). They occur twice as often in women as in men and are usually first identified in individuals between 20 and 50 years of age.

Most pigmented lesions that occur in the oral cavity are benign. Pigmented lesions that exhibit ulceration, increase in size, or change in color may be malignant.

Treatment. A biopsy and histologic examination are indicated for pigmented lesions of unknown cause, unknown duration, or recent onset. Surgical excision is the treatment of choice for intraoral nevi.

Malignant Melanoma   *MOST DISTRUCTIVE, FASTEST.*

Malignant melanoma is a malignant tumor of melanocytes (Fig. 5–37). Although the name **melanoma** suggests that this is a benign tumor, all melanomas are malignant.

[handwritten margin note: ulceration, & color ↑, ↑ size - Tumor is so malignant - dermatologist referred]

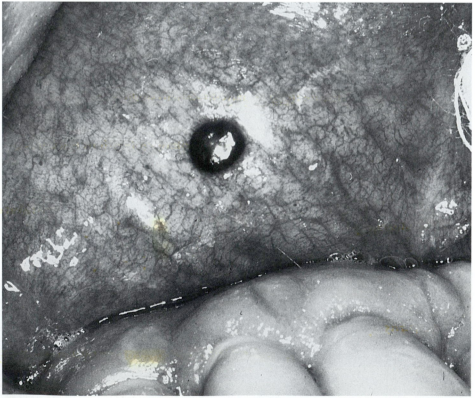

■ *f* **i g u r e** **5–36**   Clinical appearance of a melanocytic nevus showing a well-defined pigmented lesion on the buccal mucosa.

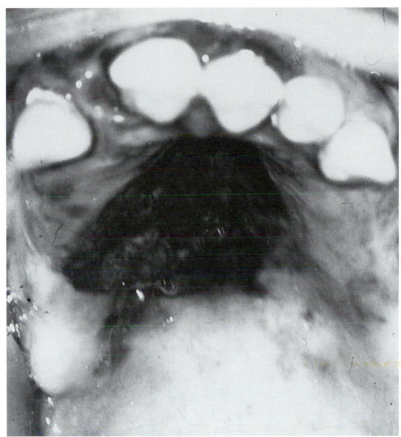

■ *f* i g u r e 5–37   Clinical appearance of a malignant melanoma showing an extensive, darkly pigmented area on the palate.

Most melanomas arise on the skin, and exposure to sunlight appears to be an important causative factor. Primary malignant melanoma within the oral cavity occurs but is rare. Melanoma of skin may metastasize to the oral cavity.

Melanoma usually presents as a rapidly enlarging bluish to black mass. Malignant melanomas are very aggressive tumors that exhibit unpredictable behavior and early metastasis. The most common intraoral locations are the palate and maxillary gingiva. Intraoral melanoma usually occurs in adults older than 40 years of age.

Treatment and Prognosis. Malignant melanomas are treated by surgical excision. Chemotherapy can be used in conjunction with surgery. The prognosis for oral melanoma is poor.

TUMORS OF BONE AND CARTILAGE

Torus

A **torus** (plural, tori) is a benign lesion composed of normal compact bone. Tori are located at either the midline of the palate (**torus palatinus** or **palatal torus**) or on the lingual aspect of the mandible in the area of the premolars (**torus mandibularis** or **mandibular torus**) (Fig. 5–38; Color Plates 53 and 61). Tori are not true tumors. They have a hereditary basis and are also discussed in Chapter 6. They are described in this chapter because of their resemblance to osteomas. Tori are covered by epithelium

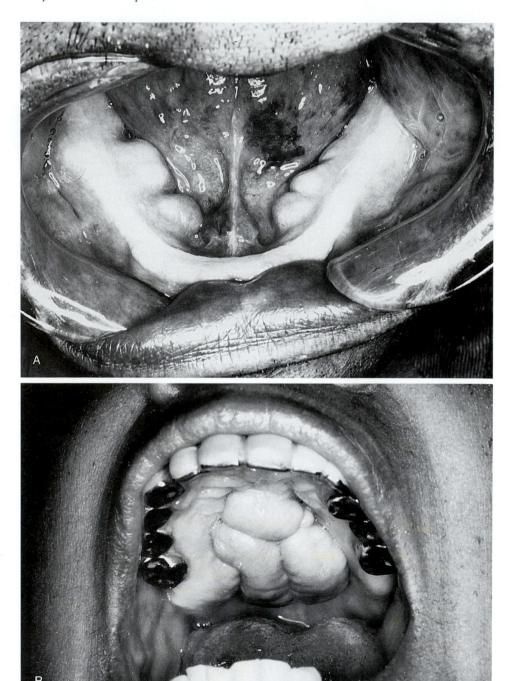

■ *figure 5–38*   *A,* Clinical appearance of bilateral mandibular tori. *B,* Clinical appearance of lobulated torus palatinus.

with very little underlying fibrous connective tissue. Surface ulceration can occur if they are traumatized, and healing may be prolonged. The presence of mandibular tori may result in a radiopacity in the mandibular premolar area. The diagnosis is confirmed by the presence of a torus on clinical examination.

Treatment. No treatment is necessary for these lesions unless they interfere with the placement of a prosthetic appliance.

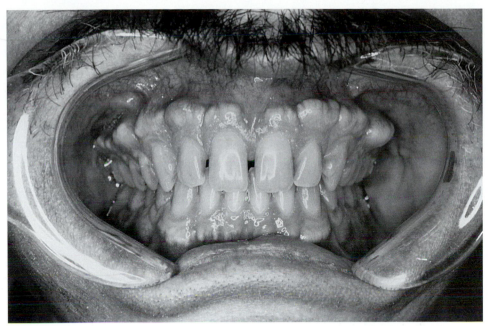

■ *f* i g u r e 5–39   Clinical appearance of exostoses present on the labial and buccal aspect of the maxilla and less prominent exostoses on the mandible.

Exostosis

An **exostosis** (plural exostoses) is a small nodular excrescence of normal compact bone (Fig. 5–39; Color Plate 75). Exostoses differ from tori only in their location. They most commonly occur on the buccal surface of the maxilla or mandible in the molar region.

Osteoma

An **osteoma** is a benign tumor composed of mature, normal-appearing bone. It is a slow-growing tumor that appears radiographically as a sharply defined radiopaque mass (Fig. 5–40). An osteoma is usually asymptomatic. When it becomes large enough, it can cause expansion of the involved bone. Osteomas are a component of Gardner's syndrome, which is genetically transmitted and is described in Chapter 6.

Treatment and Prognosis. Osteomas are treated by surgical excision and generally do not recur.

Ossifying Fibroma

The **ossifying fibroma** is a benign tumor composed of cellular fibrous connective tissue and bone (Fig. 5–41). It is similar in microscopic appearance to the cementifying fibroma, and some investigators have concluded that the ossifying fibroma and cementifying fibroma are variants of the same lesion. Ossifying fibromas are uncommon and occur in adults in the third and fourth decades of life.

Radiographically, the ossifying fibroma is well circumscribed and sharply defined and ranges from radiolucent to radiopaque, depending on the amount of calcification present in the lesion.

Treatment and Prognosis. Ossifying fibromas are treated by surgical excision or enucleation and generally do not recur.

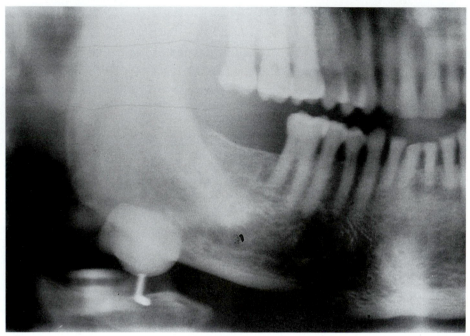

■ *figure* 5–40   Radiograph of an osteoma showing a radiopacity of the posterior mandible. (Courtesy of Dr. Sidney Eisig.)

Osteosarcoma

Osteosarcoma (**osteogenic sarcoma**) is a malignant tumor of bone-forming tissue (Fig. 5–42). It is the most common primary malignant tumor of bone in patients less than 40 years of age. Tumors that involve the long bones occur at an average age of 27 years, whereas the average age of occurrence for tumors that involve the jawbones is about 37 years of age. These tumors occur in the mandible twice as frequently as in the maxilla. Patients may present with a diffuse swelling or mass that is often painful.

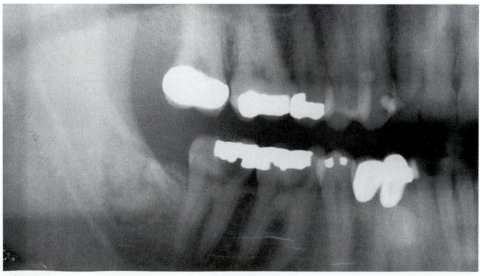

■ *figure* 5–41   Radiograph of an ossifying fibroma showing a well-defined lesion.

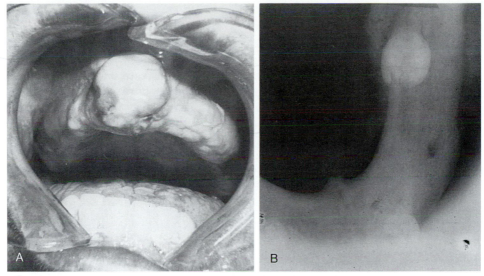

A   B

■ *figure* 5–42   *A,* Clinical appearance of an osteogenic sarcoma showing a mass on the anterior maxilla. *B,* Radiograph of an osteogenic sarcoma in another patient in the left molar area showing a poorly defined lesion.

B

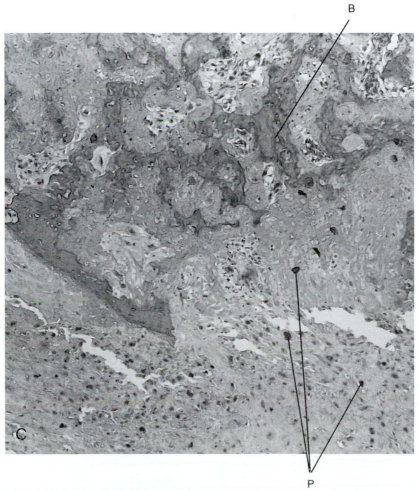

C

P

■ *figure* 5–42   *Continued C,* Microscopic appearance of an osteogenic sarcoma showing pleomorphic and hyperchromatic cells (P) and bone formation (B).

Bone expansion/distorted

Some patients present initially with a toothache or exhibit tooth mobility. Paresthesia of the lip is common in mandibular tumors.

The radiographic appearance of osteosarcomas varies from radiolucent to radiopaque (Fig. 5–42B). They are usually destructive, poorly defined lesions and may or may not involve the adjacent soft tissue. Asymmetric widening of the periodontal ligament space and a "sunburst" pattern may be seen radiographically in some cases. Microscopic examination of this tumor shows pleomorphic and hyperchromatic cells and abnormal bone formation (Fig. 5–42C).

Treatment and Prognosis. Currently, osteosarcomas are treated with preoperative multiagent chemotherapy followed by surgery. Recurrence of jaw lesions is common. Only about 20% of patients with osteosarcoma of the jaws survive 5 years.

Tumors of Cartilage *(cushion) - painful*

A **chondroma** is a benign tumor of cartilage. A **chondrosarcoma** is a malignant tumor of cartilage (Fig. 5–43). Cartilaginous tumors of the jawbones are extremely rare and are more often malignant than benign. *TMJ areas*

Treatment and Prognosis. Chondrosarcomas are treated by wide surgical excision. Radiation therapy and chemotherapy are not effective against this tumor. The prognosis is poor. Only about 30% of patients with chondrosarcoma of the jaws survive 5 years after diagnosis of the tumor. *long bones/joints*

TUMORS OF BLOOD AND BLOOD-FORMING TISSUES

Leukemia

Leukemia comprises a group of disorders characterized by an overproduction of atypical white blood cells. The normal bone marrow is replaced by a proliferation of immature white blood cells. The tumor cells appear in the circulating blood and in tissues. There are several types of leukemia, which are classified according to the kind of cells that are proliferating: myelocytes, lymphocytes, or monocytes. Leukemias are divided into two forms: acute and chronic. Acute leukemia is most common in children and young adults and is characterized by a proliferation of poorly differentiated cells. Chronic leukemia exhibits a proliferation of well-differentiated cells and most frequently occurs in middle-aged adults.

Although oral involvement can occur in any type of leukemia, the monocytic variant exhibits oral lesions most frequently. A common oral manifestation of monocytic leukemia is diffuse gingival enlargement with persistent bleeding (Fig. 5–44). (Leukemia is further described in Chapter 7.)

Treatment and Prognosis. The treatment of leukemia consists of chemotherapy, radiation therapy, and corticosteroids. The prognosis depends on the type and extent of the disease.

Lymphoma (Non-Hodgkin's Lymphoma) *(30-4 people)*

A **lymphoma** is a malignant tumor of lymphoid tissue. There are different types of lymphomas, which are differentiated on the basis of their microscopic appearance. The characteristic clinical presentation of lymphoma is the gradual enlargement of involved lymph nodes. Rarely, lymphomas can present as primary lesions in the oral soft tissue or bone. However, most lymphomas involve either lymph nodes or aggregates of lymphoid tissue, which are located along the digestive tract from the oral cavity to the

tongue, malignant, palate, adenopathy

some HIV ⊕

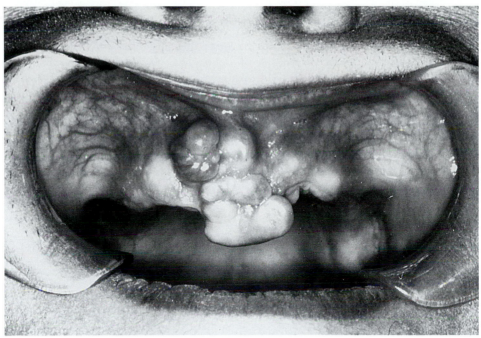

■ ***figure* 5-43**   Clinical appearance of a chondrosarcoma showing an exophytic mass on the anterior maxilla.

anus. In the oral cavity, lymphoid tissue is located at the base of the tongue, soft palate, and pharynx (Waldeyer's ring). The most common location for oral lymphoma is the tonsillar area. Lymphomas usually occur in adults and are more common in men than in women.

Treatment and Prognosis. Lymphomas are treated by radiotherapy, surgery, or chemotherapy, or a combination. The prognosis depends on the type and extent of involvement of the lymphoma.

oncologist prescribes

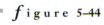
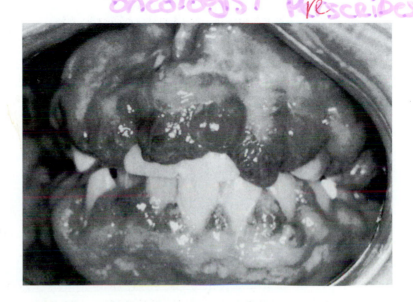

■ ***figure* 5-44**

Clinical appearance of a patient with leukemic infiltration of the gingiva resulting in diffuse enlargement. (From Regezi JA, Sciubba JJ: Oral Pathology: Clinical-Pathologic Correlations. Philadelphia, WB Saunders, 1989, p 149.)

Multiple Myeloma

Multiple myeloma is a systemic, malignant proliferation of plasma cells (Fig. 5–45), which causes destructive lesions of bone. The neoplastic plasma cells produce large amounts of immunoglobulin. Most patients are older than 40 years of age, and the disease occurs most commonly in the seventh decade of life. Men are affected more often than women. Patients usually present with bone pain and swelling. Pathologic fracture of a bone can occur because of weakening caused by destruction of the bone by disease.

Radiographically, the involved bones show multiple radiolucent lesions. The disease can involve the skull, spine, ribs, pelvis, long bones, and jaws. The mandible is affected more often than the maxilla. Most patients have an elevation of a single type

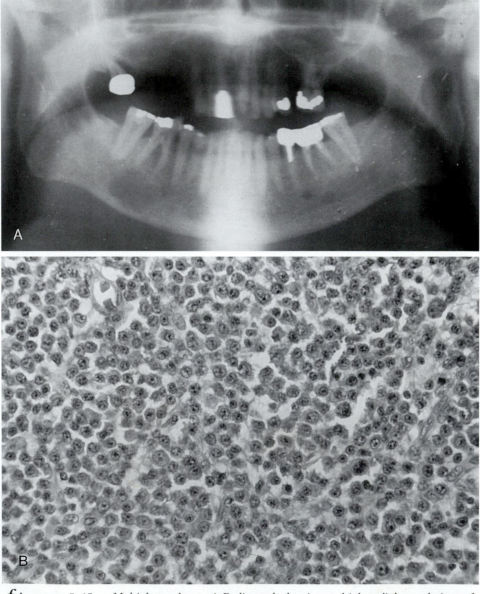

■ *figure* 5–45   Multiple myeloma. *A*, Radiograph showing multiple radiolucent lesions of the mandible in a patient with multiple myeloma. *B*, Photomicrograph showing proliferating plasma cells in multiple myeloma.

of immunoglobulin, which is detected by a process called **immunoelectrophoresis.** This elevation is called a **monoclonal spike.** Patients may have fragments of immunoglobulins present in urine. These fragments are called **Bence Jones proteins.**

The tumors are composed of sheets of well- to poorly differentiated plasma cells.

A localized tumor of plasma cells in soft tissue, not bone, is called an **extramedullary plasmacytoma.** Although these are rare tumors, they are more common in the head and neck region than anywhere else in the body. Multiple myeloma later develops in many patients with extramedullary plasmacytoma. Patients with lesions that appear to be single must be evaluated to determine if the lesion is solitary or part of multiple myeloma.

Treatment and Prognosis. Patients with multiple myeloma are treated with chemotherapy and local radiation to the lesions. The prognosis is poor, and the most common cause of death is infection followed by renal failure. Only 18% of patients survive 5 years following diagnosis.

METASTATIC TUMORS OF THE JAWS

Metastatic tumors of the jaws from primary sites elsewhere in the body are rare. The majority of these tumors arise from the thyroid, breast, lung, prostate gland, and kidney. The most frequent intraoral site for metastatic tumors is the mandible. Patients present with variable signs and symptoms, including pain, paresthesia or anesthesia of the lip, swelling, expansion of the bone, and loosening of the teeth in the involved area. Metastatic lesions usually appear several years after the primary lesion is discovered. Occasionally, the oral metastatic tumor is the first manifestation of a primary tumor elsewhere.

The radiographic appearance of metastatic tumors is variable (Fig. 5–46). Lesions are usually poorly defined and radiolucent. The roots of the involved teeth may show

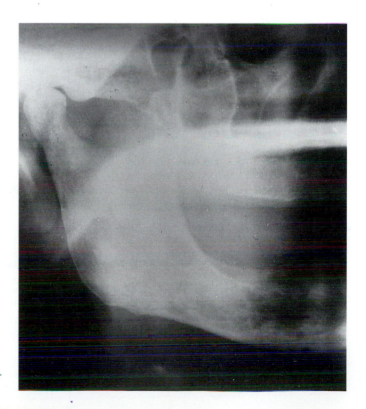

figure 5–46
Radiograph showing diffuse radiolucent-radiopaque changes resulting from metastatic carcinoma of the prostate gland.

a spiked appearance. Metastatic tumors from the breast, prostate gland, and lung may form bone and therefore may show areas of radiopacity.

Histologically, the metastatic tumor resembles the primary malignancy. The majority of metastatic tumors in the jaws are epithelial in origin and are adenocarcinomas.

Treatment and Prognosis. Chemotherapy and radiation therapy are used to alleviate the discomfort of metastatic tumors in the jaws. The prognosis for patients with tumors that have metastasized to the jaws is poor.

SELECTED REFERENCES

BOOKS

Enzinger FM, Weiss SW: Soft Tissue Tumors, 2nd ed. St. Louis, CV Mosby, 1988.
Neville BW, Damm DD, Allen CM, Bouquot JE: Oral and Maxillofacial Pathology. Philadelphia, WB Saunders, 1995.
Regezi JA, Sciubba JJ: Oral Pathology: Clinical-Pathologic Correlations. Philadelphia, WB Saunders, 1989.
Robbins SL, Kumar V: Basic Pathology. Philadelphia, WB Saunders, 1987.
Shafer WG, Hine MK, Levy BL: A Textbook of Oral Pathology. Philadelphia, WB Saunders, 1983.

JOURNAL ARTICLES

Tumors of Squamous Epithelium

Abbey LM, Page DG, Sawyer DR: The clinical and histopathologic features of a series of 464 oral squamous cell papillomas. Oral Surg Oral Med Oral Pathol 49:419, 1980.
Krutchkoff DF, Chen J, Eisenberg E, Katz RV: Oral cancer: A survey of 566 cases from the University of Connecticut Oral Pathology Biopsy Service 1975–1986. Oral Surg Oral Med Oral Pathol 70:192, 1990.
Mandez P Jr, Maves MD, Panje WR: Squamous cell carcinoma of the head and neck in patients under 40 years of age. Arch Otolaryngol 111:762, 1985.
Medina JE, Dichtel W, Luna MA: Verrucous-squamous carcinomas of the oral cavity. A clinicopathologic study of 104 cases. Arch Otolaryngol 110:437, 1984.
Padayachee A, VanWyk CW: Human papillomavirus (HPV) in oral squamous cell papillomas. J Oral Pathol 16:353, 1987.
Shibuya H, Hisamitsu S, Shioiri S, et al: Multiple primary cancer risk in patients with squamous cell carcinoma of the oral cavity. Cancer 60:3083, 1987.

Leukoplakia and Erythroplakia

Shafer WG, Waldron CA: Erythroplakia of the oral cavity. Cancer 36:1021, 1975.
Silverman S Jr, Gorsky M, Lozada F: Oral leukoplakia and malignant transformation. A follow-up study of 257 patients. Cancer 53:563, 1984.
Waldron CA, Shafer WG: Leukoplakia revisited. A clinicopathologic study of 3,256 oral leukoplakias. Cancer 36:1386, 1975.

Salivary Gland Tumors

Eveson JW, Cawson RA: Tumours of the minor (oropharyngeal) salivary glands: A demographic study of 336 cases. J Oral Pathol 14:500, 1985.
Neville B, Damm D, Weir J, et al: Labial salivary gland tumors. Cancer 61:2113, 1988.
Waldron CA, El-Mofty SK, Gnepp DR: Tumors of the intraoral minor salivary glands: A demographic and histologic study of 426 cases. Oral Surg Oral Med Oral Pathol 66:323, 1988.

Odontogenic Tumors

Ai-Ru L, Zhen L, Jian S: Calcifying epithelial odontogenic tumors: A clinicopathologic study of nine cases. J Oral Pathol 11:399, 1982.

Buchner A, Ficarra G, Hansen LS: Peripheral odontogenic fibroma. Oral Surg Oral Med Oral Pathol 64:432, 1987.

Courtney RM, Kerr DA: The odontogenic adenomatoid tumor: A comprehensive study of twenty new cases. Oral Surg Oral Med Oral Pathol 39:424, 1975.

Daley TD, Wysocki GP: Peripheral odontogenic fibroma. Oral Surg Oral Med Oral Pathol 78:329, 1994.

Kaffe I, Buchner A: Radiologic features of central odontogenic fibroma. Oral Surg Med Oral Pathol 78:811, 1994.

Kaugars GE, Miller ME, Abbey LM: Odontomas. Oral Surg Oral Med Oral Pathol 67:172, 1989.

Shamaskin RG, Svirsky JA, Kaugars GE: Intraosseous and extraosseous calcifying odontogenic cyst (Gorlin cyst). J Oral Maxillofac Surg 47:562, 1989.

Summerlin Don-John, Tomich CE: Focal cemento-osseous dysplasia: A clinicopathologic study of 221 cases. 78:611, 1994.

Ulmansky M, Hjörting-Hansen E, Paretorius F, Haque MF: Benign cementoblastoma. Oral Surg Oral Med Oral Pathol 77:48, 1994.

Waldron CA, El-Mofty SK: A histopathologic study of 116 ameloblastomas with special reference to the desmoplastic variant. Oral Surg Oral Med Oral Pathol 63:441, 1987.

Vascular Tumors

Hernandex GA, Castro A, Castro G, Amador E: Aneurysmal bone cyst versus hemangioma of the mandible. Oral Surg Oral Med Oral Pathol 76:790, 1993.

Tumors of Melanin-producing Cells

Kaugars GE, Heise AP, Riley WT, et al: Oral melanotic macules. Oral Surg Oral Med Oral Pathol 76:59, 1993.

Tumors of Bone

Forteza G, Colmenero A, Lopez-Barea F: Osteogenic sarcoma of the maxilla and mandible. Oral Surg Oral Med Oral Pathol 62:179, 1986.

Tumors of Blood and Blood-forming Tissues

Lambertenghi-Deliliers G, Bruno E, Corelezzi A, et al: Incidence of jaw lesions in 193 patients with multiple myeloma. Oral Surg Oral Med Oral Pathol 65:533, 1988.

Raubenheimer EJ, Dauth J, van Wilpe E: Multiple myeloma: A study of 10 cases. J Oral Pathol 16:383, 1987.

Metastatic Tumors

Hasimoto N, Kurihara K, Yamasaki H, et al: Pathological characteristics of metastatic carcinoma in the human mandible. J Oral Pathol 16:362, 1987.

REVIEW QUESTIONS

1. The study of tumors is called
   (A) Pathology
   (B) Neoplasia
   (C) Cytology
   (D) Oncology

2. Neoplasia involves
   (A) An irreversible change that results in an uncontrolled multiplication of cells
   (B) An abnormal proliferation of cells in response to tissue damage
   (C) A controlled proliferation of cells
   (D) A normal arrangement of proliferating cells

3. Viruses that cause neoplastic transformation of cells are called
    (A) Transformation viruses
    (B) Oncogenic viruses
    (C) Pathogenic viruses
    (D) Opportunistic viruses

4. Which one of the following is a characteristic of benign tumors?
    (A) Numerous mitotic figures
    (B) Rapid growth
    (C) Slow growth
    (D) Metastasis

5. A small exophytic lesion of the tongue that is the color of normal mucosa and is composed of papillary projections arranged in a "cauliflower-like" appearance is most likely a
    (A) Papilloma
    (B) Fibroma
    (C) Neurofibroma
    (D) Verrucous carcinoma

6. Which of the following is a histologic characteristic of squamous cell carcinoma?
    (A) Invasion of tumor cells into the connective tissue
    (B) Pleomorphic epithelial cells
    (C) Keratin pearls
    (D) All of the above

7. Which of the following are the most common locations for intraoral squamous cell carcinoma?
    (A) Upper labial mucosa, buccal mucosa, hard palate
    (B) Lower labial mucosa, maxillary gingiva, buccal mucosa
    (C) Floor of the mouth, ventrolateral tongue, soft palate
    (D) Anterior tongue, mandibular gingiva, retromolar area

8. A histologic diagnosis of epithelial dysplasia is of concern because the lesion may
    (A) Cause severe bleeding
    (B) Be cosmetically objectionable
    (C) Be premalignant
    (D) Be hyperkeratotic

9. Severe epithelial dysplasia may also be called
    (A) Epithelial hyperplasia
    (B) Carcinoma in situ
    (C) Infiltrating carcinoma
    (D) Hyperkeratosis

10. The most appropriate treatment for epithelial dysplasia is
    (A) Observation
    (B) Chemotherapy
    (C) Radiation therapy
    (D) Complete removal

11. Verrucous carcinoma is differentiated from other squamous cell carcinomas because it
    (A) Does not occur in the oral cavity
    (B) Most commonly occurs on the lower lip
    (C) Has a better prognosis
    (D) Has no keratin

12. The most common intraoral location for salivary gland tumors is the
    (A) Lower lip
    (B) Buccal mucosa
    (C) Palate
    (D) Anterior tongue

13. Which of the following is an example of a malignant salivary gland tumor?
    (A) Pleomorphic adenoma
    (B) Warthin's tumor
    (C) Monomorphic adenoma
    (D) Adenoid cystic carcinoma

14. Which of the following statements about ameloblastomas are TRUE? Ameloblastomas
    (A) Are benign, slow-growing, infiltrating tumors
    (B) Are composed of odontogenic epithelium
    (C) Most commonly occur in the mandibular molar-ramus area
    (D) All of the above

15. The odontogenic tumor that characteristically presents as a well-circumscribed radiolucency located in the anterior maxilla of an adolescent girl is an
    (A) Ameloblastic fibroma
    (B) Ameloblastoma
    (C) Odontogenic myxoma
    (D) Adenomatoid odontogenic tumor

16. The odontogenic tumor that most resembles the mesenchyme of the dental follicle histologically is
    (A) The cementifying fibroma
    (B) The odontogenic myxoma
    (C) The complex odontoma
    (D) The adenomatoid odontogenic tumor

17. A cementoblastoma can be recognized on x-ray film because
    (A) It is well circumscribed, radiopaque, and attached to the root of a tooth
    (B) It has a characteristic multilocular radiolucent radiographic appearance
    (C) It radiographically resembles a periapical granuloma
    (D) It is a rapidly growing lesion

18. Which one of the following lesions characteristically occurs on the gingiva?
    (A) Peripheral ossifying fibroma
    (B) Periapical cemental dysplasia
    (C) Odontoma
    (D) Central ossifying fibroma

19. Your patient, a 48-year-old black woman, presents with multiple asymptomatic, radiopaque masses in the mandible and maxilla. There is no expansion of bone. The most likely diagnosis is
    (A) Multiple odontomas
    (B) Cementifying fibromas
    (C) Periapical cemental dysplasia
    (D) Florid osseous dysplasia

20. A compound odontoma differs from a complex odontoma in that a compound odontoma
    (A) Is composed of tooth-like structures
    (B) Has unlimited growth potential
    (C) Is primarily composed of dental pulp tissue
    (D) Is usually located in the posterior mandible

21. "Peripheral" odontogenic tumors are located on the
    (A) Tongue
    (B) Lower lip
    (C) Buccal mucosa
    (D) Gingiva

22. A benign tumor of adipose tissue is called a
    (A) Lipoma
    (B) Schwannoma
    (C) Hemangioma
    (D) Lymphangioma

23. The most common malignant soft tissue tumor of the head and neck in children is
    (A) Squamous cell carcinoma
    (B) Malignant odontogenic tumor
    (C) Rhabdomyosarcoma
    (D) Osteogenic sarcoma

24. Malignant melanoma of the oral cavity is rare; however, the most common intraoral location is the
    (A) Palate and maxillary gingiva
    (B) Tongue
    (C) Buccal mucosa
    (D) Retromolar area

25. Osteomas are a component of
    (A) Neurofibromatosis
    (B) Gardner's syndrome
    (C) Osteosarcoma
    (D) Ossifying fibroma

26. A malignant tumor of bone-forming tissue is called
    (A) Chondrosarcoma
    (B) Angiosarcoma
    (C) Osteosarcoma
    (D) Hemangiosarcoma

27. A disorder characterized by an overproduction of atypical white blood cells is called
    (A) Hermangioma
    (B) Leukemia
    (C) Melanoma
    (D) Leukocytosis

28. A malignant tumor of lymphocytes is called
    (A) Multiple myeloma
    (B) Melanoma
    (C) Lymphoma
    (D) Angiosarcoma

29. The cell involved in multiple myeloma is the
    (A) Lymphocyte
    (B) Macrophage
    (C) Red blood cell
    (D) Plasma cell

30. The most frequent intraoral site for metastatic tumors is the
    (A) Buccal mucosa
    (B) Mandible
    (C) Soft palate
    (D) Floor of the mouth

31. Which one of the following benign tumors is associated with von Reckling-hausen's disease?
    (A) Rhabdomyoma
    (B) Lipoma
    (C) Neurofibroma
    (D) Osteoma

32. Which one of the following is the most common odontogenic tumor?
    (A) Odontoma
    (B) Ameloblastoma
    (C) Benign cementoblastoma
    (D) Odontogenic myxoma

33. Which one of the following is the most common malignant salivary gland tumor in children?
    (A) Adenoid cystic carcinoma
    (B) Monomorphic adenoma
    (C) Papillary cystadenoma lymphomatosum
    (D) Mucoepidermoid carcinoma

34. A benign tumor composed of a proliferation of capillaries is called a
    (A) Schwannoma
    (B) Hemangioma
    (C) Lipoma
    (D) Osteoma

35. A white plaque-like lesion that cannot be rubbed off or diagnosed as a specific disease is called
    (A) Speckled leukoplakia
    (B) Erythroplakia
    (C) Leukoplakia
    (D) Epithelial dysplasia

36. All of the following are benign lesions composed of mature compact bone except a(n)
    (A) Torus
    (B) Osteoma
    (C) Exostosis
    (D) Ossifying fibroma

37. Which one of the following malignant tumors may present as diffuse gingival enlargement with persistent bleeding?
    (A) Multiple myeloma
    (B) Monocytic leukemia
    (C) Chondrosarcoma
    (D) Osteosarcoma

38. Which one of the following malignancies is characterized by a monoclonal spike on immunoelectrophoresis?
    (A) Multiple myeloma
    (B) Metastatic lung carcinoma
    (C) Lymphoma
    (D) Leukemia

39. Which one of the following malignant tumors has been reported to show a characteristic "sunburst" pattern on radiographic examination?
    (A) Malignant melanoma
    (B) Osteosarcoma
    (C) Squamous cell carcinoma
    (D) Rhabdomyosarcoma

40. All of the following are malignant tumors that arise from squamous epithelium except
    (A) Basal cell carcinoma
    (B) Verrucous carcinoma
    (C) Adenoid cystic carcinoma
    (D) Squamous cell carcinoma

6

Genetics

HEDDIE O. SEDANO

Objectives

After studying this chapter, the student should be able to:

1. Define each of the words listed in the vocabulary for this chapter.
2. State the purpose of mitosis.
3. State the purpose of meiosis.
4. Explain what is meant by the Lyon hypothesis, and give an example of its clinical significance.
5. Explain what is meant by a gross chromosomal abnormality, and give three examples of syndromes that result from gross chromosomal abnormalities.
6. List the four inheritance patterns.
7. Explain what is meant by X-linked inheritance.
8. State the inheritance pattern, and describe the oral manifestations and, if appropriate, the characteristic facies for each of the following:
   Cyclic neutropenia
   Papillon-Lefèvre syndrome
   Cherubism
   Chondroectodermal dysplasia (Ellis–van Creveld syndrome)
   Mandibulofacial dysostosis (Treacher Collins syndrome)
   Osteogenesis imperfecta
   Hereditary hemorrhagic telangiectasia (Osler-Rendu-Parkes Weber syndrome)
   Peutz-Jeghers syndrome
   White spongy nevus (Cannon's disease)
   Hypohidrotic ectodermal dysplasia
   Hypophosphatasia
   Hypophosphatemic vitamin D–resistant rickets
9. State the inheritance pattern, the oral or facial manifestations, and the type and location of the malignancy associated with each of the following syndromes:
   Gardner's syndrome
   Nevoid basal cell carcinoma syndrome (Gorlin syndrome)
   Multiple mucosal neuromas, medullary carcinoma of the thyroid gland, and pheochromocytoma syndrome (MEN 2B)
   Neurofibromatosis of von Recklinghausen
10. Intestinal polyps are a component of both Peutz-Jeghers syndrome and Gardner's syndrome. State the location and malignant potential of the intestinal polyps in each of these syndromes.
11. List the four types of amelogenesis imperfecta.
12. Briefly compare and contrast dentinogenesis imperfecta, amelogenesis imperfecta, and dentin dysplasia, including the inheritance patterns and the clinical manifestations and radiographic appearance of each.

Vocabulary

Alleles (ah-lēlz′)   Genes that are located at the same level or locus in the two chromosomes of a pair and that determine the same functions or characteristics

Amino acid (ah-me′no as′id)   An organic compound containing the amino group NH_2; amino acids are the main component of proteins

Autosomes (aw′to-sōmz) (adjective, autosomal)   The non–sex chromosomes, which are identical for men and women

Barr body (bahr bod′e)   Condensed chromatin of the inactivated X chromosome, which is found at the periphery of the nucleus of cells in women

Carrier (kar′e-er)   In genetics, a heterozygous individual who is clinically normal but who can transmit a recessive trait or characteristic; also, a person who is homozygous for an autosomal dominant condition with low penetrance

Centromere (sen′tro-mēr)   The constricted portion of the chromosome that divides the short arms from the long arms

Chromatid (kro′mah-tid)   Either of the two vertical halves of a chromosome that are joined at the centromere

Chromatin (kro′mah-tin)   A general term used to refer to the material (DNA) that forms the chromosomes

Codon (ko′don)   The vertical sequence of three bases in DNA that codes for an amino acid

Consanguinity (kon″san-gwin′ĭ-te)   Blood relationship; in genetics, the term is generally used to describe a mating or marriage between close relatives

Deoxyribonucleic acid (de-ok″se-ri″bo-nu-kle′ik as′id)   DNA; a substance composed of a double chain of polynucleotides, both chains coiled around a central axis form a double helix; it is the basic genetic code or template for amino acid formation

Diploid (dip′loid)   Having two sets of chromosomes; the normal constitution of somatic cells

Dominant (dom′ĭ-nant)   In genetics, a trait or characteristic that is manifested when it is carried by only one of a pair of homologous chromosomes

Expressivity (eks″pres-siv′ĭ-te)   The degree of clinical manifestation of a trait or characteristic

Facies (fa′she-ēz)   The appearance of the face

Gamete (gam′ēt)   Spermatozoon or ovum

Genetic heterogeneity (je-net′ik het″er-o-jĕ-ne′ĭ-te)   Having more than one inheritance pattern

Haploid (hap′loid)   A cell with a single set of chromosomes; a gamete is haploid

Heterozygote (het″er-o-zi′gōt) (adjective, heterozygous)   An individual with two different genes at the allele loci

Homozygote (ho″mo-zi′gōt) (adjective, homozygous)   An individual having identical genes at the allele loci

Hypohidrosis (hi'po-hĭ-dro'sis) Abnormally diminished secretion of sweat

Hypotrichosis (hi'po-trĭ-ko'sis) Presence of less than the normal amount of hair

Karyotype (kar'e-o-tīp) A photomicrographic representation of a person's chromosomal constitution arranged according to the Denver classification

Locus (lo'kus) (plural, loci) The position occupied by a gene on a chromosome

Meiosis (mi-o'sis) The two-step cellular division of the original germ cells, which reduces the chromosomes from 4nDNA to 1nDNA

Metaphase (met'ah-fāz) The phase of cellular division in which the chromosomes are lined up evenly along the equatorial plane of the cell and in which the chromosomes are most visible

Mitosis (mi-to'sis) The way in which somatic cells divide so that the two daughter cells receive the same number of identical chromosomes

Mutation (mū-ta'shun) A permanent change in the arrangement of genetic material

Oogenesis (o"o-jen'ĕ-sis) The process of formation of female germ cells (ova)

Ovum (o'vum) (plural, ova) An egg; the mature feminine germ cell

Penetrance (pen'ĕ-trans) The frequency with which a heritable trait is manifested by individuals carrying the gene or genes that determine that trait

Phenotype (fe'noh-tīp) The entire physical, biochemical, and physiologic make-up of an individual; genotype is the genetic composition, and phenotype is its observable appearance

Recessive (re-ses'iv) A trait or characteristic that shows clinically when there is a double gene dose (homozygous) in autosomic chromosomes or a single gene dose in males if the trait is X-linked

Ribonucleic acid (ri"bo-noo-kle'ik as'id) RNA; single strands of polynucleotides found in all cells; different types of RNA have different functions in the production of proteins by the cell

Ribosome (ri'bo-sōm) The cytoplasmic organelles in which proteins are formed based on the genetic code provided by RNA

Spermatogenesis (sper"mah-to-jen'ĕ sis) The process of formation of spermatozoa (sperm)

Spermatozoon (sper"mah-to-zo'on) (plural, spermatozoa) The mature male germ cell

Syndrome (sin'drōm) A set of signs or symptoms, or both, occurring together

Translocation (trans"lo-ka'shun) A portion of a chromosome attached to another chromosome

Trisomy (tri'so-me) A pair of chromosomes with an identical extra chromosome

Genetics is the science that studies inheritance and the expression of inherited traits. The main objectives of this chapter are to introduce some of the basic concepts of genetics and present the clinical manifestations of some inherited oral disorders of interest to the dental hygienist. The descriptions of many syndromes are included. As you have learned in previous chapters, a **syndrome** is a distinctive association of signs and symptoms occurring together in the same patient. The syndromes included in this chapter are inherited. However, other syndromes, such as AIDS (acquired immunodeficiency syndrome), are acquired, not inherited. In addition, the fact that an alteration is found as part of a syndrome does not mean that it cannot also occur independently. For example, cleft lip and palate occur as components of several syndromes and can also occur independently. The classification of syndromes is difficult because they are composed of several associated anomalies and because the anomalies that compose the syndrome may not be present consistently in all patients with the same syndrome.

The term **phenotype** is used often in this chapter. It refers to the physical, biochemical, and physiologic traits of an individual. A phenotype can occur as a result of genetic factors or from a combination of genetic factors and environmental influences.

In this chapter, as in previous chapters, basic concepts are discussed first. These are followed by descriptions of specific inherited disorders.

CHROMOSOMES

The hereditary units that are transmitted from one generation to another are called **genes.** They are found on **chromosomes,** which are located in the nucleus of the cell. Using a microscope, one can see chromosomes clearly only when the nucleus and cell are dividing (Fig. 6–1*A*). At other times, the genetic material is dispersed in the nucleus (Fig. 6–1*B*). Each cell of the human body, with the exception of mature

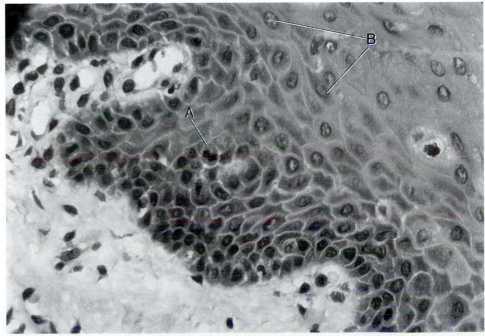

f **i g u r e 6–1**   High-power photomicrograph showing a dividing cell with visible chromosomes (A) and nuclei of cells with scattered chromatin (B).

germ cells (ova and spermatozoa), has 46 chromosomes. Half of these chromosomes are derived from the father and the other half from the mother. Chromosomes contain **deoxyribonucleic acid (DNA),** which directs the production of amino acids, polypeptides, and proteins by the cell. In addition, DNA has the ability to duplicate itself (self-replication). It creates exact copies of itself, and through the process of cell division, cells identical to the original cell are formed.

NORMAL CELL DIVISION

Mitosis

[handwritten: 23 chromosomes apiece]

All cells in the body, with the exception of ova and spermatozoa, are called **somatic cells.** Cellular division is achieved by **mitosis** during a part of the somatic cell's life span, called the **mitotic cycle.** The function of mitosis is to create an exact copy of each chromosome and, through division of the original cell, distribute an identical set of chromosomes to each daughter cell. After each cell division is completed and before the next division can occur, the cell enters a phase known as "**G₁**" **(gap 1),** which is followed by a phase called the **S phase,** in which there is replication of the DNA. The **G₂ (gap 2)** phase follows the S phase and ends when mitotic division begins. The cell cycle is illustrated in Figure 6–2.

Stages of Mitosis *[handwritten: - cell devision]*

Mitosis is composed of four stages: metaphase, prophase, anaphase, and telophase. In each of these four stages, the chromosomes are distributed in a specific arrangement. In **metaphase,** the chromosomes stain intensely and are arranged almost symmetrically at both sides of the center, or **equatorial plane,** of the cell. The appearance of a metaphase chromosome resembles the letter "X" (Fig. 6–3), having a pair of "long arms" (3 in Fig. 6–3) and a pair of "short arms" (1 in Fig. 6–3). The size of the chromosome at metaphase, as well as the length of the long and short arms, varies from chromosome to chromosome. The constriction present in all chromosomes, which joins the short and long arms, is called the **centromere** (2 in Fig. 6–3). During metaphase, chromosomes are actually formed by two identical vertical halves, each composed of either left or right short and long arms and half of the centromere. Each of these identical halves is called a **chromatid** (4 in Fig. 6–3). At metaphase, each chromatid contains one molecule of DNA, and therefore the DNA content of each chromosome is doubled (Fig. 6–4). When cell division takes place, each chromosome splits vertically at the centromere, and 46 chromatids (which now become chromosomes) form one daughter cell, while the other 46 chromatids form a second

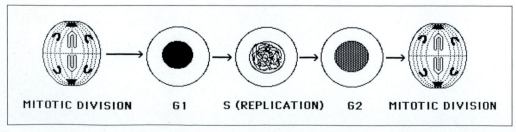

MITOTIC DIVISION   G1   S (REPLICATION)   G2   MITOTIC DIVISION

▪ *f i g u r e 6–2*   Schematic representation of the mitotic cycle showing the end of mitosis followed by the G₁, the S, and the G₂ phases and the next mitosis.

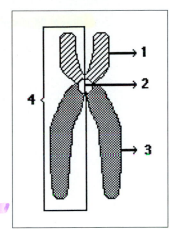

■ *figure* 6–3

Autosomal chromosome at metaphase showing short arm (1), centromere (2), long arm (3), and chromatid (4).

daughter cell. During **prophase,** the chromosomes are lining up toward metaphase; in **anaphase** and **telophase,** the chromatids are in the process of splitting.

Meiosis

Primitive germ cells (oogonia and spermatogonia) have 46 chromosomes. Mature germ cells (ova and spermatozoa) have 23 chromosomes. **Meiosis is a two-step special type of cell division in which the primitive germ cells reduce their chromosome number by half and become mature germ cells.** The primitive germ cells have two chromosomes for each pair and are called **diploid.** The suffix "ploid" refers to the number of sets of chromosomes, and the prefix it appears with refers to the degree of ploidy. In diploid "di" indicates two. The mature germ cells (or gametes) have half the number of chromosomes and are called **haploid.** During the period the cell is not in division, the DNA content of diploid cells is designated 2nDNA, and in metaphase it is double or 4nDNA. After the two stages of meiosis have been completed, the 4nDNA is reduced to 1nDNA. The two steps are called **first meiosis** and **second meiosis.** This reduction is necessary to maintain the normal number of human chromosomes. A new embryo must have 46 chromosomes per cell as did its parents. Therefore, the union of germ cells needs to result in 46 chromosomes. If two cells with 46 chromosomes were combined, the resulting cell would have 92 chromosomes.

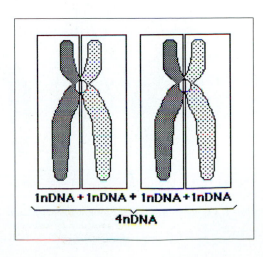

1nDNA + 1nDNA + 1nDNA + 1nDNA

4nDNA

■ *figure* 6–4

Pair of autosomal chromosomes at metaphase. Each chromatid represents 1nDNA.

First Meiosis   *nondissunctional*

Prior to the first meiosis in the primitive germ cells, there is a replication of DNA similar to that observed in the S phase of somatic cells. After replication the members of each pair of chromosomes line up next to each other in an intimate point-by-point relationship (Fig. 6–5A). This pairing does not occur in mitosis. After pairing, the two chromosomes establish actual contact at different locations. These contacts are known as **chiasmata** (meaning X-shaped) and determine points of crossing over (Fig. 6–5B). This crossing over achieves the exchange of chromosome segments between a chromatid of one chromosome and a chromatid of the other chromosome of a pair (between homologous chromosomes) (Fig. 6–5C). This special aspect of the first meiosis takes place at metaphase. After metaphase of the first meiotic division, the chromosomes separate from each other but there is no splitting of the centromere. The chromosomes remain intact, and each member of the pair migrates to one of the new cells, each of which contains 23 chromosomes but twice the final amount of DNA. During this migration, chromosomes of the paternal and maternal lines segregate at random, thus ensuring diversity of the species by creating a new combination of chromosomes.

Occasionally, the chromosomes that were crossing over do not separate and both migrate to the same cell. This is known as **nondisjunction** and results in the formation of a germ cell with an extra chromosome. If this occurs and that cell (either an ovum or a spermatozoon) participates in the formation of an embryo, three chromosomes **(trisomy)** instead of two result. An example of this type of abnormality is **Down's syndrome,** also called **trisomy 21,** in which there are three of chromosome 21 instead of two. Trisomy has been reported for several different chromosomes.

In a female embryo, **oogenesis (ovum development)** starts around the third month of prenatal life, and the future ova remain in suspended crossing over from about the time of birth until the time ovulation starts. At the beginning of ovulation, the first meiosis is completed. Nondisjunction is more prevalent in female oogenesis than in male spermatogenesis. This is probably because of the period of prolonged crossing over, and therefore the older the woman, the greater the chance of shedding a trisomic ovum and of bearing a child with Down's syndrome or other trisomy.

Second Meiosis

The second stage of meiosis is essentially a mitotic division, in which each chromosome splits longitudinally. There is no replication of DNA before the second

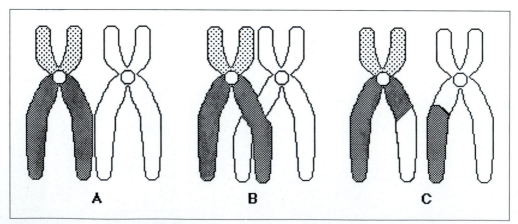

■ *f i g u r e 6–5*   *A,* Homologous autosomal chromosomes lining up in first meiosis. *B,* Crossing over during metaphase of first meiosis. *C,* Note exchange of segments after crossing over.

meiosis. After the splitting, two cells are formed, each containing the right amount of DNA (1nDNA) (Fig. 6–6). Nondisjunction can occur during the second meiosis as well as during the first meiosis. If it occurs in second meiosis, a chromosome does not split, and one daughter cell has a full chromosome and the other has none.

Immediately after fertilization, the chromosomes of the ovum and spermatozoon, each having 1nDNA, condense independently and form round structures, each known as a **pronucleus.** The DNA in these pronuclei replicates, forming a set of 23 full chromosomes for each, the maternal and paternal pronuclei. When the membranes of these pronuclei break, the 46 chromosomes mix at random, initiating the first cellular division (mitosis) that starts the development of the new embryo.

The Lyon Hypothesis

The sex chromosomes are designated XX in women and XY in men. During the early period of embryonal development (possibly by the end of the second week), the genetic activity of one of the X chromosomes in each cell of a female embryo is inactivated. The inactivation is a random process affecting either the X chromosome derived from the mother or the X chromosome derived from the father. Activated chromosomes are dispersed in the nucleus. The inactivated chromosome remains contracted when the cell is not dividing and forms a structure known as the **Barr body.** In female cells the Barr body can easily be seen under the light microscope, especially in cytologic smears, including those obtained from the oral mucosa. The Barr body appears as a dark dot at the periphery of the nucleus (Fig. 6–7).

This inactivation of one of the X chromosomes in a female embryo was postulated by Mary Lyon and is known as the **Lyon hypothesis.** This hypothesis has interesting clinical implications for female carriers of conditions caused by genes located on the X chromosome, which are explained later in this chapter.

THE MOLECULAR COMPOSITION OF CHROMOSOMES

Chromosomes contain DNA. DNA contains the basic code or template that carries all genetic information. The basic unit of DNA is called a **nucleotide,** which is formed

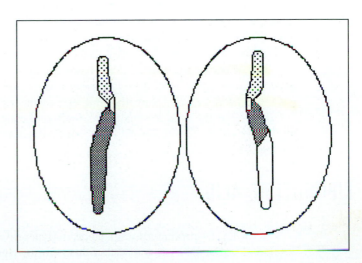

■ *f* i g u r e 6–6
Two haploid cells after second meiosis, each having 1nDNA.

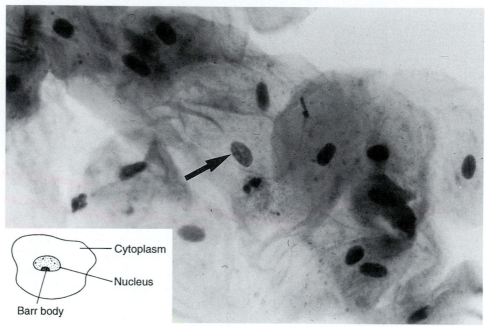

■ *f* i g u r e **6–7**   Buccal smear showing Barr body (arrow points to small dark dot on nuclear membrane) at the periphery of the nucleus of a desquamated epithelial cell from a woman's buccal mucosa. (Courtesy of Dr. Carl J. Witkop.)

by a nitrogen-containing base, a five-carbon sugar (deoxyribose), and a phosphate. There are four bases in DNA: adenine (A), guanine (G), thymine (T), and cytosine (C). These chains of polynucleotides are coiled to form a structure called a double helix (Fig. 6–8). In DNA the base adenine is always bound to the base thymine, and guanine is always bound to cytosine. This is a constant arrangement and is identical in all species from bacteria to humans, with just a few exceptions. Therefore, the ratio of adenine to thymine is always equal, and the same is true for the ratio of guanine to cytosine. In humans, G/C pairs are about four times greater than A/T pairs. The polynucleotide chains run vertically in opposite directions. Therefore, a sequence of AGC (adenine, guanine, cytosine) is always matched by the sequence TCG (thymine, cytosine, guanine).

In the linear representation shown, the nucleotide of one chain is indicated by the number 1, and the number 2 indicates the nucleotide of the other chain. Both nucleotides are bound by a molecule of hydrogen (H). This arrangement is repeated horizontally to form the polynucleotide double spiral staircase (or helix) appearance of DNA (Fig. 6–8).

The vertical sequence of three bases is called a **codon.** It codes for an amino acid. Several amino acids form a polypeptide, and one or more polypeptides form a protein. A gene is often equated with the unit that forms a polypeptide.

DNA has the unique capability of self-replication, which is achieved by unwinding its double chain (like the plaits of a braid). Each separated chain serves as a blueprint for another chain.

RIBONUCLEIC ACID

In order to produce amino acids, polypeptides, and proteins, the genetic code contained in the DNA is transcribed into **ribonucleic acid (RNA),** which differs from

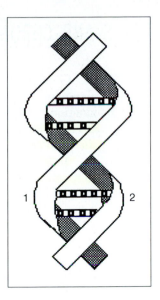

▪ *f i g u r e* 6-8   Schematic representation of the DNA double helix.

DNA in that it is a single strand (in its simplest form), its sugar is a ribose (the sugar in DNA is deoxyribose), and the base uracil (U) replaces the thymine (T) in DNA.

Types of RNA

There are four types of RNA: messenger RNA (mRNA), transfer RNA (tRNA), ribosomal RNA (rRNA), and heterogeneous RNA (hnRNA). RNA can be found in both the nucleus and the cytoplasm of a cell.

Messenger RNA is a blueprint of the genetic DNA for the coding of proteins. It carries the message for the DNA to ribosomes in the cytoplasm, in which proteins are produced. Transfer RNA transfers amino acids from the cytoplasm to the messenger RNA, positioning amino acids in the proper sequence to form polypeptides and hence proteins. Ribosomal RNA combines with several polypeptides to form ribosomes. Heterogeneous RNA is found within the nucleus and is the precursor of messenger RNA.

In the production of a protein (Fig. 6–9), the messenger RNA carries the genetic code for the formation of that protein to the ribosomes. The transfer RNA brings amino acids to the ribosomes from the cellular cytoplasm. The amino acid sequence forms proteins according to the genetic code, and these proteins exit the ribosomes as they are formed.

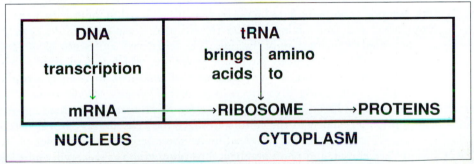

▪ *f i g u r e* 6-9   Production (synthesis) of protein from DNA.

GENES AND CHROMOSOMES

Genes in a chromosome are located in a vertical linear manner. The genes in both members of a pair of chromosomes (homologous chromosomes) govern the same functions or dictate the same characteristics. The genes that are located at the same level (or **locus**) in homologous chromosomes and that dictate the same functions or characteristics are called **alleles.**

The manifestations **(phenotype)** of a gene action are not necessarily the same from one individual to another. This is best explained with the ABO blood group system. The locus can be occupied by either the factor that determines the blood group A or the factor that determines the blood group B. If it is empty, it results in the blood group O. The locus is always the same, and the three genes govern the same function, but the clinical result is different. In this situation, the trait or condition is said to have multiple alleles. For example, if both loci are AA, or if they are AO, the person is said to have blood group A. If both loci are BB or BO, the person is said to have blood group B. If the loci are AB or BA, the person is said to have blood group AB. Only if both the loci are empty does the person have blood group O. The locus always controls blood group, but the group is dependent on the alleles that are present or lacking in each person.

When the allelic genes are identical, the person is said to be homozygous for that gene or a homozygote. Using the ABO blood group system again, for example, a person with AA, BB, and OO would be homozygous. When the genes are different (e.g., AB, AO, or BO) the person is said to be heterozygous for that gene or a heterozygote. If a gene can express its effect clinically with a single dose (heterozygous) as in the combination AO = blood group A, the characteristic is said to be dominant. If the gene needs a double dose to manifest its action (homozygous), the resulting characteristic or function is said to be recessive. For example, only the combination OO results in the blood group O.

Chromosomal Abnormalities

Abnormalities of chromosomes can be divided into two categories: molecular abnormalities and gross abnormalities. Molecular alterations occur at the DNA level and are not detectable microscopically. Most inherited disorders represent examples of molecular changes (mutations) at the level of one or both allelic genes. Examples of these conditions are presented later in this chapter.

Gross chromosomal alterations can be observed in a karyotype. A **karyotype** (Figs. 6–10 and 6–11) is a photographic representation of a person's chromosomal constitution. A karyotype can be created by culturing cells from blood, skin, or other tissues. One method uses peripheral blood by placing it in a test tube with heparin to avoid coagulation and centrifuging it. After centrifugation, the white blood cells (leukocytes) are deposited at the bottom of the tube. The leukocytes are removed and are placed in a culture medium containing phytohemagglutinin, which is a substance that enhances mitosis. Since chromosomes are best observed when cell division is arrested at metaphase, colchicine is added to the culture after 72 hours of culture at 37° C to stop mitosis at metaphase. This also prevents the centromere from dividing. A hypotonic solution is then added to the culture to make the cells swell. The cells are then fixed (preserved) and stained and observed under the microscope. Examples of well-defined mitoses are chosen and photographed. The photograph is enlarged, and each chromosome is cut out of the photographic print. When stained, the chromosomes have a

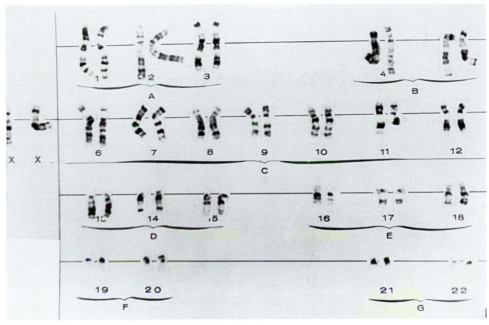

𝑓 i g u r e 6–10   Karyotype from a female showing the 22 pairs of autosomal chromosomes and the pair of X chromosomes. (Courtesy of Dr. Jaroslav Cervenka.)

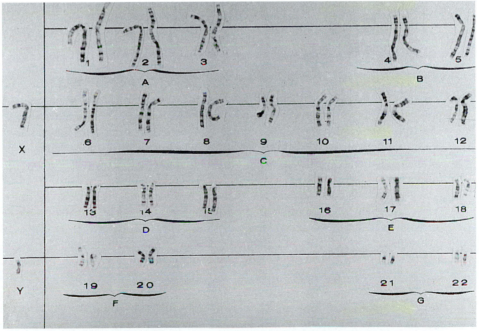

𝑓 i g u r e 6–11   Karyotype from a male showing the 22 pairs of autosomal chromosomes and the X and Y chromosomes. (Courtesy of Dr. Jaroslav Cervenka.)

band-like appearance that allows an accurate identification of each. These cutouts are then pasted on a special chart to construct the karyotype.

Gross Chromosomal Abnormalities

Alterations in Number and Structure of Chromosomes

Gross chromosomal abnormalities are caused by either alterations in chromosome number, which are almost always a result of nondisjunction (explained earlier), or alterations in structure, which develop because of chromosomal breaks or abnormal rearrangements. The following illustrate alterations in number:

Euploid: A complete second set of chromosomes, the total number being 92. This is incompatible with life.

Polyploid: Three (triploid) or four (tetraploid) complete sets of chromosomes. This has been occasionally described in humans and is incompatible with life.

Aneuploid: Any extra number of chromosomes that do not represent an exact multiple of the total chromosome complement, for example,

Trisomy: A pair with an identical extra chromosome.

Monosomy: A missing chromosome from a pair.

Examples of structural abnormalities include the following:

Deletion: The loss of part of a chromosome.

Translocation: A portion of a chromosome attached to another chromosome.

Inversion: A portion of a chromosome is upside-down.

Duplication: A chromosome is larger than normal, the extra segment being identical to a segment of the normal chromosome.

Clinical Syndromes

Trisomy 21. This condition, also known as **Down's syndrome,** is the most frequent of the trisomies. Ninety-five percent of cases of Down's syndrome are due to nondisjunction, mostly associated with late maternal age at the time of conception.

The facies (the appearance of the face) is characterized by slanted eyes. Patients are generally shorter than normal, and heart abnormalities are present in more than 30% of individuals with trisomy 21. The intelligence level varies from near normal to marked retardation.

Fissured tongue is frequently seen in patients with trisomy 21. Premature loss of teeth, especially the mandibular central incisors, caused by alveolar bone loss is frequently seen. Gingival and periodontal disease has been reported in 90% of affected individuals. Hypodontia (fewer teeth than normal), abnormally shaped teeth, and anomalies in eruption with malposition and crowding of teeth are common findings. Dental hygienists play an important role in the maintenance of oral health in these patients.

Trisomy 13. This disorder is characterized by multiple abnormalities in various organs. Seventy percent of live-born infants die within the first 7 months of life. Characteristic clinical findings include bilateral cleft lip and palate, microphthalmia or anophthalmia (small eyes or no eyes), superficial hemangioma of the forehead or nape of the neck, growth retardation, severe mental retardation, polydactyly of hands and feet (supernumerary digits), clenching of the fist with the thumb under the fingers, rocker-bottom feet, heart malformations, and several anomalies of the external genitals.

The facial appearance is quite striking because of the cleft lip, cleft palate, and ocular abnormalities (Fig. 6–12).

Turner's Syndrome. Patients with Turner's syndrome have a female phenotype, and in the majority of cases the karyotype has the normal 44 autosomic chromosomes and only one X chromosome. A normal female would have two X chromosomes—one from the mother and one from the father. Most cases of Turner's syndrome are due to nondisjunction of the X chromosome in the paternal gamete. Clinically, these women are of short stature and have webbing of the neck and edema of the hands and feet (Fig. 6–13). They frequently exhibit a low hairline on the nape of the neck. The chest is broad with wide-spaced nipples. The aorta is frequently abnormal, and body hair is sparse. The external genitals appear infantile, and generally the ovaries are not developed; therefore, these individuals have primary amenorrhea (abnormal temporary or permanent cessation of the menstrual cycle). Smears taken from the oral mucosa demonstrate the lack of Barr bodies. (condensed X chromosomes)

Klinefelter's Syndrome. This condition occurs when an ovum carrying two X chromosomes is fertilized by a spermatozoon with a Y chromosome, and therefore the fertilized ovum will have two X chromosomes plus a Y chromosome. The majority of cases result from nondisjunction of the X chromosome, generally in the ova of older females. Affected individuals have a male phenotype, and the condition cannot be detected until after puberty. These patients are taller than normal and have wide hips and a female pubic hair distribution. About 50% have gynecomastia (development of female breasts), and intelligence levels are lower than normal in 10% of affected individuals. The penis appears normal, but the testes are smaller and harder than normal and lack seminiferous tubules. *Tall, wide hips, breast developing*

The maxilla is slightly hypoplastic (underdeveloped). Buccal smears reveal the presence of one Barr body. *←sternal*

Variations of Klinefelter's syndrome also occur and they are represented by karyotypes containing XXXY or XXXXY. The greater the number of X chromosomes, the more pronounced the clinical manifestations and the lower the level of intelligence.

↑ level of retardation.

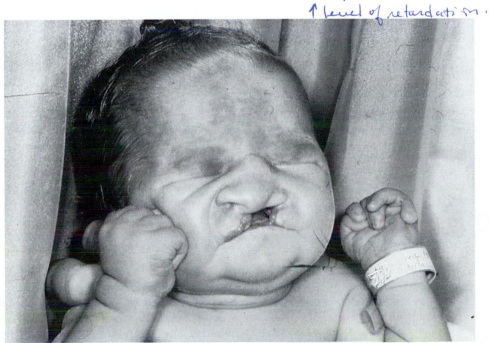

figure 6–12   Newborn with trisomy 13. Note cleft lip, frontal hemangioma, and abnormal position of fingers.

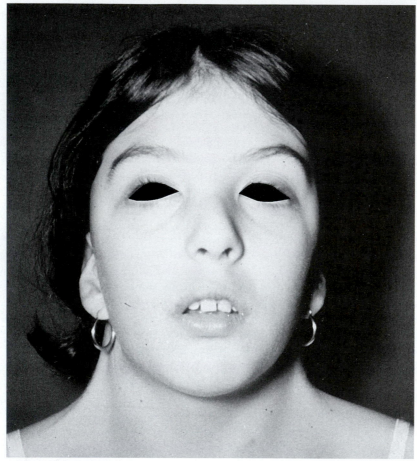

ƒ i g u r e 6–13   Patient with Turner's syndrome. Note webbing of the neck.

The maxilla becomes increasingly hypoplastic with increasing number of X chromosomes. Buccal smears show one Barr body for each extra X chromosome.

Cri du Chat (Cat-Cry) Syndrome and Wolf-Hirschhorn Syndrome. These syndromes are examples of abnormalities caused by deletions. The cri du chat syndrome results from a deletion on the short arm of chromosome 5, and the Wolf-Hirschhorn syndrome results from a deletion on the short arm of chromosome 4. Newborns with a chromosome 5 deletion exhibit a cat-like cry at birth and are mentally retarded. There are no oral abnormalities. Most newborns with the deletion in the short arm of chromosome 4 have a cleft palate and intelligence quotients of less than 30.

PATTERNS OF INHERITANCE

Because loci are present in both autosomal and X chromosomes and because of a double- and single-dose effect, there are four possible inheritance patterns. Dominant genes need only a single dose and recessive genes need a double dose. The inheritance patterns are (1) autosomal dominant, (2) autosomal recessive, (3) X-linked dominant, and (4) X-linked recessive. Autosomal chromosomes include all chromosomes except those that determine sex (X and Y). The Y chromosome participates only in the differentiation of the masculine gonads.

Autosomal Dominant Inheritance

A condition having autosomal dominant inheritance is transmitted vertically from one generation to the next. Males and females are equally affected. When a person has a gene for the condition, the risk of having an affected offspring is 50% for each pregnancy. Genetic risk is always a mathematical estimate of probability governed by chance. Therefore, none, less than half, half, more than half, or all of the offspring could be affected by a condition that is transmitted by autosomal dominant inheritance.

An individual can carry a gene with a dominant effect without presenting any clinical manifestations. This is referred to as **lack of penetrance.** This situation can be partially explained by the presence of modifying genes in the same or other chromosomes. The clinical manifestations in autosomal dominant disorders frequently vary among affected individuals. This is known as variable expressivity. **Penetrance** refers to the number of individuals affected, and **expressivity** pertains to the degree to which an individual is affected.

Autosomal Recessive Inheritance

As stated earlier, individuals manifesting an autosomal recessive trait must be homozygous for the gene. Clinically normal parents of affected children are heterozygous and are both carriers of the trait. They are not generally recognized as carriers until after the birth of an affected child. If the enzymatic defect is known, carriers can be recognized before the birth of a child by assessing levels of the responsible enzyme in clinically normal members of a family with the trait. For parents who are carriers of the same recessive trait, the risk of having an affected child is 25%; the risk of having a homozygotic normal child is 25%; and the chance of having a heterozygotic carrier is 50% for each pregnancy. As in other inheritance patterns, risk is a mathematical estimate of the probability of an event occurring. If both parents are homozygous (have two of the genes of the trait) for a recessive trait, they would be expected to be affected, and all their children would be equally affected because they would also be homozygous (have two of the same genes) for the trait. In humans this type of situation is quite rare because individuals affected by the same recessive trait usually do not mate.

In genetics, **consanguinity** means a familial relationship and is generally used to describe matings or marriages among close relatives, usually including first cousins. In the United States, marriage or mating among very close relatives (parent-offspring, brother-sister, uncle-niece, aunt-nephew) is illegal, and in most states marriage of first cousins is also illegal. However, consanguineous matings occur sporadically. The chances of having deleterious genes in common increases among close relatives. When there is consanguinity among the members of a family, the chance of the offspring being homozygous for a deleterious gene increases. The closer the degree of consanguinity, the greater the risk.

X-Linked Inheritance

Women have two X chromosomes and therefore can be either heterozygous or homozygous for a gene that is located on the X chromosome. In women, therefore, X-linked traits can be dominant or recessive. Men have only one X and one Y chromosome. If a deleterious gene occurs on the X chromosome in a male, the condition or trait will be seen clinically regardless of the dominant or recessive behavior of the same gene in women. The man's X chromosome is transmitted to all of his daughters and to none of his sons. The X chromosome in his sons comes from the mother. Consequently, there is no male-to-male (father-to-son) transmission of X-linked traits. Some X-linked dominant traits are lethal in males. Females probably survive because of the action of the allelic normal gene on the second X chromosome. All offspring, male and female, of a woman homozygotic for a dominant X-linked condition will be affected with the condition. This is because all her X chromosomes contain that gene, all offspring receive an X chromosome, and since the gene is dominant, only one of the genes is necessary for that condition to occur. A mother who is a carrier of an X-linked recessive trait has a 50% risk of having an affected son and a 50% risk of having a carrier daughter. This is because both daughters and sons have a 50% risk of getting the X chromosome with the gene for that condition. Again, remember that risk is a mathematic prediction. A male affected with an X-linked trait will have no affected sons, however, because he does not give the X chromosome to his sons. All his daughters will be carriers or affected, depending on the recessive or dominant nature of the trait, because all daughters will receive his X chromosome.

The Lyon Hypothesis and X-Linked Recessive Traits

As discussed previously, according to the Lyon hypothesis, one of the X chromosomes in the female is genetically cancelled at an early stage of embryonal development. This cancellation affects X chromosomes from both maternal and paternal lines. If a female embryo is a carrier of an X-linked recessive trait, half of the X chromosomes have the normal gene and the other half have the abnormal gene (allele) for the given trait before cancellation occurs. Classic hemophilia is a good example. Hemophilia is inherited as an X-linked recessive condition. In this disorder, blood does not coagulate because of the low or almost nonexistent levels of Factor VIII (antihemophilic globulin) in circulating blood. Males with the abnormal gene have a severe coagulation defect. In the female carrier, some of the cancelled X chromosomes have the abnormal gene, and others have the normal one. The female carrier is a **mosaic,** that is, she has both normal and abnormal X chromosomes. Because cancellation is random, the number of X chromosomes that remain genetically active and contain the normal or abnormal gene will vary. The female carrier's levels of Factor VIII are often reduced; however, this reduction and the length of coagulation time will vary, depending on the number of X chromosomes that contain the abnormal gene and remain genetically active. Although female carriers of the gene for hemophilia do not have as severe a problem as males, they tend to bleed more than usual after extraction of teeth or scaling and curettage. The variation in the bleeding problem in female carriers of the gene for hemophilia reflects the Lyon hypothesis. Other inherited disorders that reflect this hypothesis are described in detail later in this chapter. They include the X-linked type of amelogenesis imperfecta and hypohidrotic ectodermal dysplasia.

Genetic Heterogeneity

The term genetic heterogeneity is used when a condition has more than one inheritance pattern, as well as differences in the degree of clinical manifestations for each of the inherited varieties. Amelogenesis imperfecta (described further on) is a condition that illustrates genetic heterogeneity.

In general, alterations in structural proteins (complex substances formed by one or more polypeptide) are inherited as a dominant trait, whereas alterations in enzymatic proteins (a protein inducing changes in other body substances) are inherited in a recessive manner; however, there are exceptions to this rule.

Physical characteristics can be inherited either as dominant or as recessive traits. The term **recessive** does not mean deleterious or abnormal. It means instead that the individual must be homozygous for the trait for it to be seen. For example, in the ABO blood group system, blood group O is recessive, whereas groups A and B are dominant. However, no blood group is abnormal.

Genes can be codominant. Again, a good example is the ABO blood group. A and B are dominant over O, but when A and B are allelic, the result is blood group AB in which both genes are manifested. This is called **codominance.**

The four inheritance patterns refer to those characteristics that are governed by the action of one gene. This is called single-gene inheritance. **Oligogenic inheritance** refers to those characteristics or traits that are inherited by the participation of several genes. These conditions show greater clinical variation than do those inherited through single-gene action. Characteristics such as tooth shape and form, as well as eye color, are determined by oligogenic inheritance. Most physical characteristics are oligogenic. The various genes that participate in determining a trait or condition can be located in the same chromosome or in different chromosomes.

MOLECULAR CHROMOSOMAL ABNORMALITIES

All the inherited disorders in this section include oral and dental alterations and are discussed by location—gingiva and periodontium, jaw bones and facies, oral mucosa, and teeth. Patients affected with these genetic abnormalities should receive routine dental hygiene care to maintain oral health. Specific dental hygiene management considerations are included only if they are unique to the disorder described.

Inherited Disorders Affecting the Gingiva and Periodontium

Most of the disorders included here are rare. However, they are manifested by severe gingival or periodontal alterations, or both, and therefore the dental hygienist should be aware of them and their clinical manifestations.

Cyclic Neutropenia

The inheritance pattern of **cyclic neutropenia** is autosomal dominant. The disorder is characterized by a cyclic decrease in the number of circulating neutrophilic leukocytes (neutrophils); a decrease in the number of circulating neutrophils is called neutropenia. The cycles usually occur in intervals of 21 to 27 days, but in some patients the interval may be extended to several months. These episodes of neutropenia generally persist for 2 to 3 days.

The clinical manifestations are related to the decrease in neutrophils. Systemic manifestations of cyclic neutropenia include fever, malaise, sore throat, and occasional cutaneous infections. Oral manifestations consist of severe ulcerative gingivitis or gingivostomatitis (Fig. 6–14; Color Plate 86). In addition to the gingiva, areas of ulceration can also occur on the tongue and surfaces of the oral mucosa. The ulcers are of variable size and have a crater-like appearance. They are very painful and have a bleeding base. Generally, the oral lesions are secondarily infected. When neutrophils return to normal, the oral lesions tend to improve.

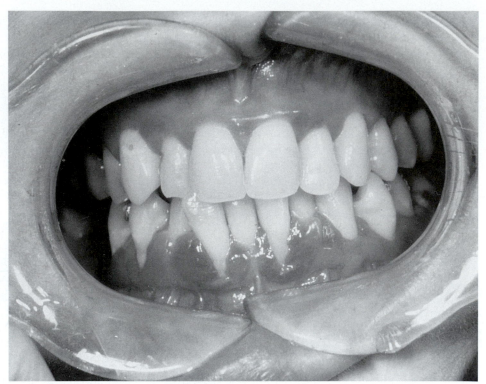

▪ *f i g u r e* 6–14   Marked hypertrophic gingivitis with areas of gingival recession in a patient with cyclic neutropenia.

Patients with cyclic neutropenia are usually managed by first determining the frequency of the cycles through periodic neutrophil counts and then by instituting preventive antibiotic therapy to protect against secondary opportunistic infections. Over time, episodes of neutropenia and associated ulcerative gingivitis lead to severe periodontal disease, with loss of alveolar bone, tooth mobility, and exfoliation of teeth. Treatment should be done when the circulating neutrophil count is normal in order to reduce the risk of complications such as gingival hemorrhage and secondary infection. Dental hygiene care, including frequent appointments for removal of local irritants and maintenance of optimal oral hygiene, reduces the risk of opportunistic infections in patients with cyclic neutropenia.

Papillon-Lefèvre Syndrome

The **Papillon-Lefèvre syndrome** has an autosomal recessive inheritance pattern and is composed of marked destruction of the periodontal tissues (periodontoclasia) of both dentitions with premature loss of teeth and hyperkeratosis of the palms of the hands and soles of the feet (palmar and plantar hyperkeratosis).

These patients are normal at birth except for a reddening of the palms of the hands and soles of the feet. Teeth erupt in normal sequence, position, and time. At about 1½ to 2 years of age, a marked gingivoperiodontal inflammatory process develops marked by edema, bleeding, alveolar bone resorption, and mobility of teeth with consequent exfoliation. A red, scaly keratosis develops on the palms and soles concurrent with these oral lesions and occasionally extends to the dorsal surfaces of the hands and feet. The oral lesions are complicated by superimposed inflammation, and radiographs reveal marked alveolar bone resorption with vertical pockets. Teeth are

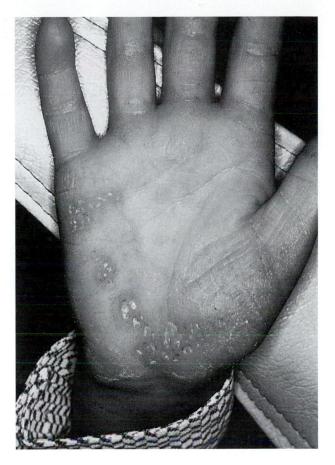

■ *f* i g u r e **6–15**
Areas of hyperkeratinization of the palms in
a patient with Papillon-Lefèvre syndrome.
(From Sedano HO, Sauk JJ, Gorlin RJ:
Oral Manifestations of Inherited Disorders.
Boston, Butterworth, 1977.)

lost in the same sequence in which they erupted. When the last tooth is lost, the
gingiva regains a normal appearance.

The lesions on the hands and feet remain as reddish-white, scaly, thick areas of
hyperkeratinization (Fig. 6–15). The permanent dentition begins to erupt at the proper
time. At about 8 or 9 years of age, the gingivoperiodontal destruction is repeated in
the same manner as occurred in the primary dentition (Fig. 6–16). All permanent teeth
are lost before age 14 years. The gingiva again resumes a normal appearance.

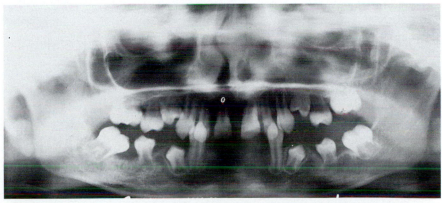

■ *f* i g u r e **6–16**   Panoramic radiograph showing marked periodontal destruction
with alveolar bone resorption in the patient in Figure 6–15. (From
Sedano HO, Sauk JJ, Gorlin RJ: Oral Manifestations of Inherited
Disorders. Boston, Butterworth, 1977.)

To date, all therapeutic attempts at preventing the gingival and periodontal destruction and subsequent loss of teeth have been unsuccessful. The basic defect that causes the condition is unknown. The skin manifestations remain for life, but treatment with retinol has proved somewhat effective in controlling the hyperkeratinization. These patients do not have any other abnormalities.

Focal Palmoplantar and Gingival Hyperkeratosis

Areas of hyperkeratinization of the palms and soles and marked hyperkeratinization of the labial and lingual gingiva characterize **focal palmoplantar and gingival hyperkeratosis.** This syndrome has an autosomal dominant inheritance pattern. The palmar and plantar hyperkeratosis starts at the tips of the fingers and toes and extends to the surface of the palms and soles. This process increases with age and also becomes localized, with calluses forming on the weight-bearing areas.

The oral hyperkeratinization is band-like and a few millimeters in width (Fig. 6–17). It follows the normal festooned contour of the gingiva. The free gingiva is not affected. Palatal and lingual mucosa can occasionally be affected with areas of hyperkeratinization. These changes start in childhood and increase with age. The rest of the oral cavity is normal.

Gingival Fibromatosis

Gingival fibromatosis is a component of several inherited syndromes. The gingival hypertrophy generally develops early in life, and within a few years the teeth are completely covered. The fibromatosis is composed of very firm tissue with a granular corrugated surface. The color is generally paler than that of the normal gingiva and

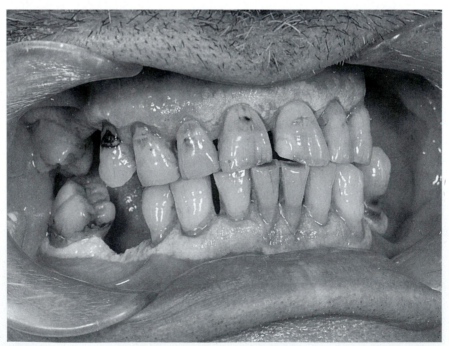

f i g u r e **6–17**   Marked hyperkeratosis following the normal contour of the gingiva in focal palmoplantar and gingival hyperkeratosis. (From Sedano HO, Sauk JJ, Gorlin RJ: Oral Manifestations of Inherited Disorders. Boston, Butterworth, 1977.)

results from the marked collagenization of the fibrous connective tissue. The extensive gingival enlargement leads to protrusion of the lips.

In addition to isolated gingival fibromatosis (Fig. 6–18), which has an autosomal dominant inheritance pattern and has no other associated abnormalities, gingival fibromatosis is a component of a number of syndromes. Because of the gingival involvement, several of these syndromes, though rare, are described here. However, only those that are well known and occur most frequently are included.

In patients with gingival fibromatosis, dental hygiene care can reduce the risk of secondary inflammation and infection.

Laband's Syndrome

The inheritance pattern of **Laband's syndrome** is autosomal dominant. In addition to gingival fibromatosis, the patients have dysplastic or absent nails and malformed nose and ears because of soft and pliable cartilage formation, hepatosplenomegaly (enlarged liver and spleen), and hypoplasia of terminal phalanges of the fingers and toes with a resultant frog-like appearance.

Gingival Fibromatosis with Hypertrichosis, Epilepsy, and Mental Retardation Syndrome

This syndrome has an autosomal dominant inheritance pattern. Hypertrichosis (excessive growth of hair), especially of the eyebrows, extremities, genitals, and sacral region, characterize gingival fibromatosis with hypertrichosis, epilepsy, and mental retardation. Epilepsy and mental retardation can also occur in this syndrome but are inconsistent features.

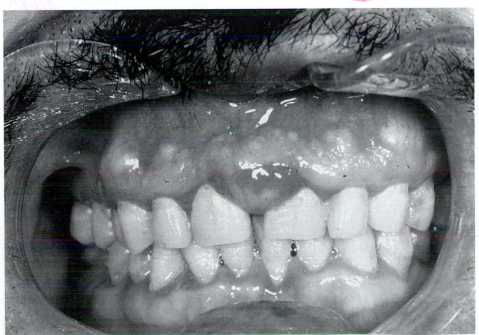

■ *figure* 6–18   Gingival hypertrophy in a patient with isolated gingival fibromatosis. (From Young WG, Sedano HO: Atlas of Oral Pathology. Minneapolis, MN, University of Minnesota Press, 1981.)

Gingival Fibromatosis with Multiple Hyaline Fibromas

Gingival fibromatosis with multiple hyaline fibromas has an autosomal dominant inheritance pattern and is also known as the Murray-Puretić-Drescher syndrome. In addition to gingival fibromatosis, it is characterized by hypertrophy of the nail beds and multiple hyaline fibrous tumors developing on the nose, chin, head, back, fingers, thighs, and legs. These tumors on the extremities can produce contractures of various joints, including hip, knee, shoulders, and elbows.

Inherited Disorders Affecting the Jaw Bones and Facies

Cherubism

The inheritance pattern of **cherubism** is autosomal dominant with marked penetrance (i.e., when the gene is present, the clinical manifestations are usually seen). The first clinical manifestation is a progressive bilateral facial swelling that appears when the patient is between 1½ and 4 years of age. This change can affect either the mandible or the maxilla, but involvement of the mandible is most common. Displacement of the eyes is evident when the maxilla is affected. This, added to the bilateral deformity, produces the characteristic cherubic facial appearance that is responsible for the name of the syndrome. Increased distance between the eyes (ocular hypertelorism) is always present in affected patients. Radiographs of the jaws show a typical "soap-bubble" or multilocular appearance (Fig. 6–19), which usually occupies the ascending ramus of the mandible and extends into the molar-premolar area. Severe cases can involve the full mandible, but the condyle is always spared. When the maxilla is affected, the changes are observed at the level of the tuberosity and involve the antrum.

These areas of bone radiolucency are occupied by fibrous connective tissue containing multinucleated giant cells. The microscopic appearance resembles the central giant cell granuloma (described in Chapter 2). The bone lesions interfere with tooth

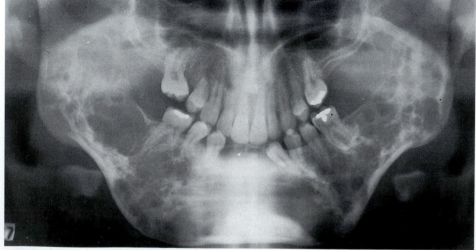

ƒigure 6–19   Panoramic radiograph of the jaws showing typical bilateral "soap-bubble" image in a patient with cherubism. (From Young WG, Sedano HO: Atlas of Oral Pathology. Minneapolis, MN, University of Minnesota Press, 1981.)

development and eruption. Most of these patients have **pseudoanodontia** (teeth falsely appear to be lacking), especially of molars and premolars, because of delayed eruption.

The size of the jaws tends to increase rapidly until about puberty and then generally remains stable. After the individual reaches age 20 or 30 years, radiographs show an almost normal bone appearance, with a few areas of increased bone density. The facial deformity remains for life, and in some patients it can be quite striking.

Chondroectodermal Dysplasia

Chondroectodermal dysplasia, also known as the **Ellis–van Creveld syndrome,** has an autosomal recessive inheritance pattern. Affected individuals are dwarfs because of distal shortening of the extremities. One third of these patients are mildly retarded. The hands show polydactyly (supernumerary digits) on the ulnar side, and fingernails and toenails are hypoplastic and deformed. Other skeletal anomalies include curvature of the legs and feet. Fifty percent of affected individuals have congenital heart defects. Anomalies of the external genitals, especially in males, are also observed.

The oral manifestations are constant and characteristic and include fusion of the anterior portion of the maxillary gingiva to the upper lip from canine to canine. The anterior maxillary vestibular sulcus is thus lacking (Fig. 6–20). This anomaly induces a V-notch appearance in the midline of the upper lip. The anterior lower alveolar ridge presents a serrated appearance caused by thick frenula, which start at the vestibular sulcus and traverse the alveolar ridge. The central incisors of both maxilla and mandible

NATAL Teeth (extraction)

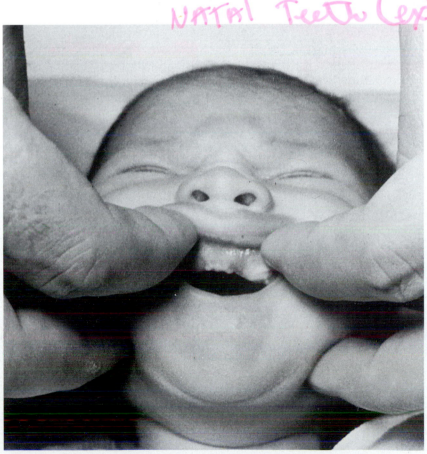

f i g u r e **6–20**   Infant with Ellis-van Creveld syndrome (chondroectodermal dysplasia). The anterior maxillary vestibular sulcus is absent.

are generally lacking and are replaced by a centrally located abnormal tooth. Most of the teeth have a conical shape and exhibit enamel hypoplasia. More than 50% of newborns with this syndrome have natal teeth.

Cleidocranial Dysplasia

The inheritance pattern of **cleidocranial dysplasia** is autosomal dominant; however, about half the cases are isolated examples due to either spontaneous mutation or a gene with poor penetrance. The cranium develops a mushroom shape because the fontanelles remain open. This makes the face appear small. Frontal, parietal, and occipital enlargement is quite noticeable. Skull radiographs reveal the open fontanelles, which are often open for life. The paranasal sinuses are lacking or hypoplastic. The neck is long and narrow because of unilateral or bilateral aplasia (lack of development) or hypoplasia of the clavicles. Affected individuals are able to approximate their shoulders to the midline because of this clavicular alteration. Various other bone anomalies can also be present.

The premaxilla is generally underdeveloped, resulting in pseudoprognathism. These patients have many supernumerary teeth, sometimes even simulating a third dentition (Fig. 6–21). These teeth are crowded in the jaws and do not erupt. They also interfere with the eruption of normal teeth, resulting in pseudoanodontia. A lack of cellular cementum has been reported in patients with this syndrome. Multiple cysts can develop in association with the impacted teeth. About 1% of affected patients have cleft lip, cleft palate, or both.

Gardner's Syndrome

Gardner's syndrome, also known as **intestinal polyposis III,** has an autosomal dominant inheritance pattern with variable expressivity and marked penetrance. One

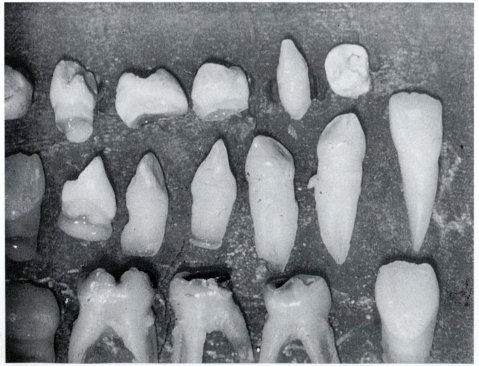

figure **6–21**   Multiple extracted supernumerary teeth from a patient with cleidocranial dysplasia.

of the basic components is the presence of osteomas in various bones, especially the frontal bones, mandible, and maxilla. Osteomas of the facial skeleton, when expanding, will obliterate the sinuses and induce facial asymmetry. Osteomas also can occur in the long bones of the skeleton but with less frequency than in the bones of the face.

In addition to osteomas, multiple odontomas can occur in the jaw bones, especially the mandible (Fig. 6–22). Teeth can exhibit hypercementosis and can fail to erupt.

The most serious component of this syndrome is the presence of intestinal polyps, which become malignant at age 30 and after. Polyposis primarily affects the colon and rectum and generally develops before puberty. Some authors advocate intestinal resection when the polyps appear because their malignant transformation into adenocarcinoma is invariable, especially with increasing age.

Mandibulofacial Dysostosis

The inheritance pattern of **mandibulofacial dysostosis** is autosomal dominant with incomplete penetrance and variable expressivity. The facies shows downward sloping of the palpebral fissures, a hypoplastic nose, hypoplastic malar bones with hypoplasia or absence of the zygomatic process, abnormal and misplaced ears, and a receding chin. The mouth appears "fish-like" with downward sloping of the lip commissures. The lower eyelids show a cleft (coloboma) of the outer third with a lack of lashes medial to it. The ears may exhibit tags, which on occasion can also be seen near the angle of the mouth. Deafness is a constant feature resulting from a lack of otic ossicles. Mental development is within normal limits; difficulty in learning arises from deafness.

Oral manifestations include a markedly hypoplastic mandible with flattened condyles and coronoid processes and an obtuse mandibular angle. Teeth are malposed, and malocclusion with open bite is quite evident. The palate is high or a cleft is present in about 30% of affected patients (Fig. 6–23). Gingival disease is common and is related to the dental abnormalities.

Nevoid Basal Cell Carcinoma Syndrome

The **nevoid basal cell carcinoma syndrome**, also known as **Gorlin's syndrome**, has an autosomal dominant inheritance pattern with high penetrance and variable expressivity. The facies is characterized by mild hypertelorism (increased distance

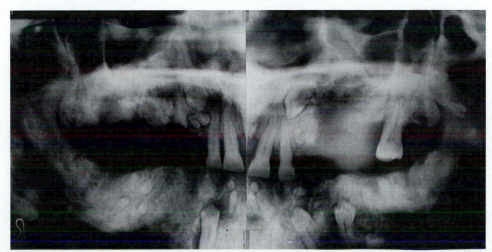

▪ *f i g u r e* **6-22**   Panoramic radiograph of a patient with Gardner's syndrome showing multiple osteomas and odontomas. (Courtesy of Dr. Carl J. Witkop.)

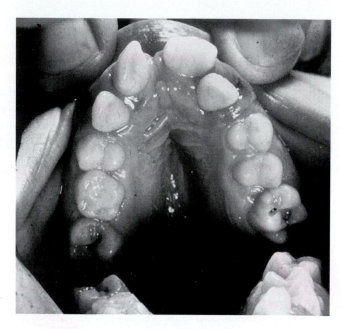

■ *f* i g u r e **6–23**
Markedly high-arched palate and malpositioned teeth in a patient with mandibulofacial dysostosis.

between the eyes) and mild prognathism, with frontal and parietal enlargement and a broad nasal root.

The cutaneous manifestations, which are called nevi, are typically basal cell carcinomas. The term nevus (plural, nevi), as defined here, is a congenital lesion characterized by skin pigmentation. These basal cell carcinomas appear early in life and continue to develop over the nose, eyelids, cheeks, neck, arms, and trunk. They can be flesh colored or pale brown and develop singly or in clusters. Histologically, they are basal cell carcinomas. The palms and soles show small pits that become filled with dirt and appear as dark spots on those surfaces.

The oral manifestations of this syndrome consist of multiple cysts of the jaws (Fig. 6–24), which histologically are odontogenic keratocysts (see Chapter 4). These cysts vary in size; they can be very large and have a marked tendency to recur after surgical removal. Occasionally, an ameloblastoma arises in these cysts as part of this syndrome.

nevoid basal cell carcinoma

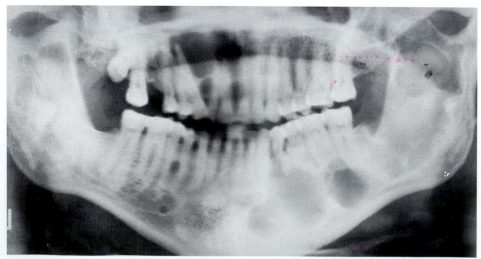

■ *f* i g u r e **6–24**   Multiple mandibular radiolucencies in a patient with nevoid basal cell carcinoma syndrome. These lesions are odontogenic keratocysts.

The cysts develop as early as 5 to 6 years of age in some affected patients and interfere with normal development of the jaw bones and teeth.

A great variety of skeletal anomalies have been reported in association with the nevoid basal cell carcinoma syndrome, the most constant being bifurcation or splaying of one or more ribs. Other frequent abnormalities of bone include shortening of the metacarpals, spina bifida occulta (defective closure of the bone encasement of the spinal cord), and kyphoscoliosis (a combination of scoliosis, which is a lateral curving of the spine, and kyphosis, which is an abnormal vertical curvature of the spine or "hunchback").

Many different neoplasms have been reported in association with this syndrome. Medulloblastoma (brain tumor) has been seen in many cases. Children surviving the medulloblastoma eventually present other manifestations of the syndrome. Other, less frequent findings include calcified ovarian fibromas and mesenteric cysts.

Osteogenesis Imperfecta

Type I

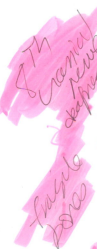

Osteogenesis imperfecta is known to have an autosomal dominant inheritance pattern with variable expressivity. However, only 30% of patients have a family history of this condition. The remaining 70% represent sporadic cases and cases suggesting autosomal recessive inheritance. The clinical manifestations are markedly variable from patient to patient. The sporadic cases tend to be more severe than those with an autosomal dominant inheritance pattern. The basic defect involves collagen and results in abnormally formed bones that fracture easily. Multiple bone fractures are the main clinical complication of this syndrome. In the congenital form, newborns can present with several fractured bones at birth. Infants with this condition have experienced fractures just by being moved. In the most severe cases, all bones can be affected, presenting a plethora of abnormalities, including bowing of the legs, curvature of the spine (kyphosis and scoliosis), deformity of the skull, shortening of arms and legs, and other abnormalities. In the mildest cases, individuals show only blue sclerae (a blue appearance of the white of the eye).

The oral manifestation of this syndrome is a dentinogenesis imperfecta–like condition (a description of dentinogenesis imperfecta follows later in this chapter). Primary teeth are affected in 80% of patients, whereas permanent teeth are affected in only 35% of these individuals (Fig. 6–25). The crowns, roots, and pulp chambers are generally smaller than normal. Teeth appear opalescent or translucent at time of eruption, but they darken with age. The enamel is lost because the abnormal dentin cannot provide adequate support.

Torus Mandibularis

Mandibular tori (singular, torus) have an autosomal dominant inheritance pattern with variable expressivity and marked penetrance. This anomaly can be unilateral or bilateral. These tori occur on the lingual aspect of the mandible at the level of the premolar teeth (Fig. 6–26; Color Plate 53). Occurrence before age 15 years is extremely rare. The size of the torus is variable, and occasionally it can be multilobulated. Mandibular tori are symptomless and generally require no treatment. Surgical removal may be necessary if the patient needs a denture. Intraoral radiographs usually show a radiopacity in the area of the mandibular premolars if mandibular tori are present. (Mandibular tori are also discussed in Chapters 1 and 5.)

Torus Palatinus

Autosomal dominance with variable expressivity and almost 100% penetrance characterizes torus palatinus. A bony overgrowth occurs at the midline of the hard

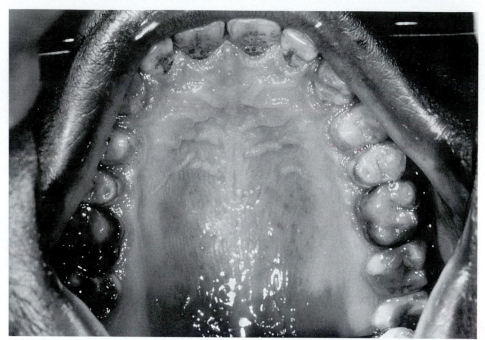

▪ *f* i g u r e **6–25**   Patient with osteogenesis imperfecta. Teeth are yellowish with chipped
enamel.

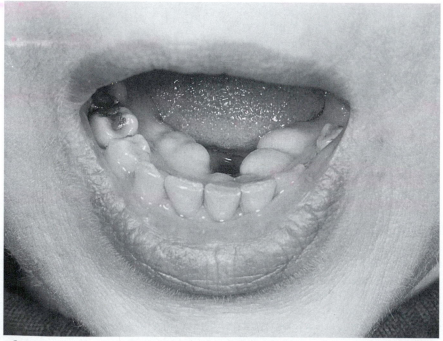

▪ *f* i g u r e **6–26**   Bilateral mandibular tori. (From Sedano HO, Sauk JJ, Gorlin RJ:
Oral Manifestations of Inherited Disorders. Butterworth, Boston,
1977.)

palate (Fig. 6–27; Color Plate 61). There is a marked predilection for women (2:1) and a higher prevalence among Native Americans, including Eskimos. Torus palatinus becomes evident around the time of puberty and is only rarely seen in children younger than 14 years of age. The size of this anomaly varies from nearly undetectable to large masses that occupy almost the entire hard palate. Some palatal tori are multilobular. Torus palatinus is symptomless. However, the surface mucosa is thin and easily traumatized. The torus may need to be removed if the patient needs a full denture. (Torus palatinus is also described in Chapters 1 and 5.)

Maxillary Exostosis

Exostoses have an autosomal dominant inheritance pattern. **Maxillary exostoses** represent tori that generally develop on the buccal aspect of the maxillary alveolar ridge, usually in the molar-premolar area (Fig. 6–28; Color Plate 75). They are generally symptomless unless traumatized. They may be single, multiple, unilateral, and bilateral and occur less frequently than either palatal or mandibular tori. (Exostoses are also described in Chapters 1 and 5.)

Inherited Disorders Affecting the Oral Mucosa

Isolated Cleft Palate and Cleft Lip With or Without Cleft Palate

The majority of cases of facial clefting are multifactorial in origin; they occur in about 1 in 800 births. A large number of inherited syndromes can include cleft lip and palate or isolated cleft palate as a component. When clefting is part of an inherited syndrome, its occurrence within affected families will be in accordance with the inheritance pattern of the syndrome. The majority of these syndromes are very rare.

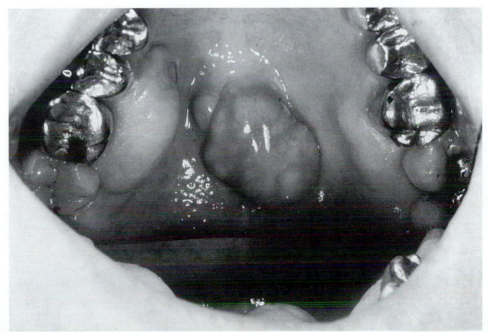

▪ *figure* 6–27 Torus palatinus.

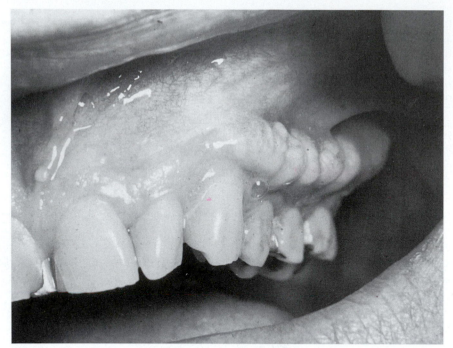

■ *figure* **6–28**   Maxillary exostoses are inherited as autosomal dominant. (From Sedano HO, Sauk JJ, Gorlin RJ: Oral Manifestations of Inherited Disorders. Boston, Butterworth, 1977.)

[handwritten: had potential for cleft]

Cleft lip-palate and congenital lip pits is the syndrome that is considered to occur most frequently and so is the only one described here. It has an autosomal dominant inheritance pattern with 80% penetrance for any of its components. The labial pits (Fig. 6–29) are bilateral and are located near the midline of the vermilion border of

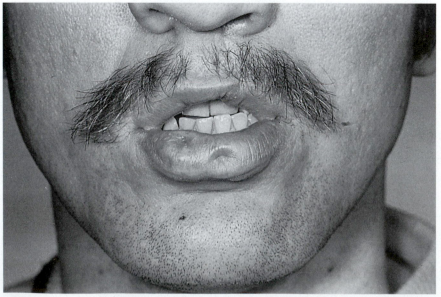

■ *figure* **6–29**   Paramedial pits in the lower lip and a scar in the upper lip resulting from correction of cleft lip. The mother of this patient was similarly affected.

the lower lip. They may be 3 mm or more in diameter and generally finish in a blind end. Occasionally, they exude saliva because of their association with a minor labial salivary gland. These pits are rarely unilateral, and the clefting is bilateral in about 80% of patients. Some patients without clefting have agenesis (lack of development) of the maxillary lateral incisors or peg lateral incisors. Other oral findings that have been seen include fibrous adhesions between the maxilla and mandible, a cleft uvula, and ankyloglossia.

Hereditary Hemorrhagic Telangiectasia

The inheritance pattern of **hereditary hemorrhagic telangiectasia,** also known as **Osler-Rendu-Parkes Weber syndrome,** is autosomal dominant. It is characterized by multiple capillary dilations of the skin and mucous membranes (Fig. 6–30). The skin of the face shows numerous pinpoint and spider-like telangiectases, especially on the lips, eyelids, and around the nose. The scalp and ears are also affected. Similar lesions are present in the nasal mucosa and are responsible for frequent and sometimes serious nosebleeds **(epistaxis)** that can last for several days. Any organ, as well as other mucous membranes, can be the site of telangiectasia.

Telangiectases of the oral mucosa are especially prominent on the tip and anterior dorsum of the tongue. The palate, gingiva, and buccal mucosa are often affected but to a lesser degree. Hemorrhage from sites in the oral cavity, mainly the lips and tongue, is second in frequency to epistaxis. Gingival bleeding has been reported and is a possible complication of dental hygiene treatment. The risk of gingival hemorrhage should be a concern of the dental hygienist when treating a patient with this syndrome.

Multiple Mucosal Neuroma Syndrome

The combination of **multiple mucosal neuromas, medullary carcinoma of the thyroid gland,** and **pheochromocytoma** is also called **multiple endocrine neoplasia,**

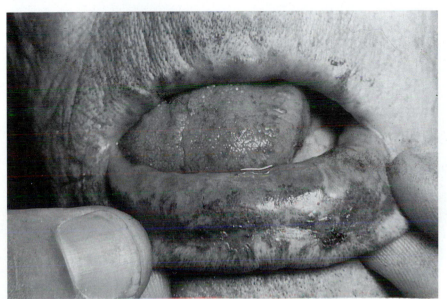

■ *f* i g u r e 6–30   Multiple telangiectases of lips and tongue in a patient with hereditary hemorrhagic telangiectasia. Gingival bleeding can be profuse in cases like this. (From Sedano HO, Sauk JJ, Gorlin RJ: Oral Manifestations of Inherited Disorders. Boston, Butterworth, 1977.)

Tall — keratinized, night sweating, hypertension, div

type 2B (MEN 2B). The inheritance pattern is autosomal dominant with decreased penetrance. Patients are tall with characteristic thick, large lips and, often, everted upper eyelids. The mucosal neuromas are prominent on the lips and the anterior dorsal surface of the tongue (Fig. 6–31). They generally appear in the first few years of life. Additionally, neuromas can occur on the buccal mucosa and also on the eyelids. The mucosal neuromas are seen as multiple, mobile, firm lumps covered by normal mucosa. Histologically, they are aggregates of nerve tissue.

Medullary carcinoma of the thyroid has been diagnosed in greater than 75% of patients with this syndrome; it generally develops in the second decade of life. Metastatic lesions develop frequently, and about 20% of patients die as a consequence of metastasis. The thyroid carcinoma produces calcitonin (a hormone normally produced by the C cells of the thyroid gland). The carcinoma can be detected by evaluating plasma levels of this hormone.

Pheochromocytoma is a benign neoplasm that generally develops in ganglia around the adrenal glands. The tumor is often bilateral and is responsible for night sweats, high blood pressure, and episodes of severe diarrhea. It generally develops in the second or third decade of life. The pheochromocytoma induces increased urinary levels of epinephrine and other substances. Other findings in this syndrome have included cutaneous pigmentation and a host of skeletal abnormalities.

Early diagnosis of this syndrome is imperative because of the high malignant potential of the thyroid carcinoma. Some authors recommend preventive thyroidectomy when this syndrome is diagnosed so that the development of carcinoma is avoided. The neuromas of the oral mucosa may be the earliest visible manifestation of this syndrome.

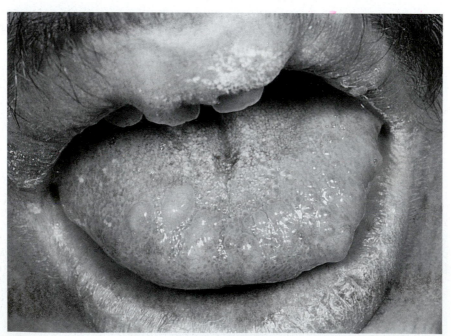

f i g u r e **6–31**   Patient with MEN 2B syndrome presenting with multiple mucosal neuromas on the tip of the tongue and upper lip. (From Sedano HO, Sauk JJ, Gorlin RJ: Oral Manifestations of Inherited Disorders. Boston, Butterworth, 1977.)

Neurofibromatosis of von Recklinghausen

Neurofibromatosis of von Recklinghausen, also called **Recklinghausen's disease,** has an autosomal dominant inheritance pattern and is probably a disorder of neural crest origin. There are several varieties. Only the classic form is described here.

Multiple neurofibromas, which appear as papules and growths of various sizes, are seen on the facial skin, especially the eyelids. The tumors can arise anywhere, including the oral cavity, and can be present at birth or develop early in life, increasing in number and size at puberty. Malignant transformation of the neurofibromas occurs in an estimated 3% to 15% of patients with neurofibromatosis. Neurofibromas also develop in the central nervous system, eyes, ears, viscera, and intraosseous locations. Mental retardation is occasionally observed, and multiple skeletal anomalies are common.

Oral involvement is seen in about 10% of patients and is characterized by single or multiple tumors at any location in the oral mucosa, the most frequent being the lateral borders of the tongue. Gingival neurofibromas can also occur in these patients (Fig. 6–32). Intramandibular neurofibromas have also been reported and present as radiolucencies in the mandible.

Café au lait (the color of coffee with milk) pigmentation of skin is present from the first decade of life in 90% of patients with neurofibromatosis. This pigmentation is quite marked in the axilla and can also affect other areas of the skin. Café au lait skin pigmentation generally precedes the development of the neurofibromas.

Peutz-Jeghers Syndrome

Autosomal dominant inheritance characterizes the **Peutz-Jeghers syndrome.** It consists of multiple melanotic macular pigmentations of the skin and mucosa, which are associated with gastrointestinal polyposis. The pigmentations occur around the eyes, nose, and mouth (Fig. 6–33). These macules are a few millimeters in diameter and vary in number and degree of pigmentation. They tend to diminish with age.

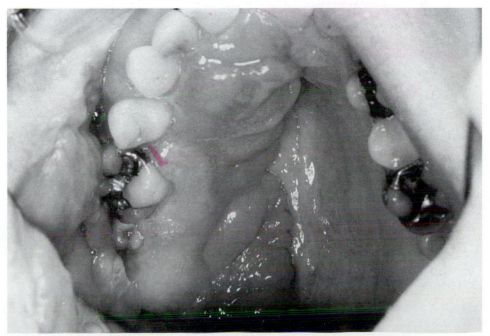

ƒ i g u r e 6-32   Multiple neurofibromas of the maxillary gingiva and palate in a patient with neurofibromatosis of von Recklinghausen.

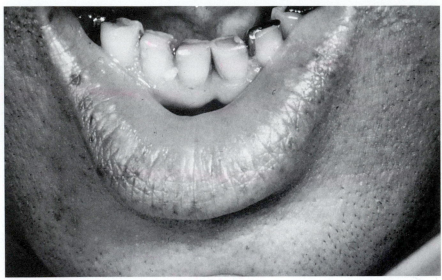

▪ *f i g u r e* 6–33   Multiple small- to medium-sized pigmented macules on the lip and perioral skin of a patient with Peutz-Jeghers syndrome. (From Young WG, Sedano HO: Atlas of Oral Pathology. Minneapolis, MN, University of Minnesota Press, 1981.)

Intraorally, larger areas of pigmentation are observed on the lips and buccal mucosa of about 98% of affected patients.

Pigmentation of the hands, nasal mucosa, and eyes can also occur. The intestinal polyps are hamartomas (an abnormal growth of normal tissue in its normal location). They develop mostly in the small intestine; only rarely do they undergo malignant transformation.

White Sponge Nevus

Autosomal dominant inheritance with complete penetrance characterizes **white sponge nevus** (Cannon's disease, or familial white folded mucosal dysplasia). The disorder can be present at birth or develop around puberty. Clinically, it is characterized by a white, corrugated, soft, folding oral mucosa (Color Plate 30). The buccal mucosa is always affected, and in most patients the lesions are bilateral. The whitening is produced by a thick layer of keratin, which at times desquamates and leaves a raw mucosal surface. Other areas of the oral mucosa can also be affected, but the free gingiva is spared.

Inherited Disorders Affecting the Teeth

Amelogenesis Imperfecta

A group of inherited conditions affecting the enamel of teeth and having no associated systemic defects characterizes **amelogenesis imperfecta.** Witkop and Sauk classified amelogenesis imperfecta into four types:

- Type I: Hypoplastic amelogenesis imperfecta
- Type II: Hypocalcified amelogenesis imperfecta
- Type III: Hypomaturation amelogenesis imperfecta
- Type IV: Hypoplastic-hypomaturation amelogenesis imperfecta

The **hypoplastic type** of amelogenesis imperfecta is characterized by tooth enamel that does not develop to a normal thickness because of failure of the ameloblasts to lay down enamel matrix properly. On radiographs, the abnormal enamel contrasts normally with dentin. There are seven varieties of this type of amelogenesis imperfecta that are further classified according to their clinical presentation: pitted, local, smooth, rough, and enamel agenesis. Combined with the clinical appearance, the classification also includes the inheritance pattern. Thus, there is an autosomal dominant and an autosomal recessive variety for the local hypoplastic type. Among this group of enamel defects, the most frequent one is the pitted autosomal dominant variety (Fig. 6–34; Color Plate 95), which is characterized by teeth that have random pits on the enamel. The size of these pits varies from pinpoint to pinhead, and the pits are observed mostly on the labial and buccal surfaces of the permanent teeth. The pits are frequently arranged in rows or columns, or both. Occasionally, more than one tooth has a normal clinical appearance.

The **hypocalcified type** of amelogenesis imperfecta (Fig. 6–35) is characterized by an enamel of normal thickness that is poorly calcified. There are two varieties of hypocalcified amelogenesis imperfecta: one is autosomal dominant and the other is autosomal recessive. The autosomal recessive pattern is more severe in its clinical manifestations. At eruption, teeth present a yellow to orange enamel that is very soft and rapidly lost, leaving exposed dentin. On radiographs, the enamel has a "moth-eaten" appearance and is less radiopaque than dentin. Cervical enamel is better calcified and generally remains on the crown. This type of amelogenesis imperfecta is frequently associated with an anterior open bite.

The **hypomaturation type** of amelogenesis imperfecta is characterized by an enamel of mottled appearance but normal thickness. This type of amelogenesis imperfecta is composed of large amounts of enamel matrix, and therefore the enamel is softer than normal. With pressure, the tip of an explorer will penetrate the enamel. The basic

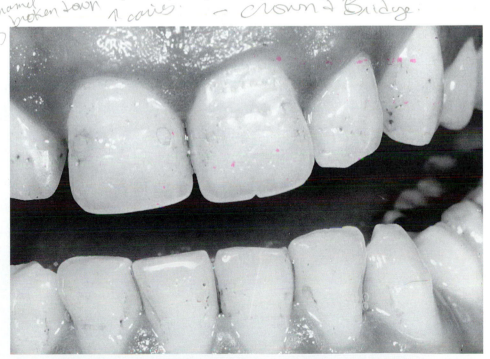

𝑓 i g u r e 6–34   Pitted autosomal dominant amelogenesis imperfecta. Note the multiple pits on the labial surface of the teeth. Some of the pits have been filled with composite. (From Young WG, Sedano HO: Atlas of Oral Pathology. Minneapolis, MN, University of Minnesota Press, 1981.)

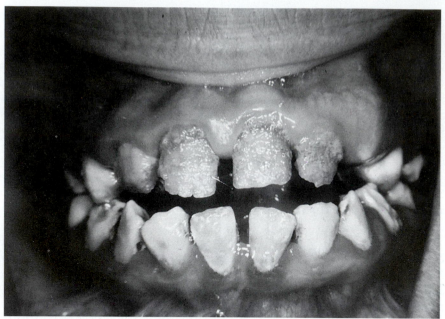

figure 6-35   Note loss of enamel in these teeth in a patient with hypocalcified amelogenesis imperfecta. (Courtesy of Dr. Carl J. Witkop.)

defect seems to be in the enamel rod sheath. The enamel chips easily from the crown. On radiographs, it has almost the same radiodensity as dentin. There are four varieties of the hypomaturation type of amelogenesis imperfecta. Only the snowcapped type is discussed here.

A type of hypomaturation amelogenesis imperfecta called **snow-capped amelo-**

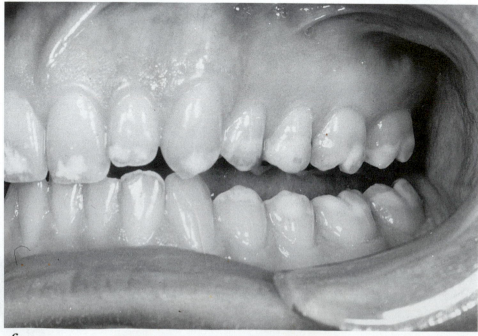

figure 6-36   Note the uniform whitening of incisal edges and occlusal cusps in a case of snowcapped amelogenesis imperfecta.

genesis imperfecta apparently has an X-linked recessive inheritance pattern in some families and an autosomal dominant pattern in others. Clinically, both varieties are identical and are characterized by a hypomaturation of the surface enamel of the occlusal third of all the teeth of both dentitions. The maxillary teeth are more severely affected with this whitish discoloration (Fig. 6–36). The enamel in those areas is of regular hardness and smooth. It does not fracture or chip from the crown.

The **hypoplastic-hypomaturation type** of amelogenesis imperfecta is characterized by its association with taurodontic teeth (described later in this chapter and also in Chapter 4). The thin enamel is yellow to brown and pitted. On radiographs, the enamel has a radiodensity similar to dentin, and single-rooted teeth have large pulp chambers.

Dentinogenesis Imperfecta

Dentinogenesis imperfecta is usually subdivided into three types. One type is dentinogenesis imperfecta associated with osteogenesis imperfecta (previously described in this chapter). The other two types are not associated with osteogenesis imperfecta. The teeth in all three types have a similar clinical appearance.

Dentinogenesis imperfecta type II is also known as hereditary opalescent dentin. The inheritance pattern is autosomal dominant. Teeth have bulbous crowns with a color that varies from opalescent brown to brownish blue (Fig. 6–37; Color Plate 96). The primary teeth are usually affected more severely than the permanent teeth. Twenty percent of patients present with enamel hypoplasia as well. The dentin is very soft, which produces chipping of enamel that results in tooth attrition. Occasionally, this

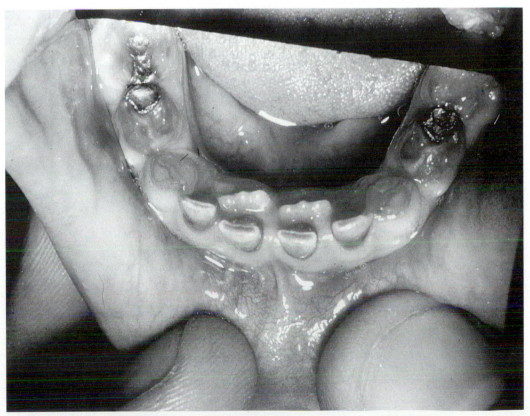

f i g u r e 6–37   Opalescent bluish hue in the anterior teeth typical of dentinogenesis imperfecta. The yellow color seen in the molars is from exposed abnormal dentin due to loss of enamel.

attrition can cause the teeth to be worn down to the alveolar process. Radiographically, no pulp chambers or root canals are seen (Fig. 6–38). Roots are short and thin with periapical radiolucencies. Patients may lose teeth prematurely because of complications produced by the attrition and the short roots. The basic defect lies with the odontoblasts, which lay down an abnormal matrix and then degenerate. These odontoblasts are later replaced by cells derived from the dental pulp, which lay down abnormal dentin.

Dentin Dysplasia

Dentin dysplasia is subdivided into type I, radicular dentin dysplasia, and type II, coronal dentin dysplasia.

Radicular Dentin Dysplasia. This condition, which has an autosomal dominant inheritance pattern, is characterized by teeth with normal crowns and abnormal roots. The basic defect seems to lie in a disturbance in the epithelial root sheath of Hertwig, which guides the formation of the root. Radiographs show total or partial lack of pulp chambers and root canals (Fig. 6–39). Primary and secondary dentitions are affected equally. The color of the teeth is normal. Because of the short roots, the teeth are generally exfoliated prematurely, especially in the event of even minor trauma. The pulp chambers of the permanent teeth generally are not obliterated fully and have a half-moon appearance on the radiograph. Occasionally, periapical cysts can be associated with this condition.

Coronal Dentin Dysplasia. Dentin dysplasia type II has an autosomal dominant inheritance pattern. The basic defect in this condition is unknown. The primary dentition is characterized by translucent teeth with an amber color. Radiographs show a lack of pulp chambers and small root canals. Primary teeth are quite similar to those observed in dentinogenesis imperfecta. Permanent teeth present normal crown formation with normal color. Radiographs show "thistle-shaped" pulp chambers in single-rooted teeth and a "bow-tie" appearance of the pulp chambers of permanent molars (Fig. 6–40). Permanent teeth may or may not have pulp stones.

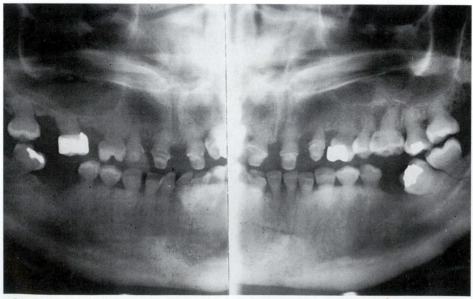

■ *figure 6–38*   Panoramic radiograph of a patient with dentinogenesis imperfecta showing marked short roots and almost complete lack of pulp chambers. (From Young WG, Sedano HO: Atlas of Oral Pathology. Minneapolis, MN, University of Minnesota Press, 1981.)

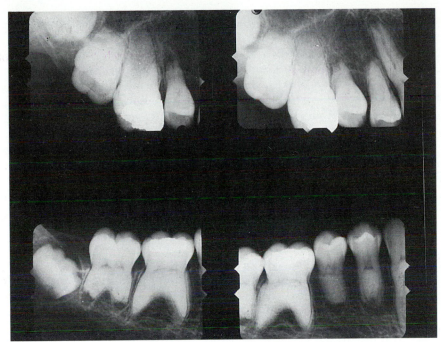

= *f* i g u r e **6–39** Radiographs of a patient with radicular dentin dysplasia showing blunted and short tooth roots. Note that the few remaining pulp chambers have a half-moon appearance. (Courtesy of Dr. Carl J. Witkop.)

Hypohidrotic Ectodermal Dysplasia. This syndrome usually has an X-linked recessive inheritance pattern. However, affected females have been reported. In these cases, there has been parental consanguinity, suggesting autosomal recessive inheritance. The syndrome has genetic heterogeneity. The clinical manifestations for both the X-linked and autosomal recessive forms are identical.

This entity represents the most severe form of ectodermal dysplasia. Its major components are hypodontia (partial anodontia), hypotrichosis (less than the normal amount of hair), and hypohidrosis (abnormally diminished secretion of sweat). Affected children are born without lanugo (body hair present at birth), and many have episodes of "fevers of unknown cause" because of the almost complete lack of sweat glands. Some patients die of hyperthermia (greatly increased body temperature) after prolonged

die from hyperthermia

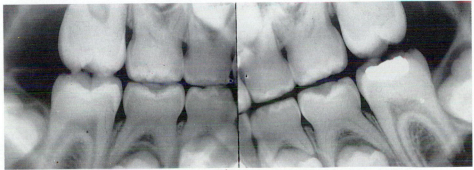

= *f* i g u r e **6–40** Note obliteration and partial lack of coronal pulp chambers and small root canals in these teeth in a patient affected with coronal dentin dysplasia. (Courtesy of Dr. Carl J. Witkop.)

exposure to the sun or heavy exercise. The clinical characteristics may not be apparent until the second year of life.

The facies is quite typical, with marked frontal bossing, depressed nasal bridge (saddle nose), protuberant lips, and almost complete lack of scalp hair. The hair that is present is usually blond, short, fine, and stiff. The skin is soft, thin, and very dry. Sebaceous glands are also lacking. Linear wrinkles and increased pigmentation are seen around the eyes and mouth. The eyelashes and eyebrows are often missing entirely. After puberty, the beard is generally normal, but axillary and pubic hair is scanty.

The oral manifestations of hypohidrotic ectodermal dysplasia consist of hypodontia or, rarely, anodontia. When present, incisors and canines have small, conical crowns (Fig. 6–41). The alveolar bone is formed only when teeth are present, and therefore patients lacking alveolar processes have loss of vertical dimension with markedly protruding lips. There may also be partial lack and aplasia of minor salivary glands in the buccal, labial, and lower respiratory tract mucosa.

Female carriers of the X-linked form of hypohidrotic ectodermal dysplasia have minor clinical manifestations, such as thin and slightly sparse hair, cone-shaped teeth, hypodontia, and variable degrees of reduced sweating. This is in accordance with the Lyon hypothesis of variability of expression.

Hypophosphatasia. The inheritance pattern of this disorder is autosomal recessive. The basic defect in this condition is a decrease in serum alkaline phosphatase levels with increased urinary and plasma levels of phosphoethanolamine. Alkaline phosphatase participates in the process of calcification of bone and cementum; therefore, those two tissues will be altered in patients with hypophosphatasia. Agenesis or abnormal formation of cementum in these patients leads to spontaneous premature

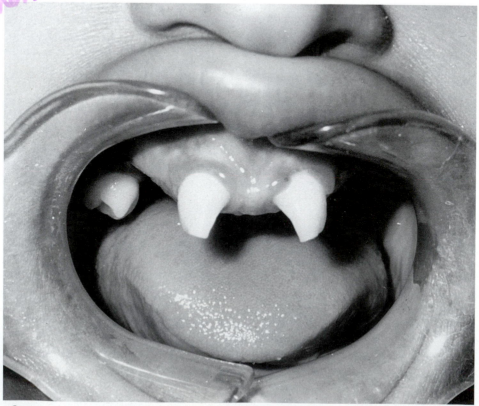

■ *figure* **6–41**   This patient with hypohidrotic ectodermal dysplasia has only three abnormally shaped teeth. Note also marked dryness of skin.

shedding of primary teeth, especially mandibular incisors (Fig. 6–42). Teeth are exfoliated without evidence of periodontal or gingival disease. The primary molars, as well as permanent teeth, are rarely if ever affected, which is probably associated with the greater mechanical fixation resulting from the larger size of their roots. The total lack of cementum observed in exfoliated teeth implies a lack of periodontal fiber attachment, with consequent exfoliation of single-rooted teeth. The most important alteration in this syndrome is the improper formation of mature bone. Therefore, individuals who survive the neonatal period present with rachitic-like changes, such as bowing of legs and multiple fractures.

Hypophosphatemic Vitamin D–resistant Rickets. This condition, which is quite common, has an X-linked dominant inheritance pattern. It consists of low serum levels of phosphorus, which are produced by low absorption of inorganic phosphate in the renal tubules; rickets or osteomalacia; resistance to treatment with usual doses of vitamin D; and a lack of other abnormalities. Affected individuals are generally of short stature and have bow legs, especially if the condition is present from childhood. Adult-onset forms also exist, and the clinical manifestations in these patients are minor or even lacking, with the exception of low serum levels of inorganic phosphate.

The characteristic radiographic oral findings are large pulp chambers with very long pulp horns. Additionally, the dentin exhibits pronounced cracks that extend to the dentinoenamel junction. These cracks induce fracture of the enamel with microexposure of the pulp and subsequent pulpal infection. Eventually, there is periapical abscess formation associated with the progress of the infectious-inflammatory pulpal disease.

■ *f* i g u r e 6-42

Histologic section of a tooth from a patient with hypophosphatasia showing only dentin. Cementum is entirely lacking.

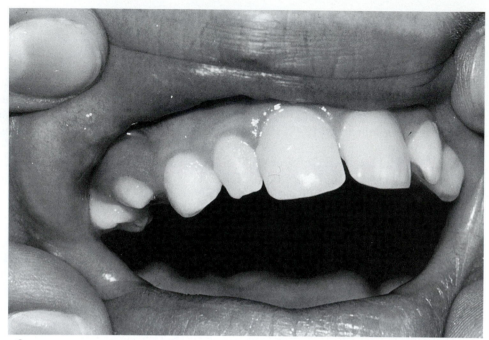

■ *f i g u r e* **6–43**   Pegged maxillary lateral incisor. Note conical shape.

Gingival abscesses are also frequent. Regional lymphadenitis accompanies these processes.

Pegged or Absent Maxillary Lateral Incisors. The inheritance pattern of this trait is generally autosomal dominant with variable expressivity. The lateral incisor can be small, peg shaped, or congenitally lacking, either unilaterally or bilaterally (Fig. 6–43). Both primary and secondary dentitions can be affected, but mostly the latter. This condition has a prevalence of 1% to 3% in the white population and about 7%

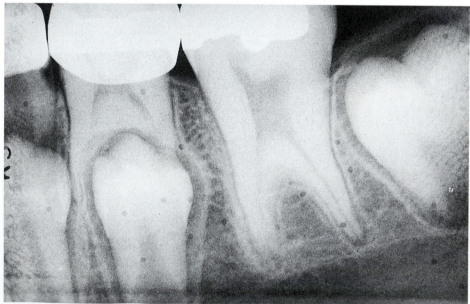

■ *f i g u r e* **6–44**   Intraoral radiograph of taurodontic teeth showing large pulp chambers and low bifurcation of the roots in this pyramid-shaped molar.

in Asians. In addition, the premolar teeth are congenitally lacking in 10% to 20% of affected individuals.

Taurodontism. This is a genetic heterogeneous condition with dominant and recessive inheritance. It is characterized by very large, pyramidally shaped molars with large pulp chambers (Fig. 6–44). (Taurodontic teeth [bull teeth] are also described in Chapter 4.) Taurodontism is most frequent among Native Americans, including Eskimos. The furcation of the roots is displaced apically, and these teeth are classified according to the degree of furcation displacement. It is frequently found in Klinefelter's syndrome and is associated with many other syndromes as well.

SELECTED REFERENCES

BOOKS

Cummings MR: Human Heredity: Principles and Issues. St. Paul, MN, West Publishing, 1988.

Gorlin RJ, Cohen MM, Levin LS: Syndromes of the Head and Neck, 3rd ed. New York, Oxford University Press, 1990.

Larsen WJ: Human Embryology. New York, Churchill Livingstone, 1933.

Sadler TW: Langman's Medical Embryology, 5th ed. Baltimore, Williams & Wilkins, 1985.

Thompson MW: Thompson and Thompson Genetics in Medicine, 5th ed. Philadelphia, WB Saunders, 1991.

Witkop CJ Jr, Sauk JJ Jr: Dental and Oral Manifestations of Hereditary Disease (Monograph). Washington, DC, American Academy of Oral Pathology, 1971.

Witkop CJ Jr, Sauk JJ Jr: Heritable defects of enamel. In Stewart RE, Prescott GH (eds): Oral Facial Genetics. St. Louis, CV Mosby, 1976, pp 151–226.

Young WG, Sedano HO: An Atlas of Oral Pathology. Minneapolis, MN, University of Minnesota Press, 1981.

JOURNAL ARTICLES

Barnet ML, Friedman D, Kastner T: The prevalence of mitral valve prolapse in patients with Down's syndrome: Implications for dental management. Oral Surg Oral Med Oral Pathol 66:445–447, 1988.

Bozzo L, Scully C, Aldred MJ: Hereditary gingival fibromatosis. Oral Surg Oral Med Oral Pathol 78:452–454, 1994.

Chadwick B, Hunter L, Aldred M, Wilkie A: Laband syndrome: Report of two cases, review of the literature, and identification of additional manifestations. Oral Surg Oral Med Oral Pathol 78:57–63, 1994.

Crawford PJM, Aldred MJ: Clinical features of a family with X-linked amelogenesis imperfecta mapping to a new locus (AIH3) on the long arm of the X chromosome. Oral Surg Oral Med Oral Pathol 76:187–191, 1993.

Koury ME, Stella JP, Epker BN: Vascular transformation in cherubism. Oral Surg Oral Med Oral Pathol 76:20–27, 1993.

Yuasa K, Yonetsu K, Kanda S, et al: Computed tomography of the jaws in familial adenomatosis coli. Oral Surg Oral Med Oral Pathol 76:251–255, 1993.

REVIEW QUESTIONS

1. The constriction present in all chromosomes, which joins the short and long arms, is called
   (A) Equatorial plate
   (B) Chromatid
   (C) Centromere
   (D) Chiasmata

2. The process by which a primitive germ cell becomes a gamete is called
   (A) Meiosis
   (B) S phase
   (C) Haploid
   (D) Mitosis

3. Trisomy means
   (A) Three times the amount of chromosome complement
   (B) The presence of an extra chromosome in a pair
   (C) The presence of two extra X chromosomes in a male
   (D) One extra chromosome in each pair

4. The Lyon hypothesis is applied to
   (A) Autosomal dominant traits
   (B) Autosomal recessive traits
   (C) X-linked dominant traits
   (D) X-linked recessive traits

5. Barr bodies are seen at the
   (A) Cytoplasm periphery of all human cells
   (B) Nuclear periphery of all cells from women
   (C) Nuclear periphery of all human cells
   (D) Cytoplasm periphery of all cells from women

6. The karyotype of a patient with Klinefelter's syndrome shows
   (A) 44 autosomes and 1X
   (B) 43 autosomes and XYY
   (C) 44 autosomes and XXY
   (D) 44 autosomes and XYY

7. Hypothetically, an autosomal recessive trait would be clinically present in
   (A) 25% of the offspring of carrier parents
   (B) 50% of the offspring of carrier parents
   (C) 75% of the offspring of carrier parents
   (D) Only in males, never in female offspring

8. Patients with an X-linked hereditary condition
   (A) Are always men
   (B) Have cells with many Barr bodies
   (C) Are always women
   (D) If men, are generally affected more severely

9. The major concern for a dental hygienist when treating a patient with cyclic neutropenia should be
   (A) Hemorrhage
   (B) Severe infections
   (C) Chipping away of enamel
   (D) Exfoliation of teeth due to short roots

10. A 9-year-old boy presents with markedly swollen red and bleeding gingiva. Additionally, he has tooth mobility and the intraoral radiographs show marked alveolar bone atrophy with vertical periodontal pockets. Which of the following will be found in this child if he were to have the Papillon-Lefèvre syndrome?
    (A) Diminished sweating
    (B) Lack of anterior vestibular sulcus
    (C) Blue sclerae
    (D) Palmoplantar hyperkeratosis

11. The inherited varieties of gingival fibromatosis have in common that the gingival enlargement is produced by a marked
    (A) Collagenization of the connective tissue
    (B) Hyperplasia of the covering epithelium
    (C) Chronic inflammatory cellular infiltrate
    (D) Alveolar bone hypertrophy

12. A 14-year-old boy is seen in consultation because of bilateral mandibular swelling. Radiographs show a bilateral multilocular lesion in the ascending mandibular rami. The mother of this patient has similar findings. The most likely diagnosis is
    (A) Ellis–van Creveld syndrome
    (B) Gorlin's syndrome
    (C) Cleidocranial dysplasia
    (D) Cherubism

13. A 19-year-old woman is diagnosed with cleidocranial dysplasia. She has absent clavicles and a mushroom-shaped skull; additionally, which one of the following is she most likely to have?
    (A) Taurodontism
    (B) Pegged lateral incisors
    (C) Supernumerary teeth
    (D) Large pulp chambers

14. Which one of the following is the most serious component of Gardner's syndrome?
    (A) Mandibular osteomas
    (B) Multiple odontomas
    (C) Intestinal polyposis
    (D) Teeth hypercementosis

15. Two of the characteristic clinical components of mandibulofacial dysostosis are
    (A) Lack of clavicles and delayed teeth eruption
    (B) Hypoplastic mandible and deafness
    (C) Hypodontia and dysplastic nails
    (D) Cleft lip and fistulas of lower lip

16. Odontogenic keratocysts are a clinical component of
    (A) Nevoid basal cell carcinoma syndrome
    (B) Neurofibromatosis of von Recklinghausen
    (C) MEN 2B syndrome
    (D) Cherubism

17. Torus mandibularis and torus palatinus are similar in that both are
    (A) Inherited as an autosomal dominant trait
    (B) More prevalent in females
    (C) Inherited as an autosomal recessive trait
    (D) Manifested during the first years of life

18. The etiology for all forms of labial and palatal clefting is considered to be
    (A) Genetic
    (B) Multifactorial
    (C) Environmental
    (D) Drug induced

19. The major concern for a dental hygienist when treating a patient with Osler-Rendu-Parkes Weber syndrome should be
    (A) Severe infections
    (B) Spontaneous ulcerations
    (C) Gingival hemorrhage
    (D) Epithelial desquamation

20. The most serious clinical manifestation of the MEN 2B syndrome is considered to be
    multiple endocrine neoplasia
    (A) Carcinoma of the colon
    (B) Carcinoma of the thyroid gland
    (C) Pheochromocytoma
    (D) Basal cell carcinomas

21. Which one of the following is FALSE for Recklinghausen's disease?
    (A) It is inherited as an autosomal dominant trait
    (B) Patients present with multiple neurofibromas
    (C) There is café au lait pigmentation of the skin
    (D) There is generalized whitening of the oral mucosa

22. Teeth in snowcapped amelogenesis imperfecta have
    (A) A thin brown enamel
    (B) Obliterated pulp chambers
    (C) Short, blunted roots
    (D) White hypocalcified enamel at the incisal and occlusal thirds

23. In dentinogenesis imperfecta type II, teeth have roots that are
    (A) Shorter than normal
    (B) Normal in length
    (C) Markedly brittle
    (D) Larger than normal

24. The characteristic finding in permanent teeth affected with coronal dentin dysplasia is
    (A) Crowns with amber color
    (B) "Thistle-shaped" pulp chambers on radiographs
    (C) Markedly short roots
    (D) Large, square pulp chambers

25. Patients with hypohidrotic ectodermal dysplasia characteristically present with
    (A) Diminished salivary flow
    (B) Lack of anterior vestibular sulcus
    (C) Hypodontia
    (D) Blue sclerae

26. Patients with hypophosphatasia characteristically present with
    (A) Absence of root cementum
    (B) Obliterated pulp chambers
    (C) Gangrenous gingivitis
    (D) Marked gingival keratinization

27. Taurodontic teeth
    (A) Are supernumerary
    (B) Have long roots
    (C) Have no pulp chambers
    (D) Are pyramidal in shape

28. Which one of the following is not inherited as an autosomal dominant trait?
    (A) Torus mandibularis
    (B) Cleidocranial dysplasia
    (C) Papillon-Lefèvre syndrome
    (D) Dentin dysplasia type II

29. Which one of the following is not inherited as an autosomal recessive trait?
    (A) Papillon-Lefèvre syndrome
    (B) Hypophosphatasia
    (C) Dentinogenesis imperfecta type II
    (D) Chondroectodermal dysplasia

30. Which one of the following is usually inherited as an X-linked recessive trait?
    (A) Hypohidrotic ectodermal dysplasia
    (B) White sponge nevus
    (C) Peutz-Jeghers syndrome
    (D) Hereditary hemorrhagic telangiectasia

7

Oral Manifestations of Systemic Diseases

OLGA A. C. IBSEN
·

JOAN A. PHELAN
·

ANTHONY T. VERNILLO
·

Objectives

After studying this chapter, the student should be able to:

1. Define each of the words in the vocabulary list for this chapter.
2. Describe the difference between gigantism and acromegaly, and describe the physical characteristics of each.
3. State the oral manifestations of hyperthyroidism.
4. Describe the difference between primary and secondary hyperparathyroidism.
5. Define diabetes mellitus, and describe the oral manifestations.
6. Describe the differences between type I and type II diabetes.
7. Define Addison's disease, and describe the changes that occur on the skin and oral mucosa in a patient with Addison's disease.
8. Compare and contrast monostotic fibrous dysplasia with polyostotic fibrous dysplasia.
9. Compare and contrast the radiographic appearance, histologic appearance, and treatment of fibrous dysplasia of the jaws with those of ossifying fibroma of the jaws.
10. Compare and contrast the three types of polyostotic fibrous dysplasia.
11. Describe the histologic appearance of Paget's disease of bone, and describe its clinical and radiographic appearance when the maxilla or mandible is involved.
12. State the cause of osteomalacia and rickets.
13. Compare and contrast the cause, laboratory findings, and oral manifestations of each of the following: iron deficiency anemia, pernicious anemia, folic acid deficiency, and vitamin B_{12} deficiency.
14. Compare and contrast the definitions and oral manifestations of thalassemia and sickle cell anemia.
15. Define celiac sprue.
16. Describe the difference between primary and secondary aplastic anemia.
17. Explain why platelets may be deficient in polycythemia vera.
18. Describe the oral manifestations of polycythemia.
19. Describe the most characteristic oral manifestations of agranulocytosis.
20. Describe and contrast acute and chronic leukemia.
21. State the purpose of each of the following laboratory tests: platelet count, bleeding time, prothrombin time, partial thromboplastin time.
22. List two causes of thrombocytopenic purpura.
23. Describe the oral manifestations of thrombocytopenia and nonthrombocytopenic purpura.
24. Define hemophilia, and describe its oral manifestations and treatment.
25. Describe the difference between primary and secondary immunodeficiency.
26. Describe the spectrum of HIV disease, including initial infection and the development of AIDS.
27. List five oral manifestations of HIV infection.

Vocabulary

Agranulocytosis (ah-gran″u-lo-si-to′sis)   A marked decrease in the number of granulocytes, particularly neutrophils

Anemia (ah-ne′me-ah)   Reduction of the number of red blood cells, quantity of hemoglobin, or volume of packed red blood cells to less than normal

Aplasia (ā-pla′zhe-ah) (adjective, aplastic)   Lack of development

Arthralgia (ar-thral′-jĭ-ah)   Severe pain in a joint

Autoimmunity (aw″to-ĭ-mu′nĭ-te)   Immune-mediated destruction of the body's own cells and tissues; immunity against self

Coagulation (ko-ag″u-la′shun)   Formation of a clot

Ecchymosis (ek″ĭ-mo′sis)   A small, flat, hemorrhagic patch, larger than a petechia, on the skin or mucous membrane

Fibrin (fi′brin)   An insoluble protein that is essential to the clotting of blood

Hematocrit (he-mat′ah-krit)   The volume percentage of red blood cells in whole blood

Hemolysis (he-mol′ĭ-sis)   The release of hemoglobin from red blood cells by destruction of the cells

Hemostasis (he″mo-sta′sis)   The stoppage or cessation of bleeding

Hepatomegaly (hep″ah-to-meg′ah-le)   Enlargement of the liver

Hormone (hor′mōn)   A chemical substance produced in the body that has a specific regulatory effect on certain cells or a certain organ or organs

Hypercalcemia (hi″per-kal-se′me-ah)   An excess of calcium in the blood

Hyperglycemia (hi″per-gli-se′me-ah)   An excess of glucose in the blood

Hypochromic (hi″po-kro′mik)   Stained less intensely than normal

Hypophosphatemia (hi″po-fos″fah-te′me-ah)   Deficiency of phosphates in the blood

Insulin (in′sū-lin)   A hormone produced in the pancreas by the beta cells in the islets of Langerhans; insulin regulates glucose metabolism and is the major fuel-regulating hormone

Ketoacidosis (ke″to-ah″sĭ-do′sis)   An accumulation of acid in the body resulting from the accumulation of ketone bodies

Microcyte (mi′kro-sīt)   A red blood cell that is smaller than normal

Myalgia (mi-al′-jē-ah)   muscle pain

Neutropenia (nu″tro-pe′ne-ah)   A decreased number of neutrophils in the blood

Osteoporosis (os″te-o-po-ro′sis)   Abnormal rarefaction of bone

Parathormone (par″ah-thor′mōn)   Parathyroid hormone

Petechia (pe-te′ke-ah)   A minute red spot on the skin or mucous membrane caused by escape of a small amount of blood

Platelet (plāt′let)   A disc-shaped structure, also called a thrombocyte, found in the blood; it plays an important role in blood coagulation

Polycythemia (pol″e-si-the′me-ah)   An increase in the total red blood cell mass in the blood

Purpura (pur′pu-rah)   Blood disorders characterized by purplish or brownish-red discolorations caused by bleeding into the skin or tissues

Receptor (re-sep′ter)   A cell surface protein to which a specific hormone can bind; such binding leads to biochemical events

Splenomegaly (sple″no-meg′ah-le)   Enlargement of the spleen

Thrombocyte (throm′bo-sīt)   A platelet

Thrombocytopenia (throm″bo-si″to-pe′ne-ah)   Decrease in the number of platelets in circulating blood

---

Many diseases that affect the body as a whole are associated with alterations of the oral mucosa, maxilla, and mandible. Systemic diseases can cause mucosal changes such as ulceration or mucosal bleeding. Generalized immunodeficiency can lead to the development of opportunistic diseases such as infection and neoplasia. Bone disease can affect the maxilla and mandible, and systemic disease can cause dental and periodontal changes. Drugs prescribed for a systemic disease can affect the oral tissues.

Local factors are frequently involved in manifestations of systemic disease in the oral mucosa. In some systemic diseases the mucosa is more easily injured; therefore, mild irritation and chronic inflammation can cause lesions that would not occur without the presence of the systemic disease.

This chapter discusses systemic diseases that have oral manifestations. There is a great deal of overlap among the diseases included in this chapter and those included in other chapters, and some of the diseases in this chapter could have been included in other chapters. Included here are endocrine disorders, bone diseases, disorders of red and white blood cells, disorders of platelets and other bleeding and clotting disorders, and immunodeficiency disorders. Oral changes can be similar for several different systemic diseases, and similar oral lesions can occur without the presence of systemic disease. Because of this, many oral lesions described in this chapter are also described elsewhere in this text.

ENDOCRINE DISORDERS

The endocrine system consists of a group of integrated glands and cells that secrete hormones. The secretion of hormones by these glands is controlled by feedback mechanisms in which the amount of hormone circulating in blood triggers factors that control production. Diseases of this system can result from conditions in which either too much or too little hormone is produced and from either dysfunction of the glands themselves or a problem in the mechanism that controls hormone production. Some of the endocrine gland diseases in which there are oral changes are included here.

Hyperpituitarism

Hyperpituitarism is excess hormone production by the anterior pituitary gland. It is caused most often by a benign tumor **(pituitary adenoma)** that produces growth hormone. If the increase in growth hormone production occurs during development, before the closure of the long bones, **gigantism** results. **Acromegaly** results when the hypersecretion occurs in adult life.

In gigantism there is excessive growth of the overall skeleton. Affected individuals can be more than 8 feet tall and weigh several hundred pounds, and as adults they experience headaches, chronic fatigue, and muscle and joint pain.

Acromegaly affects both men and women and most commonly presents in the fourth decade of life. The onset is slow and insidious. Patients experience poor vision, sensitivity to light, enlargement of the hands and feet, and an increase in rib size. The facial changes include enlargement of the maxilla and mandible, frontal bossing (an enlargement of the bones of the forehead), and enlargement of the nasal bones. There is also an enlargement of the maxillary sinus, which causes a characteristically deep voice. The enlargement of the maxilla and mandible causes separation of teeth and malocclusion. Mucosal changes such as thickened lips and **macroglossia** (enlarged tongue) have also been described in patients with acromegaly (Fig. 7–1).

Diagnosis and Treatment

The diagnosis of hyperpituitarism involves measurement of growth hormone, and treatment often involves pituitary gland surgery.

Hyperthyroidism

Hyperthyroidism, also called **thyrotoxicosis,** is characterized by excessive production of thyroid hormone. It is much more common in women than in men. There are several different causes of hyperthyroidism. These include hyperplasia of the gland,

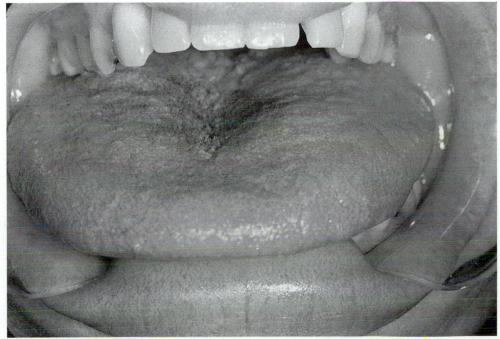

▪ *f i g u r e 7–1*   Enlarged tongue (macroglossia) in a patient with acromegaly.

benign and malignant tumors of the thyroid, pituitary gland disease, and metastatic tumors.

Clinical Features

The clinical features of hyperthyroidism include rosy complexion, erythema of the palms, excessive sweating, fine hair, and softened nails. Exophthalmus (protrusion of the eyeballs) may be seen in hyperthyroidism. Anxiety, weakness, restlessness, and cardiac problems may be associated with the disorder.

Oral Manifestations

Hyperthyroidism in children may lead to premature exfoliation of deciduous teeth and premature eruption of permanent teeth. Osteoporosis may also occur, which may affect alveolar bone. Dental caries and periodontal disease appear to develop and progress more rapidly in these patients than in other patients. Burning discomfort of the tongue has also been reported in patients with hyperthyroidism.

Treatment

Treatment of hyperthyroidism may include surgery, medications to suppress thyroid activity, or the administration of radioactive iodine.

Hypothyroidism

Hypothyroidism is characterized by decreased output of thyroid hormone. When hypothyroidism is present during infancy and childhood, it is known as **cretinism.** In older children and adults, the condition is known as **myxedema.** Causes include developmental disturbances, autoimmune disease, iodine deficiency, drugs, and pituitary disease. In infants, facial and oral changes include thickened lips, enlarged tongue, and delayed eruption of teeth. Adults with hypothyroidism may present with an enlarged tongue.

Hyperparathyroidism

Hyperparathyroidism results from excessive secretion of parathyroid hormone (parathormone or PTH), which is secreted by the parathyroid glands. The four parathyroid glands are located near the thyroid gland. Parathyroid hormone plays an important role in calcium and phosphorus metabolism. Hyperparathyroidism is characterized by elevated blood levels of calcium **(hypercalcemia),** low levels of blood phosphorus **(hypophosphatemia),** and abnormal bone metabolism.

The most frequent cause of hyperparathyroidism is a benign tumor of one or more of the parathyroid glands (parathyroid adenoma). The disease is found in middle-aged adults and is far more common in women than in men.

Calcium is obtained mainly from dairy products and plays an important role in the contraction of all types of muscle. Parathyroid hormone maintains normal blood levels of calcium through its effects on the kidney, gastrointestinal tract, and bone. It increases the uptake of dietary calcium from the gastrointestinal tract and is able to move calcium from bone to circulating blood when necessary. The hormone appears to be able to remove calcium from bone through the action of osteoclasts.

Hyperparathyroidism that results from an abnormality of the parathyroid glands is called **primary hyperparathyroidism. Secondary hyperparathyroidism** occurs when calcium is abnormally excreted by the kidneys, and the parathyroid glands increase their production of parathyroid hormone to maintain adequate blood levels of calcium.

Clinical Manifestations

The clinical manifestations of hyperparathyroidism are varied. Patients with mild cases can be asymptomatic. Joint pain or stiffness may be seen. The disease can affect the kidneys, skeletal system, and gastrointestinal system. In severe disease, lethargy and coma can occur.

Oral Manifestations

The oral manifestations of hyperparathyroidism include changes in the bone of the mandible and maxilla. The chief oral manifestation is the appearance of well-defined unilocular or multilocular radiolucencies (Fig. 7–2A). Microscopically, these lesions appear indistinguishable from central giant cell granulomas (described in Chapter 2) (Fig. 7–2B). There have also been reports of a few cases of peripheral giant cell granulomas associated with hyperparathyroidism. Other radiographic changes that occur in hyperparathyroidism include a generalized mottled appearance of the bone and partial loss of the lamina dura. Loosening of teeth can also occur.

Diagnosis and Treatment

The diagnosis of hyperparathyroidism involves the measurement of parathyroid hormone blood levels and can also include serum calcium and phosphorus measurements. Treatment is directed at correcting the cause of the increased production of the hormone. Causes of increased production of hormone can include tumors, renal disease, and vitamin D deficiency. Bone lesions resolve when the hyperparathyroidism is successfully treated.

Diabetes Mellitus

hypo – lack of glucose control!

Diabetes mellitus involves the beta cells of the pancreas. It is a chronic disorder of carbohydrate (glucose) metabolism and is characterized by abnormally high blood glucose levels **(hyperglycemia),** which result from a lack of the hormone insulin, defective insulin that does not work effectively to lower blood glucose levels, or increased insulin resistance due to obesity. Normally, glucose signals the beta cells of the pancreas to make insulin. This hormone is then directly secreted into the blood stream to facilitate the uptake of glucose into fat and skeletal muscle cells. In the presence of insulin, fat and skeletal muscle cells can use glucose as an energy source. When insulin is lacking, these cells are starved of energy. Without insulin to meet the body's demand for carbohydrate, tissues are broken down and weight loss occurs. Furthermore, the production of ketone acid from the breakdown of fatty tissue is a life-threatening condition and is a common metabolic disturbance in type I diabetes. These ketone acids (e.g., acetone) can lower the pH of the blood **(ketoacidosis),** which can lead to coma and death. White blood cell function is affected in patients with diabetes mellitus. Phagocytic activity is reduced, and chemotaxis is delayed. In addition, collagen production is abnormal.

acid breath fruity/sweet

The precise cause of diabetes mellitus is unknown. Genetic and environmental factors have been implicated in its onset. Fourteen million Americans have been diagnosed with diabetes mellitus. It is estimated that an additional 7 million Americans

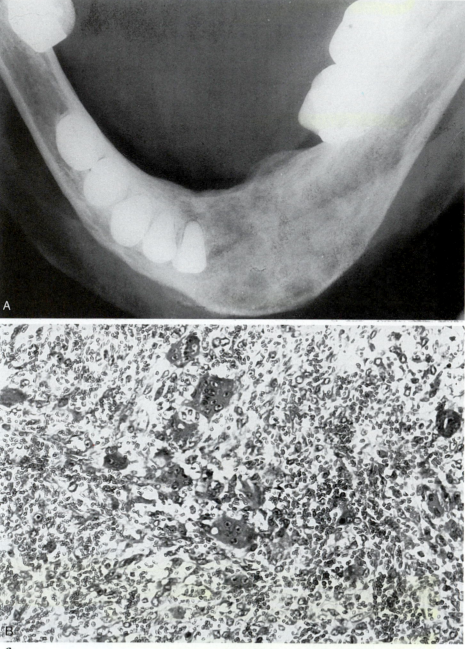

■ *f* i g u r e 7–2   *A*, Radiograph of a mandibular lesion in a patient with hyperparathyroidism. (Courtesy of Drs. Paul Freedman and Stanley Kerpel.) *B*, Micro-
scopic appearance of a jaw lesion occurring in a patient with hyperparathyroidism. The histologic appearance is identical to that of a central giant
cell granuloma.

have undiagnosed diabetes and, therefore, are at risk for life-threatening complications of untreated diabetes.

Types of Diabetes

Insulin-dependent Diabetes Mellitus. Two major types of diabetes have been recognized and classified. The first type is called insulin-dependent diabetes mellitus (IDDM or type I). Autoimmunity appears to play a key role in the development of type I diabetes, leading to the destruction of the insulin-producing beta cells of the pancreas and, ultimately, profound insulin deficiency. Five percent to 10% of all diabetic patients have this type of diabetes. IDDM can occur at any age, but its time of onset is usually at a peak age of 20 years. The onset is abrupt and can present with the three Ps: (1) **polydipsia** (excessive thirst and intake of fluid), (2) **polyuria** (excessive urination), and (3) **polyphagia** (excessive appetite). Complications can occur in 90% of individuals with type I diabetes within 20 years of diagnosis. Difficulty in controlling blood glucose levels is a major problem for patients with IDDM. In recent years it has become increasingly evident that long-term, rigorous control of blood glucose levels is important in minimizing the extent of complications (especially those of the eye, kidney, and nerves) in patients with IDDM. Rigorous control of glucose is more likely achieved with multiple injections of insulin throughout the day to simulate physiologic conditions rather than with a single daily injection. Multiple insulin injections, proper diet, exercise, and frequent determinations of blood glucose levels at home constitute the current approach to the management of the patient with IDDM. The disease is controlled by replacement of the hormone insulin; however, insulin injections are not a cure for diabetes. All patients with IDDM remain insulin-dependent for their entire lives.

Noninsulin-dependent Diabetes Mellitus. The second type of diabetes is noninsulin-dependent diabetes mellitus (NIDDM or type II). Increased insulin resistance, rather than profound insulin deficiency, is characteristic of type II diabetes. Approximately 90% of all diabetic patients have type II diabetes. The onset of this type of diabetes is gradual and usually occurs in patients who are 40 years of age or older. Obesity is a common finding in these individuals. Obesity probably decreases the number of receptors for insulin binding in sensitive tissues (e.g., fat), thereby leading to the development of the diabetic state. Complications are less common in this type of diabetes than in type I diabetes. Some patients achieve control of blood glucose levels with diet and weight reduction alone, whereas others require oral hypoglycemic agents. These medications also lower blood glucose levels, but unlike insulin are not given by injection. However, approximately 25% to 30% of patients with type II diabetes require insulin injections to obtain control of blood glucose levels.

Clinical Manifestations

The vascular system is the most severely affected in diabetes. Accelerated atherosclerosis (thickening of the blood vessel wall from fibrofatty plaques) can occur and lead to impaired circulation of blood, resulting in impaired transport of oxygen and nutrients to tissues. This increases the risk of ulceration and gangrene of the feet, high blood pressure, kidney failure, and stroke. Blood vessel changes in the eye (diabetic retinopathy) can lead to hemorrhage, which can result in blindness. The nervous system can also be affected in diabetes, resulting in a variety of neurologic complaints. Decreased resistance to infection is seen, particularly in uncontrolled diabetes. Skin infections, especially furuncles (boils), urinary tract infections, and tuberculosis are common.

Oral Complications

The oral complications of diabetes are most severe when blood glucose levels are not controlled. In some patients, control is difficult even with careful monitoring of these levels and insulin injections. These patients are said to have **brittle diabetes.**

Increased colonization of the oral mucosa by *Candida albicans* and an increased prevalence of oral candidiasis have been reported in patients with diabetes mellitus, as has mucormycosis, a rare fungal infection that affects the palate and maxillary sinuses. (Both oral candidiasis and mucormycosis are described in Chapter 3.)

Bilateral, asymptomatic parotid gland enlargement occurs in some patients and results from a deposition of fat and hypertrophy of the salivary gland tissue.

Xerostomia (dry mouth) is usually associated with uncontrolled diabetes mellitus. Dehydration of the oral tissues can result, increasing the risk of the development of oral candidiasis.

Altered subgingival flora have been described in diabetes and may be due to immunologic or salivary changes.

Patients with diabetes mellitus have an accentuated response to plaque. The gingiva can be hyperplastic and erythematous, and acute and fulminating gingival abscesses can occur. Excessive periodontal bone loss, tooth mobility, and early tooth loss can also be associated with diabetes mellitus (Fig. 7–3).

Slow wound healing and increased susceptibility to infection occur as a result of the immunologic changes and defective collagen production.

The diabetic patient who is receiving good medical management and whose glucose levels are controlled can receive any indicated dental treatment. Early identification of oral infections is important. Infection aggravates diabetes because it often results in the loss of blood glucose control. Therefore, elimination of infection is important in diabetic patients. Antibiotic medication, calculus and plaque removal, and effective oral hygiene care are especially important in the management of the diabetic patient.

Addison's Disease "hypofunction" of adrenal cortex

Addison's disease, also known as **primary adrenal cortical insufficiency,** is characterized by an insufficient production of adrenal steroids. A malignant tumor or tuberculosis may be responsible for destruction of the adrenal gland. However, in most cases, the cause of the destruction of the adrenal cortex is unknown. In these patients the condition may be an autoimmune disease.

As a result of the decreased production of adrenal steroids, the pituitary gland increases its production of adrenocorticotropic hormone (ACTH), which would normally increase the production of adrenal steroids. This hormone is similar to melanin-stimulating hormone and causes stimulation of melanocytes. Brown pigmentation (bronzing) of the skin occurs, and melanotic macules can develop on the oral mucosa. Treatment involves steroid administration (replacement therapy).

DISEASES OF BONE

Fibrous Dysplasia

Fibrous dysplasia is a disease that is characterized by the replacement of bone with abnormal fibrous connective tissue containing varying amounts of calcification.

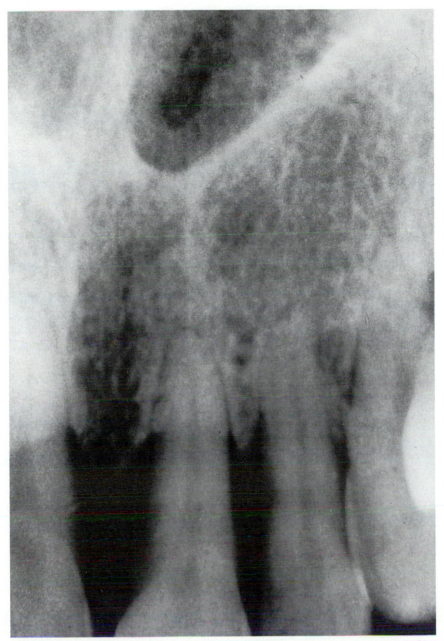

figure 7-3   Periapical radiograph of a patient with diabetes mellitus showing severe bone loss.

Although the cause is unknown, several theories have been proposed. One of the most widely accepted is that the unusual fibrous growth results from abnormal mesenchymal cell function. There are several types of fibrous dysplasia. The microscopic features of each are the same, but the clinical and associated systemic signs and symptoms differ. Histologically, fibrous dysplasia is a benign fibro-osseous lesion. It is composed of cellular fibrous connective tissue that is usually quite vascular with irregular trabeculae of bone emerging from the connective tissue.

Monostotic Fibrous Dysplasia

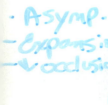

Monostotic fibrous dysplasia, the most common form of fibrous dysplasia, is characterized by the involvement of only one bone. The mandible and maxilla are commonly affected—the maxilla more frequently than the mandible. Other bones frequently affected include the ribs, femur, and tibia. Monostotic fibrous dysplasia is most commonly diagnosed in children and young adults, and there is no sex predilection. Clinically, there is a painless swelling or bulging of the jaws involving the buccal plate. The expanding nature of the lesion can lead to malocclusion, tipping, or displacement of teeth.

Polyostotic Fibrous Dysplasia

Polyostotic fibrous dysplasia is characterized by involvement of more than one bone. It is also most commonly diagnosed in children, and there is a definite predilection for females. Bones of the face, skull, clavicles, and long bones are most often affected. The lesions are often asymptomatic. When long bones are affected, there may be bowing and aching pain. Skin lesions in polyostotic fibrous dysplasia appear as light-brown skin macules called **café au lait spots.** There are several forms of polyostotic fibrous dysplasia. **Craniofacial fibrous dysplasia** is the term used for the form in which the maxilla is involved and the lesions extend into the sinuses and adjacent bones such as the zygoma, sphenoid bone, and occipital bone. Another form of polyostotic fibrous dysplasia is called **Jaffe's type (or Jaffe-Lichtenstein type).** It involves lesions in multiple bones, and there are associated café au lait macules on the skin. The most severe type of polyostotic fibrous dysplasia is called **Albright's syndrome.** This condition is characterized by endocrine abnormalities, which include precocious puberty in females, stunting or deformity of skeletal growth because of early epiphyseal closure in both sexes, and other complications that can include diabetes and hyperthyroidism. Precocious puberty is manifested by menses, pubic hair, and breast development by two years of age. The bone involvement is progressive and can involve all the bones in the body. Café au lait skin macules occur in this type of polyostotic fibrous dysplasia as well as in Jaffe's type.

Clinical Manifestations

Clinically, fibrous dysplasia appears as a painless enlargement of the involved bone or bones. The maxilla is involved more frequently than the mandible. Jaw lesions appear as painless, progressive enlargements, usually unilateral, of the maxilla or mandible. When fibrous dysplasia involves the maxilla, the disease usually extends into the maxillary sinus. Involvement of the jaws can occur in all types of fibrous dysplasia.

The classic radiographic appearance of fibrous dysplasia is a diffuse radiopacity, which has been described as looking like ground glass (Fig. 7–4A). The abnormal bone blends into the normal adjacent bone. Unilocular and multilocular radiolucencies, patchy radiolucency and radiopacity, and dense radiopacity have also been described in fibrous dysplasia.

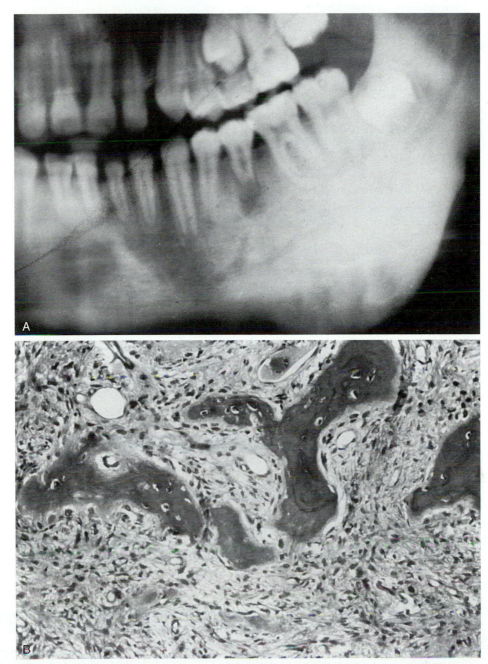

▪ *f i g u r e* 7-4   Fibrous dysplasia. *A,* Radiograph of fibrous dysplasia illustrating the indistinct borders of the lesion, which blends into adjacent normal bone. (Courtesy of Drs. Paul Freedman and Stanley Kerpel.) *B,* Microscopic appearance (high power) of fibrous dysplasia showing cellular fibrous connective tissue and irregular trabeculae of bone.

Histologically, fibrous dysplasia is a benign fibro-osseous lesion (Fig. 7–4B). The microscopic appearance is characterized by cellular fibrous connective tissue and irregularly shaped bone trabeculae. Other fibro-osseous lesions include ossifying fibroma, periapical cemental dysplasia, and florid osseous dysplasia (Table 7–1).

Diagnosis and Treatment

The diagnosis of fibrous dysplasia is made by a combination of microscopic examination, radiographic appearance, and clinical features. Fibrous dysplasia of the maxilla or mandible is distinguished from other fibro-osseous lesions such as ossifying fibroma on the basis of its radiographic appearance. The radiographic changes blend into the surrounding normal bone. Ossifying fibroma, a tumor that can appear the same microscopically, is a well-defined lesion. The radiolucent or radiopaque appearance depends on the degree of calcification of the lesion. Other fibro-osseous lesions, such as periapical cemental dysplasia (cementoma) and florid osseous dysplasia, have distinct radiographic features (described in Chapter 5), which are important in establishing the diagnosis. Examination of the skin and entire skeleton is necessary to determine if the fibrous dysplasia is polyostotic.

Fibrous dysplasia can be treated surgically. Often the bone is recontoured for cosmetic reasons. There is no treatment for severe and progressive polyostotic fibrous dysplasia. Radiation treatment of fibrous dysplasia has been associated with malignant transformation and therefore is not used.

Paget's Disease of Bone

Paget's disease of bone, also called **osteitis deformans** and **leontiasis ossea,** is a chronic metabolic bone disease. It is characterized by resorption, osteoblastic repair, and remineralization of the involved bone. The cause is unknown. Several theories have been proposed, and a viral cause is suspected. The disease is most common in men older than 50 years of age. It typically involves the pelvis and spinal column. When found in the jaws, the maxilla is more commonly affected than the mandible.

Clinical Manifestations

Clinically, enlargement of the bone is seen (Fig. 7–5A). The alveolar ridges are significantly enlarged, and in a patient with teeth, spacing is obvious. Edentulous patients may complain that their dentures no longer fit. Clinical manifestations depend on the bone involved and include severe headache, dizziness, and deafness when other bones of the skull are involved. The patient often complains of pain. The classic radiographic appearance described for Paget's disease is a patchy radiolucency and

TABLE 7–1 Benign Fibro-Osseous Lesions of the Jaws
Fibrous dysplasia
Monostotic type
Polyostotic types (Jaffe's and Albright's)
Craniofacial type
Central ossifying fibroma
Cemento-ossifying fibroma
Cementifying fibroma
Peripheral ossifying fibroma
Periapical cemental dysplasia (cementoma)
Florid osseous dysplasia

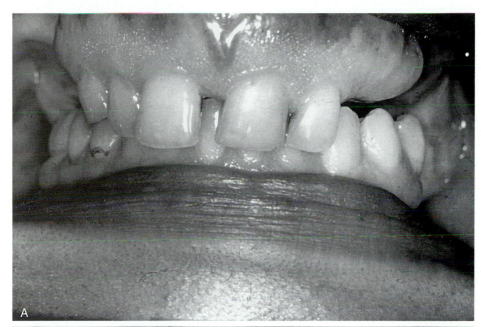

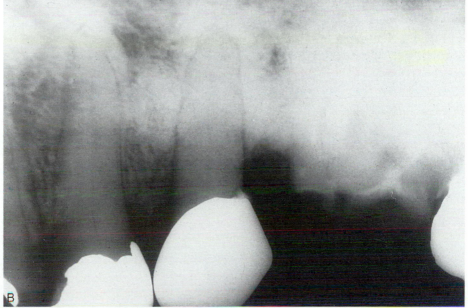

■ *f i g u r e* **7–5**   Paget's disease. *A*, In this patient with Paget's disease, the maxilla has enlarged and spaces have formed between teeth. *B*, Radiograph of a patient with Paget's disease showing irregular opacification, called "cotton-wool" appearance. The lamina dura is obliterated.

giantism Aachromaglia

radiopacity that has been referred to as a cotton-wool appearance (Fig. 7–5B). However, this occurs in the later stages of Paget's disease. In earlier stages the radiographic appearance is not as unique. Hypercementosis, loss of the lamina dura, and obliteration of the periodontal ligament may also be seen. *Denture doesn't fit*

hypercementosis

Histologically, Paget's disease is characterized by the appearance of osteoclasts and osteoblasts (Fig. 7–6). Involved bone shows prominent reversal lines that result from the resorption and deposition of bone; it has been described as **mosaic bone.** The connective tissue between the trabeculae of bone is so well vascularized in active Paget's disease that the bone feels warm when touched.

Diagnosis and Treatment

Laboratory tests are important in the diagnosis of Paget's disease. Biopsy results show the histologic changes described previously. The serum alkaline phosphatase level is significantly elevated in active Paget's disease. (Two different measurements are used for alkaline phosphatase. In Bodansky units, the normal serum alkaline phosphatase value is 1.5 to 5.0. In Paget's disease, the serum alkaline phosphatase value can be as high as 250 Bodansky units. Another measurement used for evaluating serum alkaline phosphatase is the King-Armstrong unit [KAU]. Normal values are 5 to 10 KAU. In patients with Paget's disease, KAU values may be as high as 200 KAU.)

Treatment of Paget's disease is experimental. The disease is slowly progressive. Complications include fracture of the involved bone and development of malignant tumors, particularly osteogenic sarcoma. Heart disease is a rare complication.

Osteomalacia

Osteomalacia is a disease of bone caused by a deficiency of calcium over a long period. When found in young children, the disease is usually caused by a nutritional

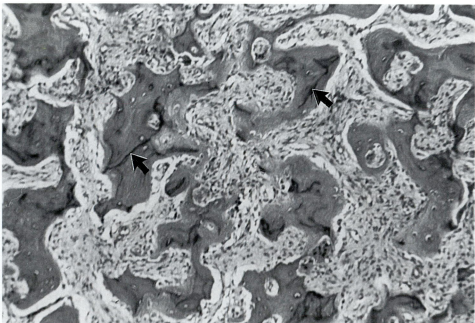

■ *figure 7–6*   Microscopic appearance (low power) of Paget's disease. The prominent reversal lines (*arrows*) seen here characterize the "mosaic bone" pattern of Paget's disease.

deficiency of vitamin D and is called **rickets.** Delayed tooth eruption and periodontal disease have been associated with osteomalacia. Treatment includes nutritional supplements of vitamin D and dietary calcium. In adults the disease may be related to various problems such as malabsorption syndromes, drugs, liver and kidney disease, and chronic use of antacids. Changes in bone trabeculation that occur in patients with osteomalacia may be subtle and difficult to detect. Pathologic fractures may occur in patients with osteomalacia.

BLOOD DISORDERS

The **complete blood count (CBC)** is important in the diagnosis of blood disorders. The CBC is a series of tests that examines the red blood cells, white blood cells, and platelets. It provides information about the number of each type of cell, the ratio of types of cells, and the appearance of the cells. The information included in a complete blood count and normal values are included in Table 7–2.

TABLE 7–2. Complete Blood Count (CBC) Normal Adult Values

Red Blood Cells (RBCs)

RBC Count: The total number of RBCs/mm^3 of whole blood
   Males $4.6–6.2 \times 10^6$
   Females $4.2–5.4 \times 10^6$

Hemoglobin (Hgb): The amount of hemoglobin contained in 100 ml of whole blood
   Males   13.5–18 g
   Females   12.0–16 g

Hematocrit (Hct): The volume of packed RBCs in 100 ml of whole blood
   Males   40–54%
   Females   38–47%

RBC Indices
   Mean corpuscular (cell) volume (MCV): Describes the average size of an individual RBC

   80–96 μm^3 (cubic microns)

   Mean corpuscular (cell) hemoglobin (MCH): Indicates the amount of hemoglobin present in an RBC by weight

   27–31 pg (picogram)

   Mean corpuscular (cell) hemoglobin concentration (MCHC): Indicates the proportion of each cell occupied by hemoglobin

   32–36%

White Blood Cells (WBCs)

Total WBC Count: 4000–11,000/mm^3
Differential WBC Count: The number of each type of WBC expressed as a percentage of the total number of WBCs

Mature neutrophils (granulocytes)	50–60%
Immature neutrophils (bands)	2–4%
Lymphocytes	30–40%
Monocytes	1–9%
Basophils	0–1%
Eosinophils	2–3%

Disorders of Red Blood Cells and Hemoglobin

Anemia

Anemia is defined as a reduction in the oxygen-carrying capacity of the blood. There are many different types and causes of anemia.

Nutritional anemias occur when a substance necessary for the normal development of red blood cells is in scant supply in the bone marrow. The most common deficiencies are of iron, folic acid, or vitamin B_{12}. These deficiencies can occur when the intake of the nutrient is insufficient or when disorders of absorption prevent its uptake. Anemia can also occur when there is suppression of the bone marrow stem cells, resulting in an inability of the bone marrow to produce red blood cells.

Oral Manifestations. Oral manifestations are similar for all types of anemia and include skin and mucosal pallor, angular cheilitis, erythema and atrophy of the oral mucosa, and loss of filiform and fungiform papillae on the dorsum of the tongue. Circumvallate papillae and foliate papillae are not affected.

Iron Deficiency Anemia

Iron deficiency anemia occurs when there is an insufficient amount of iron supplied to the bone marrow for red blood cell development. This type of anemia can occur as a result of a deficiency of iron intake, blood loss from heavy menstrual bleeding or chronic gastrointestinal bleeding, poor iron absorption, or an increased requirement for iron, as in pregnancy or infancy.

The Plummer-Vinson syndrome can develop as a result of long-standing iron deficiency anemia. This syndrome includes dysphasia (difficulty swallowing), atrophy of the upper alimentary tract, and a predisposition to the development of oral cancer.

Clinical Manifestations. Iron deficiency anemia is most often asymptomatic. Nonspecific symptoms such as weakness and fatigue can occur. Oral mucosal signs in severe cases include angular cheilitis, pallor of the oral tissues, and an erythematous, smooth, painful tongue (Fig. 7–7; Color Plate 89). The changes in the oral mucosa occur as a result of a lack of nutrients to the epithelium. The filiform papillae on the dorsum of the tongue disappear first because they have the highest metabolic requirements. Disappearance of the fungiform papillae can also occur in chronic and severe cases.

Diagnosis and Treatment. The diagnosis of iron deficiency anemia is made by laboratory tests, which show a low hemoglobin content of red blood cells and a reduced hematocrit value. The red blood cells are smaller than normal (**microcytic**) and lighter than normal (**hypochromic**). Iron deficiency anemia is treated by increasing the intake of iron. Dietary supplements are usually used. The oral lesions resolve when the deficiency is corrected.

Pernicious Anemia

Pernicious anemia is caused by a deficiency of **extrinsic factor,** a substance secreted by the parietal cells of the stomach. Extrinsic factor is necessary for the absorption of vitamin B_{12}. Normally, vitamin B_{12} is transported across the intestinal mucosa by **intrinsic factor.** An autoimmune mechanism is the most likely cause of pernicious anemia. Antibodies to components of gastric mucosa have been identified in patients with pernicious anemia. Vitamin B_{12} is needed for DNA synthesis; when it is lacking, the development of rapidly dividing cells, such as bone marrow cells and epithelial cells, is affected.

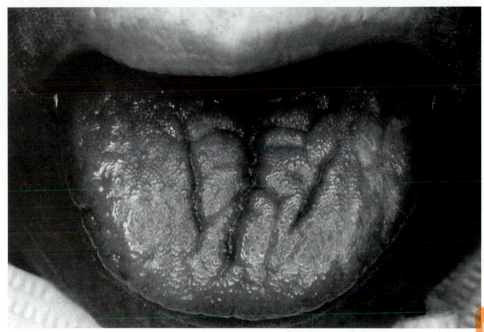

f i g u r e 7–7   Iron deficiency anemia. The tongue is devoid of filiform papillae. Angular cheilitis was also present in this patient.

Clinical Manifestations. Pernicious anemia is clinically manifested by the clinical signs of anemia—weakness, pallor, and fatigue on exertion. Other constitutional signs can include nausea, dizziness, diarrhea, abdominal pain, loss of appetite, and weight loss. Neurologic changes such as severe paresthesia may also occur in patients with pernicious anemia.

Oral manifestations of pernicious anemia include angular cheilitis; mucosal pallor; painful, atrophic and erythematous mucosa; mucosal ulceration; loss of papillae on the dorsum of the tongue, or burning; and painful tongue (Fig. 7–8; Color Plate 41).

Diagnosis and Treatment. The diagnosis of pernicious anemia is made by laboratory testing. The diagnostic features include low serum vitamin B_{12} levels, gastric achlorhydria (lack of hydrochloric acid), and megaloblastic anemia (abnormally large red blood cells). The Schilling test, which detects an inability to absorb an oral dose of vitamin B_{12} (cobalamin), is another method used in the diagnosis of pernicious anemia. The treatment consists of injections of vitamin B_{12}. The oral mucosa improves in time, but the papillae on the dorsum of the tongue may not completely regenerate.

Folic Acid and Vitamin B_{12} Deficiency Anemia

Dietary deficiencies of folic acid and vitamin B_{12} can result in anemia and can occur in association with malnutrition and increased metabolic requirements. Malnutrition can occur in association with alcoholism, and pregnant women can experience a deficiency because of increased metabolic demands. Folic acid is essential for DNA synthesis, as is vitamin B_{12}. Therefore, the oral manifestations are indistinguishable from those of pernicious anemia.

Diagnosis and Treatment. The diagnosis of these anemias is based on laboratory test results that include abnormally large red blood cells (megaloblastic) and serum assays of folic acid and vitamin B_{12}. Treatment involves dietary supplements.

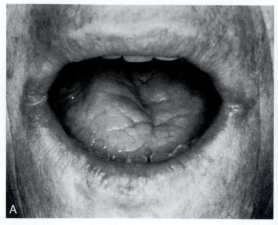
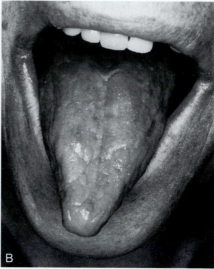

▪ *f i g u r e 7–8*   Pernicious anemia. *A,* Angular cheilitis in a patient with pernicious anemia. *B,* The tongue is completely devoid of both filiform and fungiform papillae, and the mucosa is atrophic. Note the ulcer on the left lateral aspect.

Thalassemia

Thalassemia, also called **Mediterranean** or **Cooley's anemia,** is the name of a group of inherited disorders of hemoglobin synthesis. It has an autosomal dominant inheritance pattern, and therefore there is no predilection for either sex. The heterozygous form (see Chapter 6), in which only one gene at a locus is involved, is called **thalassemia minor** and can be asymptomatic or only mildly symptomatic. The homozygous form, in which the genes on both chromosomes are involved, is called **thalassemia major** and is associated with severe hemolytic anemia, which results from damage to the red blood cell membranes and destruction of the red blood cells.

Clinical Manifestations. The severe form of the disease begins early in life. The child has a yellowish skin pallor, fever, malaise, and weakness. An enlarged liver and spleen are common. The characteristic facies includes prominent cheekbones, depression of the bridge of the nose, an unusual prominence of the premaxilla, and protrusion or flaring of the maxillary anterior teeth. Intraoral radiographs show a peculiar trabecular pattern of the maxilla and mandible. There is a prominence of some trabeculae and a blurring and disappearance of others, resulting in a "salt-and-pepper" effect. Thinning of the lamina dura and circular radiolucencies in the alveolar bone have also been described.

Treatment. Treatment of thalassemia major is experimental. Blood transfusions and splenectomy have provided periods of remission. The prognosis is poor. However, these supportive therapies have extended life from early childhood to about 20 years of age.

Sickle Cell Anemia

Sickle cell anemia is an inherited disorder of the blood that is found predominantly in black individuals and those of Mediterranean origin. Persons who are heterozygous for the disease are generally asymptomatic. This is called **sickle cell trait.** Those that are homozygous are much more severely affected. The disease presents before age 30 years and is more common in women than in men. Sickle cell anemia occurs as a result of abnormal hemoglobin in red blood cells. Because of this abnormal hemoglobin, the cells develop a sickle shape when there is decreased oxygen; hence, the name sickle cell anemia. Exercise, exertion, administration of a general anesthetic, pregnancy, or even sleep can trigger a sickling of the red blood cells. Because of the change in their shape, the red blood cells are no longer able to pass through small blood vessels and are destroyed more rapidly than normal.

Clinical and Oral Manifestations. The patient with sickle cell anemia experiences weakness, shortness of breath, fatigue, joint pain, and nausea.

Oral manifestations are seen on dental radiographs (Fig. 7–9). There is a loss of trabeculation, with the appearance of large, irregular marrow spaces. This change is most prominent in the alveolar bone. Changes in the skull have been described as a "hair-on-end" pattern because the trabeculae radiate outward.

Diagnosis and Treatment. The sickle-shaped cells are seen on a blood smear (Fig. 7–10). The number of red blood cells is usually low, as is the hemoglobin content. Management of sickle cell anemia is largely symptomatic and supportive and involves the administration of oxygen and intravenous and oral fluids. Sickle cell anemia can result in profound changes of the heart, such as enlargement, and lead to cardiac failure.

Celiac Sprue

Celiac sprue is a chronic disorder associated with a sensitivity to dietary gluten, a protein found in wheat and wheat products. When gluten is ingested, injury to the intestinal mucosa results. Malabsorption of other nutrients, such as vitamin B_{12} and folic acid, occurs because of mucosal injury, and, as a result, anemia develops and the oral and clinical signs associated with it.

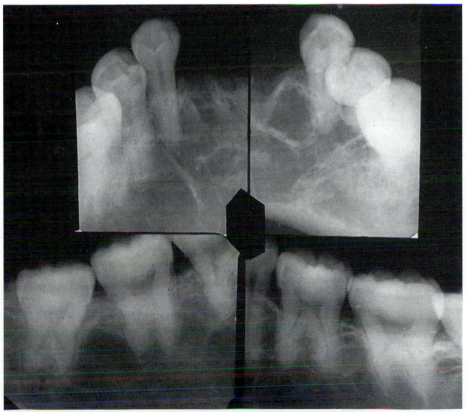

■ *f* i g u r e **7-9**   Sickle cell anemia. Radiograph shows abnormal trabeculation. (Courtesy of Dr. Edward V. Zegarelli.)

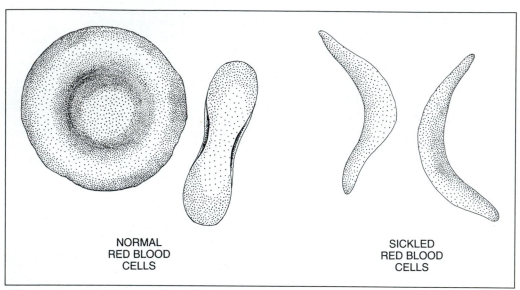

NORMAL
RED BLOOD
CELLS

SICKLED
RED BLOOD
CELLS

▪ *f i g u r e* **7–10**   Sickled red blood cells compared with normal red blood cells.

Clinical and Oral Manifestations. Systemic symptoms include diarrhea, nervousness, and paresthesia of the extremities.

Oral manifestations include glossitis, a painful burning tongue, atrophy of the papillae of the tongue, and ulceration of the oral mucosa.

Diagnosis and Treatment. Patients should adhere to a gluten-free diet. Oral manifestations resolve when the systemic disease is under control.

Aplastic Anemia

In aplastic anemia there is a dramatic decrease in all the circulating blood cells because of a severe depression of bone marrow activity. All the blood cells are produced in the marrow (Fig. 7–11). The cause of **primary aplastic anemia** is unknown. In **secondary aplastic anemia** the bone marrow failure is a result of a drug or chemical agent. Chemotherapy, radioactive isotopes, radium, or radiant energy have been associated with the development of aplastic anemia. Primary aplastic anemia occurs most frequently in young adults.

Oral Manifestations. These are related to the generalized decrease in white blood cells and platelets and include infection, spontaneous bleeding, petechiae, and purpuric spots (Fig. 7–12).

Diagnosis and Treatment. In both forms of aplastic anemia there is a generalized decrease of circulating blood cells. In addition to anemia there is also **leukopenia** (a decrease in white blood cells) and **thrombocytopenia** (a decrease in platelets). White blood cells are essential in the defense against infection (see Chapters 2 and 3), and platelets are essential in the clotting of blood. Primary aplastic anemia is usually progressive and fatal. Treatment of secondary aplastic anemia involves removing the cause.

Polycythemia

Polycythemia is characterized by an abnormal increase in the number of circulating red blood cells. Normal red blood cell production is carefully regulated and involves

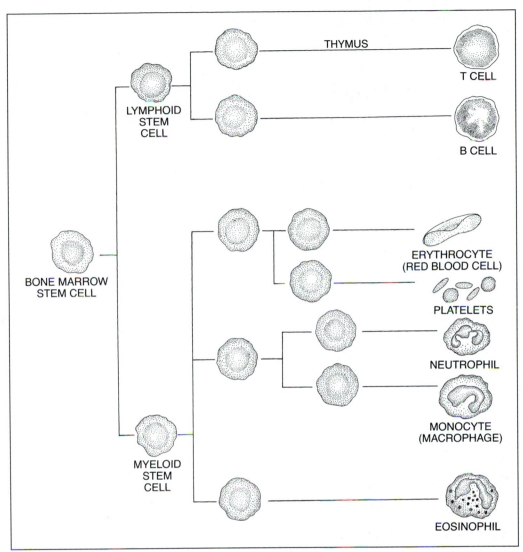

■ ƒ i g u r e 7–11   Blood cells are derived from stem cells in the bone marrow.

both the precursor cells in the bone marrow and the hormone erythropoietin, which is produced by the kidney.

Oral Manifestations. The oral mucosa in patients with polycythemia may appear deep red to purple, and the gingiva may be edematous. The gingiva may bleed easily, and submucosal petechiae, ecchymosis, and hematoma formation can be present. There can be excessive bleeding after oral surgical procedures. Abnormalities of the oral mucosa result from an increase in circulating red blood cells, the impaired blood flow, and thrombocytopenia.

Types of Polycythemia

There are three forms of polycythemia: (1) polycythemia vera (primary polycythemia), (2) secondary polycythemia, and (3) relative polycythemia.

Polycythemia Vera (Primary Polycythemia). In polycythemia vera there is a neoplastic proliferation of bone marrow stem cells that results in an abnormally high number of circulating red blood cells. The production of red blood cells is uncontrolled.

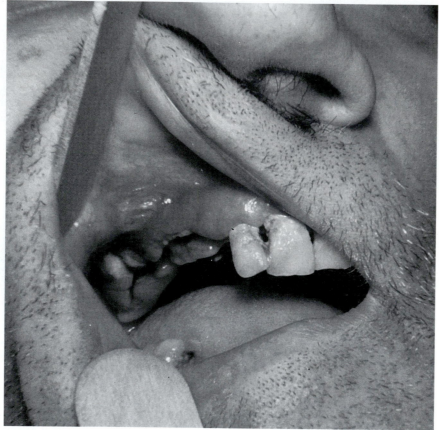

▪ *f i g u r e* **7–12**   Aplastic anemia. Severe oral infection occurred following extraction of teeth in this patient with aplastic anemia. (Courtesy of Dr. Harry Lumerman.)

The cause of this disorder is unknown. It is somewhat more common in men than in women, and the age of onset is usually between 40 and 60 years. It is generally seen in white individuals and is extremely rare in black individuals. The symptoms of polycythemia vera include headache, dizziness, and itching of the skin (pruritus). The increase in red blood cells leads to impaired blood flow, vascular stasis, and poor circulation. The formation of thrombi can cause a disruption of the blood supply to the brain, heart, or peripheral vessels. A decrease in platelets (thrombocytopenia) can occur because of the disruption of the marrow from which they are derived.

Secondary Polycythemia. In secondary polycythemia, the increase in red blood cells is caused by a physiologic response to decreased oxygen. A decrease in oxygen in the blood triggers an increase in erythropoietin by the kidneys, which results in increased production of red blood cells. A number of factors can cause a decrease in oxygen, including pulmonary disease, heart disease, living in high altitudes, and an elevation in carbon monoxide. The increase in carbon monoxide has been associated with tobacco smoking.

Relative Polycythemia. This is due to a decreased plasma volume and not to an increase in red blood cells. In acute forms the cause is usually easily recognized. Causes of acute relative polycythemia include diuretic use, vomiting, diarrhea, or excessive sweating. A chronic form of relative polycythemia has been called **stress polycythemia.** Most patients with this type of polycythemia are middle-aged white men who are under physiologic stress, mildly overweight, hypertensive, and heavy smokers. There is an increased incidence of cardiovascular accidents in these patients.

Diagnosis and Treatment. Diagnosis of the different forms of polycythemia involves laboratory testing and measurement of the hemoglobin content and the hematocrit. Treatment is related to the type of polycythemia and may include removal of causative factors, chemotherapy, and phlebotomy (blood-letting). Oral lesions generally do not require local treatment. However, there is a tendency toward increased bleeding following oral surgery.

Disorders of White Blood Cells

Three groups of white blood cells are found in the circulation: granulocytes, lymphocytes, and monocytes. There are three types of granulocytes: polymorphonuclear leukocytes (neutrophils), eosinophils, and basophils. The primary function of the neutrophils is to defend the body against foreign invaders (e.g., bacteria, viruses, and fungi) (described in Chapter 3). These cells, which participate in the first line of defense against infection—the inflammatory response—are produced primarily in the bone marrow and are released into the circulating blood (see Fig. 7–11).

Agranulocytosis

In **agranulocytosis** there is a marked reduction in circulating neutrophils, which has serious consequences. An abnormally low white blood cell count is called **leukopenia.** Any of the white blood cells can be involved, but leukopenia most commonly involves the neutrophils. A reduction in the number of circulating neutrophils is called **neutropenia;** it can be seen in a variety of circumstances and is usually temporary and of little significance.

Agranulocytosis can result from either a problem in the development of neutrophils or a problem in accelerated destruction of neutrophils. Primary and secondary forms of agranulocytosis have been described. The cause of the primary form is unknown and may be an immunologic disorder. The secondary form of agranulocytosis is most commonly produced by drugs and other chemicals. Secondary agranulocytosis is most commonly seen in women.

Clinical and Oral Manifestations. Clinically, there is a sudden onset of high fever, chills, jaundice, weakness, and sore throat. Orally, the most characteristic feature is the presence of infection. Necrotizing ulcerations, excessive bleeding from the gingiva, and rapid destruction of the supporting tissue of the teeth have been described. Regional lymphadenopathy can accompany the oral problems.

Diagnosis and Treatment. The diagnosis is made by laboratory testing. The white blood cell count, which is normally 5000 to 10,000 cells/mm^3, is dramatically reduced to less than 1000 cells/mm^3. Treatment includes transfusions, antibiotics to control infection, and, in the secondary form, removal of the causative agent. Infections can become overwhelming and cause death. All surgical procedures, including dental hygiene procedures, are contraindicated.

Cyclic Neutropenia

Cyclic neutropenia is a form of agranulocytosis. A severe depression of granulocytes (neutrophils) occurs at periodic intervals. Cyclic neutropenia is described in detail in Chapter 6. (See also Color Plate 86.)

Leukemia

Leukemias are malignant neoplasms of the hematopoietic (blood-forming) stem cells. They are primarily disorders of the bone marrow. However, the most dramatic feature of leukemias is the excessive number of abnormal white blood cells in the circulating blood. The pathogenesis is unknown. However, current investigations are concentrating on oncogenic viruses (see Chapter 5). There are many different types of leukemias, which are classified by the cell type involved and the maturity of the neoplastic cells (Table 7–3). Leukemias are described in this chapter with other abnormalities of blood. They could also have been included in Chapter 5, in which other neoplasms are described. Many different types of leukemias are known, and this text gives only an overview of them in order to discuss the oral manifestations. The student is encouraged to use other texts for a more complete description of leukemias. The two general categories of leukemias described here are acute leukemias and chronic leukemias. Oral lesions are most common in acute leukemias but also occur in chronic forms of leukemia.

Acute Leukemias

Acute leukemias are characterized by the presence of very immature cells (**blast cells**) and by a rapidly fatal course if not treated. Acute leukemias can involve immature lymphocytes **(acute lymphoblastic leukemia)** or immature granulocytes **(acute myoblastic leukemia).** Acute lymphoblastic leukemia primarily affects children and young adults and has a good prognosis. Acute myoblastic leukemia involves adolescents and young adults (age range, 15 to 39 years), and the prognosis is not as good. The onset of acute leukemia is sudden and dramatic.

Clinical Manifestations. Clinically, there is weakness, fever, enlargement of lymph nodes, and bleeding. There is a general loss of cells produced by the bone marrow. The fatigue mainly results from anemia, the fever from infection, and the bleeding from a decrease in platelets (thrombocytopenia). Enlargement of the spleen **(splenomegaly)** and liver **(hepatomegaly)** occurs when those organs are infiltrated by the leukemic cells.

Oral Manifestations. Oral manifestations can include gingival enlargement (which can be severe) caused by infiltration of leukemic cells (Fig. 7–13) and oral infections (including acute necrotizing ulcerative gingivitis) because white blood cells are not functioning. In addition, if there is a decrease in platelets, bleeding gums, petechiae, and ecchymoses may be present. Toothache due to invasion of the pulp by leukemic cells has been reported.

Diagnosis and Treatment. In acute leukemia, laboratory findings include an elevated white blood cell count with the presence of many immature cells, anemia, and a low platelet count. In young children with acute lymphocytic leukemia, the prognosis with treatment is very good. In adolescents and adults with acute myelocytic leukemia, the prognosis is poor. Remissions occur with chemotherapy, and then relapses occur. Bone marrow transplantation is a treatment for this form of leukemia.

Chronic Leukemias

There are also several different types of chronic leukemias. They are all characterized by a slow onset and they all primarily affect adults. The disease can be present for

TABLE 7–3 Classification of Leukemias	
Acute Leukemias	**Chronic Leukemias**
Acute lymphoblastic leukemia (lymphocytes)	Chronic granulocytic (myeloid) leukemia
Acute nonlymphoblastic leukemia (granulocytes, monocytes, erythrocytes)	Chronic lymphocytic leukemia

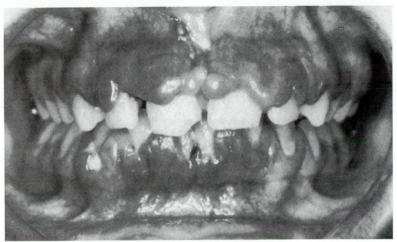

_f_ igure 7–13   Generalized gingival hyperplasia in a patient with leukemia. (From Regezi JA, Sciubba JJ: Oral Pathology: Clinical-Pathologic Correlations. Philadelphia, WB Saunders, 1989, p 190.)

months before a diagnosis is made, and occasionally the diagnosis is made during a routine physical examination on the basis of laboratory testing. One of the forms of chronic leukemia, **chronic myeloid leukemia,** is associated with a distinctive chromosomal abnormality, the Philadelphia chromosome. Another form of chronic leukemia, **chronic lymphocytic leukemia,** is the most common form and accounts for about one quarter of the total cases of leukemia. It may be asymptomatic for a long time. About half the patients with this type of leukemia have abnormal karyotypes; however, the abnormality is different from the Philadelphia chromosome.

Clinical and Oral Manifestations. The clinical onset is slow. The symptoms are nonspecific and include easy fatigability, weakness, weight loss, and anorexia. Oral manifestations include pallor of the lips and gingiva, gingival enlargement, petechiae and ecchymosis, gingival bleeding, and atypical periodontal disease.

Diagnosis and Treatment. The white blood cell count can increase to 500,000/mm³, and most of the total cells can be leukemia cells. Remissions occur with chemotherapy; however, they are of short duration, and the long-term prognosis is poor. Bone marrow transplantation is used to treat chronic leukemia as well as acute leukemia.

BLEEDING DISORDERS

Hemostasis

Patients with bleeding disorders can have one of a number of different defects. **Hemostasis** (the cessation of bleeding) is a complex process that involves a number of events (Fig. 7–14). When a blood vessel is damaged, marked constriction of the vessel **(vasoconstriction)** occurs in an attempt to stop the flow of blood. Platelets (thrombocytes) that are produced by the bone marrow and are circulating in blood adhere to the damaged surface and aggregate to form a temporary clot. In order to stop the bleeding permanently, it is necessary for fibrin to be produced. Fibrin tightly binds the aggregating platelets to form a clot. A cascade of 11 circulating plasma proteins called **clotting factors** or **coagulation factors** is necessary to convert the precursor fibrinogen to fibrin (Table 7–4; Fig. 7–15). Finally, anticlotting mechanisms

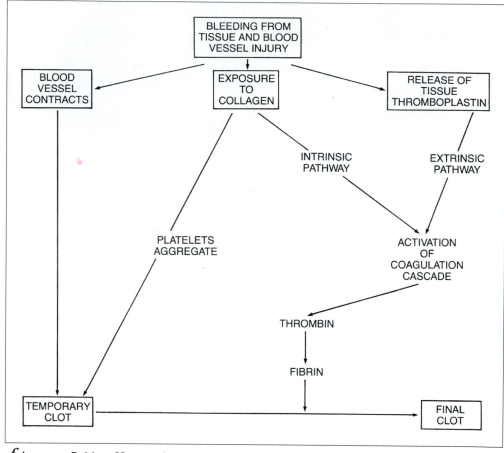

■ *f* i g u r e **7-14**   Hemostasis.

are activated to prevent the spread of more clots and to allow the clot to dissolve so that the damaged vessel can be repaired. This complexity is necessary to prevent inappropriate clotting. Successful hemostasis is dependent on the walls of the blood vessels, adequate numbers of functioning platelets, and adequate levels of properly functioning clotting factors.

TABLE 7-4 Factors Involved in Coagulation*	
Factor	**Name**
I	Fibrinogen
II	Prothrombin
III	Tissue factor
IV	Calcium ions
V	Proaccelerin
VII	Convertin
VIII	Antihemophilic factor
IX	Plasma thromboplastin
X	Stuart factor
XI	Plasma thromboplastin antecedent
XII	Fibrin stabilizing factor

*Factors are numbered in the order in which they were discovered and not in the order in which they function. (There is no Factor VI.)

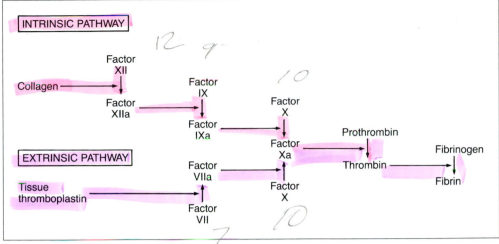

f i g u r e 7-15 Coagulation cascade. Coagulation factors remain inactive until needed. As each coagulation factor becomes activated (a), it is responsible for the activation of another factor until all have been activated and the final clot is formed. There are two pathways by which this cascade is activated: the intrinsic pathway and the extrinsic pathway.

Diagnosis. Defects in hemostasis are caused by abnormalities of either platelets or coagulation factors. These defects can be diagnosed with a few laboratory tests (Table 7–5). Normal values may differ according to the specific test used and the individual laboratory.

Platelet Count

The **platelet count,** which is usually requested with a CBC, provides a quantitative or numeric evaluation of platelets. A normal platelet count should be 150,000 to 400,000/mm³. A platelet count less than 100,000/mm³ is considered thrombocytopenia. In addition, a physician can request specific clotting factor assays, which can also be performed in patients with suspected or known clotting factor deficiencies. Nearly all bleeding disorders are caused by abnormalities of either platelets or clotting factors. Rarely, bleeding disorders result from capillary fragility or weakness of the blood vessel walls.

Bleeding Time

The **bleeding time** provides an assessment of the adequacy of platelet function, not platelet number. The test measures how long it takes a standardized skin incision to stop bleeding by the formation of a temporary hemostatic plug or clot. The normal

TABLE 7–5 Laboratory Tests for Hemostasis	
Test	**Normal Values***
Platelet count (number of platelets)	150,000–400,000/mm³
Bleeding time (platelet function)	1–6 minutes
PT (prothrombin time; fibrin clot formation—extrinsic pathway)	11–16 seconds
PTT (partial thromboplastin time; fibrin clot formation—intrinsic pathway)	25–40 seconds

Normal values may differ according to the specific test used and the individual laboratory.

range of bleeding time is dependent on the way the test is performed but is usually between 1 and 6 minutes. The bleeding time is prolonged, or greater than 5 to 10 minutes, in patients with platelet abnormalities.

Prothrombin Time

The **prothrombin time (PT)** measures the patient's ability to form a clot. It is performed by measuring the time it takes for a clot to form when calcium and a tissue factor are added to the patient's plasma. A normal PT is usually between 11 and 16 seconds. The value is usually compared with a normal control, which is generated daily by the laboratory using standardized plasma. A prolonged or greater than normal PT can be associated with postoperative bleeding because of abnormal clot formation. A prolonged PT is usually not associated with bleeding unless it is longer than one and one-half times the control. PT is used most often by physicians to monitor anticoagulant therapy (e.g., coumarin or warfarin sodium) for preventing myocardial infarction.

Partial Thromboplastin Time

The **partial thromboplastin time (PTT)** also measures the effectiveness of clot formation. There are two different pathways by which clot formation occurs. PT measures one of these, and PTT measures the other. The test is performed by measuring the time it takes for a clot to form after the addition of kaolin, a surface-activating factor, and cephalin, a substitute platelet factor, to the patient's plasma. A normal PTT is usually 25 to 40 seconds. Prolongation of the PTT to 45 to 50 seconds can be associated with mild bleeding problems. With further prolongation (>50 seconds), severe bleeding can occur. PTT is also used by physicians to monitor heparin therapy, which is commonly used for kidney hemodialysis in patients with renal failure.

Purpura

Purpura is a reddish-blue or purplish discoloration of the skin or mucosa that results from spontaneous extravasation of blood. It can be caused by a defect or deficiency in blood platelets or an increase in capillary fragility. A significant oral clinical finding is the oozing of blood at the gingival margins in several sites without the presence of gingivitis or inflammation. Petechiae, ecchymoses, and hemorrhagic blisters can also be present.

Thrombocytopenic Purpura

Thrombocytopenic purpura is a bleeding disorder that results from a severe reduction in circulating platelets. The normal platelet level is 150,000 to 400,000/mm³ of blood. Spontaneous bleeding occurs when platelet levels fall to less than 50,000/mm³. When the cause is unknown, the condition is called **idiopathic thrombocytopenic purpura.** An autoimmune type of process has been identified for thrombocytopenia, and therefore it is sometimes called **immune thrombocytopenia.** The condition can also be secondary to an existing disease or condition. **Secondary thrombocytopenic purpura** is often associated with drugs, including those used for cancer chemotherapy. The idiopathic or primary form is usually seen in young patients, with the greatest incidence occurring before the age of 10 years. There is no age predilection for the secondary type and no sex predilection for either.

Clinical and Oral Manifestations. Clinically, spontaneous purpuric or hemorrhagic lesions of the skin develop that can vary in size and severity. Additionally, these patients bruise easily, can have blood in the urine, and have frequent nosebleeds (epistaxis). Oral manifestations include gingival bleeding when there is no inflammation and clusters of petechiae or purpuric spots.

Diagnosis and Treatment. Laboratory tests show a significant decrease in platelets. Bleeding time can be prolonged to an hour or more, and the capillary fragility test result is positive. Treatment depends on the cause and includes transfusions, corticosteroids, and splenectomy. Any dental surgical procedure, including scaling, is contraindicated until laboratory test results confirm sufficient improvement in the patient's bleeding problem.

Nonthrombocytopenic Purpura

Nonthrombocytopenic purpuras are bleeding disorders that can result from either a defect in the capillary walls or disorders of platelet function. Vascular wall alterations occur in vitamin C deficiency and infections and can also result from chemicals and allergy. Many factors can cause disorders of platelet function, including drugs, allergy, and autoimmune disease. By far the most common reason for a prolonged bleeding time is the ingestion of drugs that affect platelet function. Ingestion of small doses of aspirin (0.3 to 1.5 g) produces an impairment of platelet function for 7 to 10 days. The nonsteroidal anti-inflammatory drugs (e.g., ibuprofen, naproxen, indomethacin) can also adversely affect platelet function. Patients with kidney failure and those with leukemia can have impaired platelet function. **Von Willebrand's disease** is an inherited disorder of platelet function.

Oral Manifestations. The oral manifestations in nonthrombocytopenic purpura are the same as those that occur in thrombocytopenic purpura and include spontaneous gingival bleeding, petechiae, ecchymoses, and hemorrhagic blisters.

Diagnosis and Treatment. The platelet count is normal in nonthrombocytopenic purpura. The bleeding time is prolonged. Treatment includes systemic corticosteroids, splenectomy, and permanent or temporary discontinuation of the causative agent.

Hemophilia

Hemophilia is a disorder of blood coagulation that results in severely prolonged clotting time. The problem results from a deficiency of one of the plasma proteins involved in the coagulation cascade that is necessary for the conversion of fibrinogen to fibrin (see Fig. 7–15).

Types of Hemophilia

There are three types of hemophilia. Two of these types, called types A and B, are inherited as X-linked diseases and are therefore transmitted through an unaffected (carrier) daughter to a grandson. The carrier daughter can have a mildly prolonged coagulation time. The other type is called type C and is not sex-linked and therefore affects women as well as men. (Inheritance patterns, including sex-linked inheritance, are described in Chapter 6.)

Type A hemophilia is the classic and most common type and is caused by a deficiency of the clotting factor called **plasma thromboplastinogen** or **Factor VIII.** This deficiency is characterized by severe hemorrhage following even mild to moderate injury or surgery. Type B, or Christmas disease, is less common. The clotting defect is in **plasma thromboplastin** or **Factor IV.** In type C, there is less severe bleeding and the deficiency is in **plasma thromboplastin antecedent** or **Factor IX.**

Oral Manifestation. The oral manifestations of hemophilia are spontaneous gingival bleeding, petechiae, and ecchymoses. There is a risk of hemorrhage after oral surgery procedures and scaling.

Diagnosis and Treatment. The bleeding time and PT in hemophilia are normal, and the PTT is prolonged. Diagnosis involves identifying the missing factor, and treatment involves replacing it.

IMMUNODEFICIENCY

Immunity is described in Chapter 3. Immunodeficiency can involve the different parts of the immune system either alone or together. Immunodeficiency can involve the cell-mediated (T cell) response or the humoral (B cell or antibody) response. Deficiencies in phagocytosis can also be considered deficiencies in immunity. Immunodeficiency diseases are divided into primary and secondary immunodeficiencies. Primary immunodeficiencies are those of genetic origin, and secondary immunodeficiencies result from some other underlying disorder. The signs and symptoms that occur in a person with immunodeficiency depend on the degree of the deficiency and the type of immune response involved.

Primary Immunodeficiencies

Primary immunodeficiencies are immunodeficiencies of genetic origin and can involve B cells or T cells, or both. These primary immunodeficiencies have provided much information about the functions of the different immunologic responses and are extremely rare.

Three examples are included here. The first is **Bruton's disease,** also called **X-linked congenital agammaglobulinemia** (lack of immunoglobulins), which is a disorder in which B cells do not mature. There is a lack of plasma cells throughout the body; T cells are normal. Autoimmune diseases are common in these patients.

The second example is **DiGeorge's syndrome,** which is also called **thymic hypoplasia.** It is a disorder in which the thymus is deficient or lacking and therefore T lymphocytes do not mature. Infants and children with this syndrome are extremely susceptible to fungal and viral infections, as well as bacterial infections, which require T- and B-cell cooperation. B lymphocytes and immunoglobulins are not affected.

The third example is **severe combined immunodeficiency.** Most infants with this type of immunodeficiency die within the first year of life and are vulnerable to all forms of viral, fungal, and bacterial infections.

Secondary Immunodeficiencies

Secondary immunodeficiencies are those that occur as a result of an underlying disorder. They are much more common than the primary immunodeficiency disorders. Disorders that can have accompanying immunodeficiency include malnutrition, which can lead to inadequate synthesis of antibodies; viral infection; cancer; renal diseases in which antibodies are excreted abnormally; and Hodgkin's disease. They can also occur with the use of immunosuppressive drugs, including corticosteroids; drugs that are used, along with radiation, to suppress the immune system in organ and bone marrow transplantation and to treat autoimmune diseases; and drugs used for cancer chemotherapy. Table 7–6 lists some of the most common drugs that can cause immunodeficiency and the reasons they are generally used. Acquired immunodeficiency syndrome (AIDS),

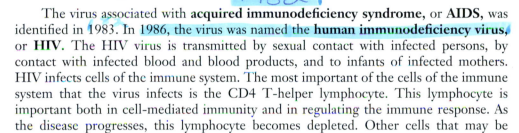

TABLE 7–6 Examples of Drugs That Can Cause Immunosuppression	
Name	**Use**
Azathioprine	Prevention of rejection of renal transplants
	Treatment of rheumatoid arthritis
Cyclosporine	Prevention of rejection of renal transplants
Cyclophosphamide	Cancer chemotherapy
Methotrexate	Cancer chemotherapy
Prednisone	Treatment of autoimmune diseases, e.g., rheumatoid arthritis, pemphigus vulgaris, Behçet's syndrome, lupus erythematosus

which occurs as a result of infection with the human immunodeficiency virus (HIV), is described here, both as an example of a secondary immunodeficiency and because of the number and significance of the oral lesions that occur in this disease.

HIV Infection and AIDS

The virus associated with **acquired immunodeficiency syndrome,** or **AIDS,** was identified in 1983. In 1986, the virus was named the **human immunodeficiency virus,** or **HIV.** The HIV virus is transmitted by sexual contact with infected persons, by contact with infected blood and blood products, and to infants of infected mothers. HIV infects cells of the immune system. The most important of the cells of the immune system that the virus infects is the CD4 T-helper lymphocyte. This lymphocyte is important both in cell-mediated immunity and in regulating the immune response. As the disease progresses, this lymphocyte becomes depleted. Other cells that may be infected with HIV include macrophages, Langerhans cells, and cells of the nervous system.

The Spectrum of HIV Disease

Following infection with HIV, many individuals experience an acute disease that occurs shortly after infection and other individuals remain asymptomatic. The acute disease resolves, and infected individuals may have no signs or symptoms of disease for some time. In most patients infected with HIV, a progressive immunodeficiency eventually develops. As the immune system begins to fail, the number of CD4 lymphocytes decreases, patients have nonspecific problems such as fatigue, and opportunistic infections such as oral candidiasis may develop. As the immune system becomes profoundly deficient, life-threatening opportunistic infections and cancers occur. The most severe result of infection with HIV is AIDS.

Diagnosing AIDS

The diagnosis of AIDS is well defined. The definition of AIDS has been established by the Centers for Disease Control and Prevention (CDC) and is given in Table 7–7. Since it was identified in the early 1980s, the definition of AIDS has been changed several times as knowledge of the disease has grown. The most recent definition of AIDS in adults and adolescents includes HIV infection with severe CD4 lymphocyte depletion (less than 200 CD4 lymphocytes per microliter [μl] of blood). The normal CD4 lymphocyte count is between about 550 and 1000 lymphocytes/μl. The revised definition continues to include a number of opportunistic diseases, such as *Pneumocystis carinii* pneumonia, esophageal candidiasis, and Kaposi's sarcoma. Also included is HIV-

Handwritten annotations (margins): ARC = AIDS Related Complex; Primary; Full Blown aids; ① lesion most common on palate; Fungal; Bilat.

TABLE 7–7 Definition of AIDS*

AIDS is an illness characterized by one or more of the following diseases or conditions:

HIV Laboratory Tests Not Performed or Results Inconclusive and the Patient Has No Other Cause of Immunodeficiency

 1. Candidiasis of the esophagus, trachea, bronchi, or lungs
 2. Cryptococcosis, extrapulmonary
 3. Cryptosporidiosis with diarrhea persisting longer than 1 month
 4. Cytomegalovirus disease of an organ other than liver, spleen, or lymph nodes in a patient older than 1 month of age
 5. Herpes simplex virus infection causing a mucocutaneous ulcer that persists longer than 1 month, or bronchitis, pneumonitis, or esophagitis for any duration affecting a patient older than 1 month of age
 6. Kaposi's sarcoma affecting a patient less than 60 years of age
 7. Lymphoma of the brain affecting a patient less than 60 years of age
 8. Lymphoid interstitial pneumonia or pulmonary hyperplasia, or both, affecting a child less than 13 years of age
 9. *Mycobacterium avium* or *Mycobacterium kansasii* disease, disseminated
10. *Pneumocystis carinii* pneumonia
11. Progressive multifocal leukoencephalopathy
12. Toxoplasmosis of the brain affecting a patient older than 1 month of age

With Laboratory Evidence for HIV Infection
Less than 200 CD4+ T lymphocytes/μl, or a CD4+ T-lymphocyte percentage of total lymphocytes of less than 14

Any of the preceding diseases listed or those that follow:
 1. Multiple bacterial infections of certain types affecting a child less than 13 years of age
 2. Coccidioidomycosis, disseminated
 3. HIV encephalopathy (HIV dementia)
 4. Histoplasmosis, disseminated
 5. Isosporiasis with diarrhea persisting longer than 1 month
 6. Lymphoma of the brain at any age
 7. Kaposi's sarcoma at any age
 8. Certain types of lymphoma
 9. Mycobacterial disease, other than tuberculosis, disseminated
10. Extrapulmonary tuberculosis
11. *Salmonella* septicemia, recurrent
12. HIV wasting syndrome
13. Pulmonary tuberculosis
14. Recurrent pneumonia
15. Invasive cervical cancer

Even if HIV laboratory test results are negative, if other causes of immunodeficiency are ruled out, a diagnosis of AIDS can be made if certain of these diseases are diagnosed.

*Adapted from Centers for Disease Control and Prevention: 1993 Revised classification system for HIV infection and expanded surveillance case definition for AIDS among adolescents and adults. MMWR 41(RR-17), 1992.

related wasting syndrome. In addition to including the CD4 lymphocyte count, the revised definition includes pulmonary tuberculosis, recurrent pneumonia, and invasive cervical cancer.

HIV Testing

Two antibody tests are now generally used to determine if a person has been infected with HIV. The first test is often called an **enzyme-linked immunosorbent assay (ELISA or EIA)**. When this test is positive twice, it is followed by a more specific test called the **Western blot test.** In order to be considered seropositive for HIV, a person must have two positive ELISA test results followed by a positive Western blot test result. Other tests, such as the **polymerase chain reaction (PCR),** are now available. The PCR identifies virus rather than antibody and thereby enables the identification of infection earlier than antibody tests. Although not used for routine testing, these tests are used in the management of some patients. Informed consent by the patient and pretest counseling may be required before HIV testing can be done.

Clinical Manifestations

As mentioned, the initial infection with HIV may be completely asymptomatic. In some individuals lymphadenopathy may develop, and in still others an acute illness, resembling infectious mononucleosis and lasting 8 to 14 days, can occur. When this acute illness develops, the patient may have sore throat, general malaise, myalgia and arthralgia, lymphadenopathy, and fever. Patients with acute infection can also have a skin rash, nausea, and diarrhea. Following this acute illness, some individuals have persistent lymphadenopathy, but many become completely asymptomatic.

The virus infects cells of the immune system, and as a result this system stops protecting the individual against certain infections and tumors. In time, as the immune system becomes deficient, a variety of signs and symptoms can develop, signaling changes in the immune system. Several of these signs and symptoms occurring together are sometimes called AIDS-related complex (ARC). These symptoms include oral candidiasis, fatigue, weight loss, and lymphadenopathy. HIV can also infect cells of the nervous system, resulting in dementia in some patients.

Antibodies to HIV generally begin to be detectable in blood about 6 weeks after the initial infection. However, in some individuals antibodies may not be detectable for 6 months and occasionally for up to 1 year or more.

The spectrum of HIV infection includes the full range of problems that result from infection with this virus—from asymptomatic infection to AIDS (Fig. 7–16). It is not yet known how many of the persons who become infected with HIV go on to experience immunodeficiency, opportunistic diseases, or dementia. Some patients who are HIV-seropositive appear to remain immunocompetent for many years. Cofactors that can contribute to the development of the immunodeficiency are being studied. Each year the results of natural history studies show an increase in the percentage of HIV-infected individuals in whom AIDS develops. The time from initial infection with HIV to the development of AIDS ranges from 2 years to more than 10 years.

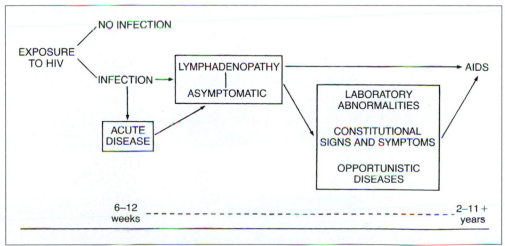

■ *figure* 7–16   Spectrum of HIV disease. (Courtesy of the American Dental Association, Division of Scientific Affairs, Speakers Bureau.)

Oral Manifestations

Oral lesions are prominent features of AIDS and HIV infection (Table 7–8). Some of these lesions are known to be indicators of developing immunodeficiency and predictors of the development of AIDS in individuals who are HIV-seropositive. The oral lesions that occur develop because of the deficiency in cell-mediated immunity and because of the deregulation of immunologic responses that occurs when the T-helper cells become depleted. Oral lesions include opportunistic infections, tumors, and autoimmune-like diseases.

Oral Candidiasis. This oral lesion, described in Chapter 3, occurs frequently in individuals with cell-mediated immunodeficiency and is one of the most common oral lesions seen in persons with HIV infection (Fig. 7–17). It is also called **thrush.** All of the different types of oral candidiasis described in Chapter 3, as well as skin and nail involvement, can occur. It is important to remember that candidiasis can be associated with a variety of conditions other than HIV infection, such as uncontrolled diabetes, other immunodeficiency diseases, antibiotic treatment, and xerostomia. Both topical and systemic antifungal treatment can be used to control oral candidiasis in the patient with immunodeficiency caused by HIV infection. Recurrence is common.

In persons who are known to be infected with HIV, the development of oral candidiasis is worrisome because it generally signals the beginning of a progressively severe immunodeficiency. Persons with unexplained oral candidiasis should be referred to a physician for evaluation if the cause of the candidiasis cannot be determined. Studies have shown oral candidiasis to be a very early sign of developing immunodeficiency and predictive of the development of AIDS in a person who is infected with HIV.

Other fungal infections, such as histoplasmosis and coccidiodomycosis, have also been reported in persons with HIV infection, but they are rare.

Herpes Simplex Infection. Ulcers caused by the herpes simplex virus occur in persons with HIV infection (Fig. 7–18). Herpes labialis and lesions consistent with intraoral recurrent herpes simplex infection can develop in persons with HIV infection. The clinical characteristics of these lesions are the same as those occurring in immunocompetent individuals. However, when the immune system, particularly cell-mediated immunity, becomes deficient, HIV-infected individuals are at risk for the development of ulcers caused by the herpes simplex virus that do not have the same clinical

TABLE 7–8 Oral Lesions Associated with HIV Infection

Candidiasis
Herpes simplex infection
Herpes zoster
Hairy leukoplakia
HPV (human papillomavirus) lesions
Atypical gingivitis and periodontitis
Other opportunistic infections reported
 Mycobacterium avium, Mycobacterium intracellulare
 Cytomegalovirus
 Cryptococcus neoformans
 Klebsiella pneumoniae
 Enterobacter cloacae
 Histoplasma capsulatum
Kaposi's sarcoma
Non-Hodgkin's lymphoma
Aphthous ulcers
Mucosal pigmentation
Bilateral salivary gland enlargement and xerostomia
Spontaneous gingival bleeding resulting from thrombocytopenia

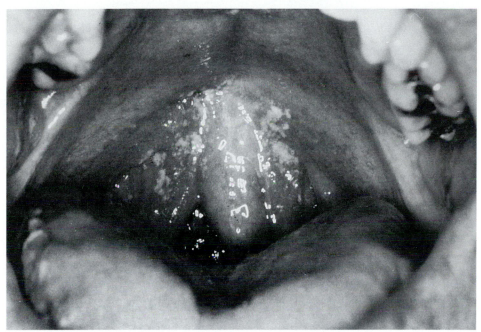

■ *f i g u r e* **7–17** Candidiasis in a patient with HIV infection.

characteristics as those seen in non–HIV-infected persons. These appear as persistent, superficial, painful ulcers that can be located anywhere in the oral cavity. Small, characteristic herpes simplex–like ulcers can be seen surrounding larger ulcers, but their presence cannot be depended on for diagnosis. The diagnosis of these ulcers is made by several methods, including viral culture, cytologic smear, biopsy, and response to the antiviral medication acyclovir.

Ulceration of the oral mucosa from herpes simplex infection that has been present for more than a month is an oral lesion that meets the criteria for the diagnosis of AIDS. This can occur only when a person has profound immunodeficiency.

Oral ulcers caused by **cytomegalovirus** may also occur in HIV-infected individuals who are severely immunodeficient. These ulcers are much rarer than those caused by herpes simplex virus.

Herpes Zoster. Herpes zoster is caused by the varicella-zoster virus and is described in Chapter 3. When herpes zoster occurs in a person with HIV infection, it generally follows the usual pattern. Although the infection can disseminate, most cases are self-limited. In the facial and oral area, the lesions appear as distinctly unilateral ones following the distribution of one or more branches of the trigeminal nerve.

The development of herpes zoster in a person infected with HIV is a sign of developing immunodeficiency.

Hairy Leukoplakia. Hairy leukoplakia usually occurs on the lateral borders of the tongue in individuals with HIV infection (Fig. 7–19; Color Plate 47). It appears as an irregular, white lesion that often has a corrugated surface. Histologically, this lesion shows hyperkeratosis, often with hair-like projections, and epithelial hyperplasia, vacuolated epithelial cells, and little or no inflammatory infiltrate in the underlying connective tissue.

Other white lesions, such as those resulting from chronic tongue chewing and hyperplastic candidiasis, can resemble hairy leukoplakia clinically. Biopsy of the lesions can reveal a histologic appearance that is consistent with hairy leukoplakia. However, the most reliable method of diagnosis is identification of the Epstein-Barr virus in the lesion.

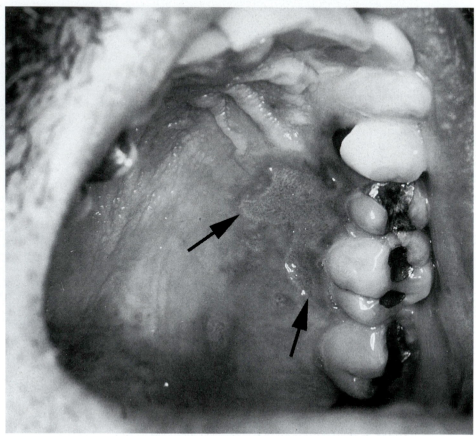

■ *f i g u r e* **7–18**   Herpes simplex ulceration of the hard palate in a patient with HIV infection. Arrows point to the periphery of the ulcer.

Generally, hairy leukoplakia is not treated. Lesions may respond to antiviral medication (acyclovir or zidovudine) but recur when treatment is discontinued. The development of hairy leukoplakia in individuals who are known to be infected with HIV is worrisome. Studies have shown hairy leukoplakia to be predictive of the development of AIDS in these persons.

Papillomavirus Infections. Lesions caused by papillomaviruses are described in Chapter 3. Papillary oral lesions resulting from several different papillomaviruses have been described in persons with HIV infection. They present with either normal color or slightly erythematous mucosa (Fig. 7–20). These lesions may be persistent and may occur in multiple oral mucosal locations. Diagnosis of these lesions is made by biopsy and histologic examination with special tests to identify papillomavirus.

Kaposi's Sarcoma. Kaposi's sarcoma is one of the opportunistic neoplasms that occur in patients with HIV infection. Oral lesions appear as reddish-purple flat or raised lesions and are seen anywhere in the oral cavity. The most common locations are the palate and gingiva (Fig. 7–21; Color Plates 90 and 91).

The diagnosis is made by biopsy. However, the clinical appearance of the lesion can be used when it is characteristic and the diagnosis of Kaposi's sarcoma has been made at another site.

At present, there is no effective treatment for Kaposi's sarcoma. Surgical excision to decrease the size of the lesion is sometimes attempted, as are radiation treatment and chemotherapy.

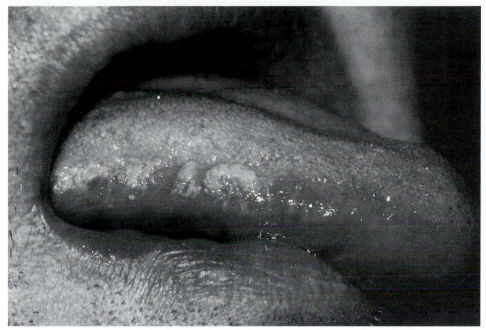

■ *f* **i g u r e** **7–19**   Hairy leukoplakia.

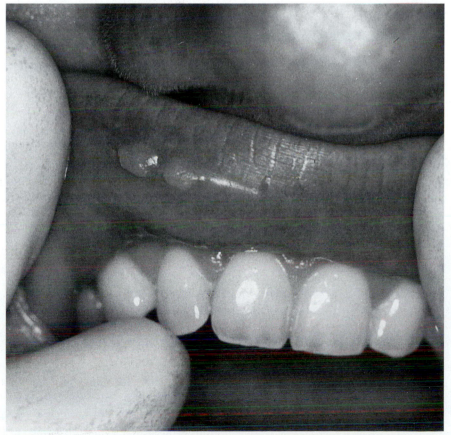

■ *f* **i g u r e** **7–20**   Papillary lesion of the upper lip caused by human papillomavirus in a patient with HIV infection.

Kaposi's sarcoma is one of the intraoral lesions that may fulfill the criteria for the diagnosis of AIDS.

Lymphoma. Non-Hodgkin's lymphoma is another of the tumors that occur in association with HIV infection. It occasionally occurs in the oral cavity. These tumors have appeared as nonulcerated, necrotic, or ulcerated masses and have been surfaced by either normal-color or erythematous mucosa (Fig. 7–22).

The diagnosis is made by biopsy and histologic examination. Treatment involves several different chemotherapeutic drugs.

Oral lymphoma is another oral lesion that may meet the criteria for the diagnosis of AIDS.

Periodontal Disease. In patients with HIV infection, unusual forms of gingival and periodontal disease can develop. These occur in HIV-infected individuals whose immune system has become deficient. These have been called linear gingival erythema (LGE) and necrotizing ulcerative periodontitis (NUP). A condition resembling acute necrotizing ulcerative gingivitis (ANUG) also occurs in individuals with HIV infection.

LGE has three characteristic features: spontaneous bleeding; punctate or petechiae-like lesions on the attached gingiva and alveolar mucosa; a band-like erythema of the gingiva that does not respond to therapy.

LGE is different from typical gingivitis in that gingivitis is generally not characterized by spontaneous bleeding, and the erythema of typical gingivitis responds within a few days to a week to scaling, root planning, and improvement of oral hygiene. LGE occurs independently of oral hygiene status.

Some patients experience gingivitis that resembles ANUG, and it can be either generalized or localized to specific areas.

NUP resembles ANUG in that there is pain, spontaneous gingival bleeding, interproximal necrosis, and interproximal cratering (Fig. 7–23; Color Plate 77). There is also intense erythema and, most characteristically, extremely rapid bone loss. **Necrotizing stomatitis** is characterized by extensive focal areas of bone loss along with the features of NUP.

The specific causes of these atypical gingival and periodontal diseases remain

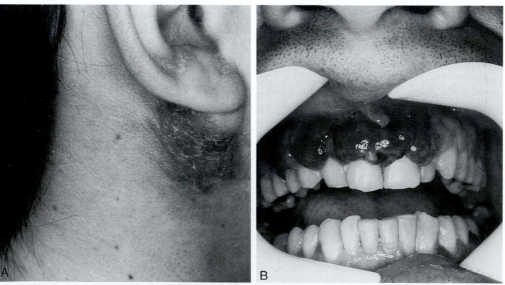

f i g u r e 7–21   Kaposi's sarcoma in a patient with AIDS. *A,* Skin. *B,* Gingiva. (Courtesy of Dr. Fariba Younai.)

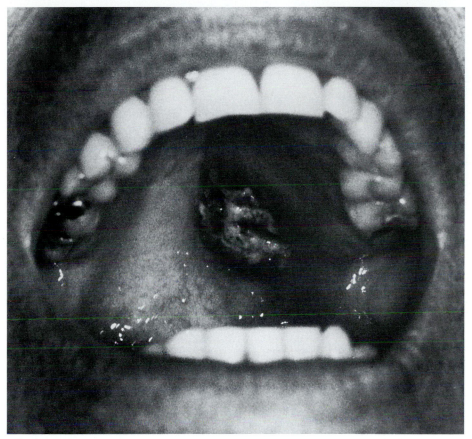

■ *f* **i g u r e** 7–22   Intraoral lymphoma in a patient with AIDS.

unclear. The microbiota associated with these diseases are being studied and have not been found to be distinctly different from those of inflammatory periodontal disease. These atypical gingival and periodontal conditions are not common in HIV-infected individuals and appear to occur in those patients whose immune system has become severely compromised.

Treatment of HIV gingivitis and periodontitis involves scaling, root planing, and soft tissue curettage. In addition, intrasulcular lavage with povidone-iodine, use of chlorhexidine mouth rinse, and short-term systemic metronidazole administration have been helpful in the treatment of these conditions. Good oral hygiene, including the use of smaller toothbrushes and interproximal cleaning devices, has been a component of management.

Not all HIV-infected patients have periodontal problems. However, recognition of early lesions is essential to prevent extensive bone loss, and frequent recall is helpful in early identification of gingival and periodontal disease. Lack of response to periodontal treatment is a clue to the recognition of HIV-associated gingivitis and periodontitis.

Spontaneous Gingival Bleeding. A decrease in the number of platelets resulting from an autoimmune type of thrombocytopenic purpura is occasionally seen in patients with HIV infection. These patients can present with bleeding gums or mucosal petechiae.

Gingival bleeding not related to thrombocytopenia has also been described in LGE and NUP.

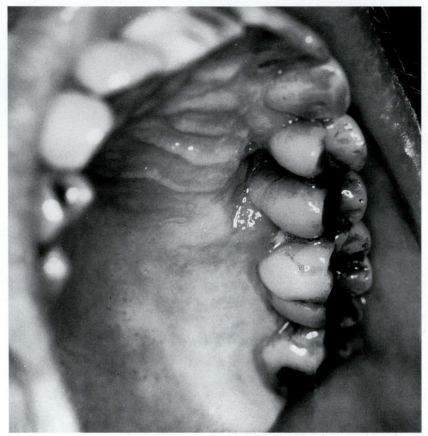

▪ *figure* **7–23**   Atypical periodontal disease in a patient with HIV infection.

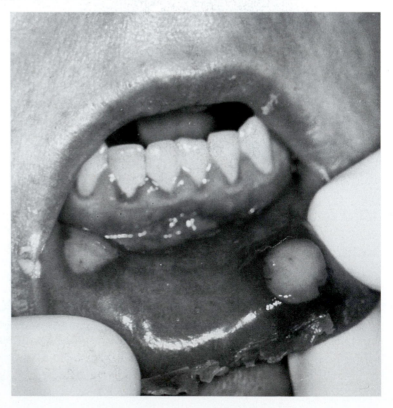

▪ *figure* **7–24**
Major aphthous-like ulcers in
a patient with HIV infection.
(Courtesy of Dr. Sidney Eisig.)

A platelet count and bleeding time should be considered before deep scaling procedures are performed.

Aphthous Ulcers. Characteristic minor aphthous ulcers occur in patients with HIV infection and AIDS. Studies have suggested that there is an increase in the incidence of these ulcers in patients with HIV infection. Minor aphthous ulcers are diagnosed on the basis of their clinical appearance.

Ulcers that resemble major aphthous ulcers also occur in patients with HIV infection (Fig. 7–24). They appear as deep, persistent, painful ulcers and must be differentiated from infectious ulcers. Biopsy and histologic examination of these ulcers does not show any evidence of an infectious cause. These ulcers respond to topical steroid application. Topical application of tetracycline has also been used in the management of these ulcers. Similar ulcers have been seen in the esophagus of patients with HIV infection.

Salivary Gland Disease. Xerostomia has been reported to be associated with HIV infection. The cause is not clear. It may be related to medication administration or salivary gland disease. Bilateral parotid gland enlargement has been reported to occur in patients who are HIV-positive (Fig. 7–25). The histologic appearance is reported to be that of a benign lymphoepithelial lesion, often with a prominent cystic component.

Mucosal Melanin Pigmentation. Macular areas of melanin pigmentation of unknown cause also occur in patients with HIV infection.

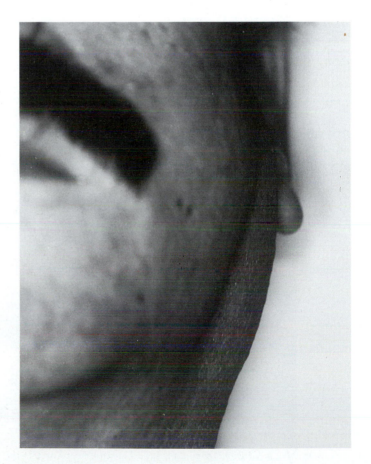

■ *f* i g u r e 7–25
Salivary gland enlargement was bilateral in this patient with HIV infection.

ORAL MANIFESTATIONS OF THERAPY FOR ORAL CANCER

Oral cancer can be treated by surgery, radiation therapy, or chemotherapy, or any combination of the three. Radiation therapy and chemotherapy can result in the development of several different oral manifestations.

Radiation Therapy

During radiation therapy the patient often experiences mucositis (Fig. 7–26), which begins about the second week of therapy and subsides a few weeks after its completion. The mucositis is painful and appears as erythematous and ulcerated mucosa. Difficulty in eating, pain on swallowing, and loss of taste can occur as a result of the mucositis. If the radiation affects the major salivary glands, irreversible salivary gland destruction can occur, resulting in severe xerostomia. As a result, the mucosal tissues are easily irritated and the patient is prone to the development of rampant caries and oral candidiasis (Fig. 7–27). A patient who has received radiation therapy for oral cancer is also at risk for the development of osteonecrosis (necrosis of bone) because of the decreased blood supply to the bone following radiation therapy. Osteonecrosis develops

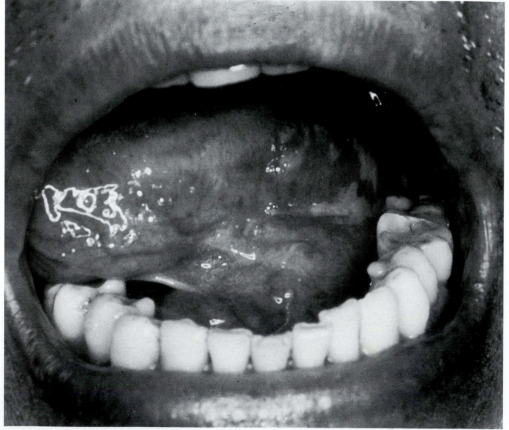

■ *figure* **7-26**   Radiation mucositis.

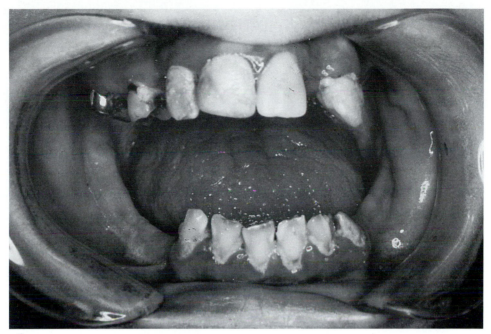

■ *figure* **7-27**   Radiation caries.

in the mandible more frequently than in the maxilla, and the increased risk for its development does not decrease with time.

Chemotherapy

The complications of cancer chemotherapy are predictable and differ for the various types of chemotherapy used. Mucositis and oral ulceration are frequent complications because drugs used for cancer chemotherapy affect rapidly dividing cells and therefore affect the basal cells of the epithelium. The epithelium becomes atrophic and ulcerated with minor irritation. In addition, cells of the bone marrow are also affected, and therefore a decrease in all blood cells (red blood cells, white blood cells, and platelets) can result. Therefore, the patient can experience anemia because of a decrease in red blood cells; and is at increased risk for opportunistic infections (e.g., candidiasis) because of a decrease in white blood cells; and is at increased risk for bleeding problems because of a decrease in the number of platelets.

EFFECTS OF DRUGS ON THE ORAL CAVITY

Many drugs can cause changes in the oral tissues. Xerostomia can be caused by drugs used to control blood pressure. Xerostomia can also be caused by antianxiety medications, antipsychotic medications, and antihistamines (Fig. 7–28). Drugs such as prednisone that suppress the immune system can increase the risk of candidiasis and other oral infections (Fig. 7–29; Color Plate 68). Antibiotics can also increase the risk of candidiasis. Tetracycline taken when teeth are forming can cause tooth discoloration (Fig. 7–30). Phenytoin (Dilantin) and nifedipine (Procardia) can cause gingival hypertrophy (Fig. 7–31; Color Plates 87 and 88).

The complete medical history should include a listing of the medications taken by a patient and is useful in establishing the diagnosis of drug-induced oral lesions.

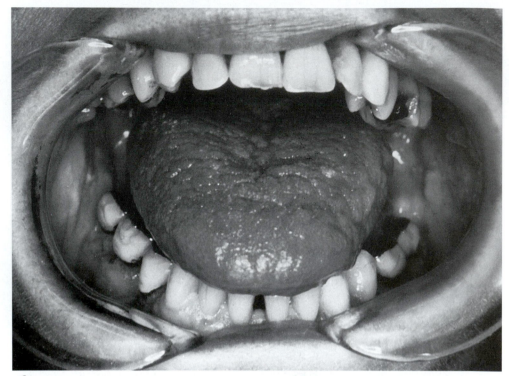

▪ *f* i g u r e **7–28**   Xerostomia caused by chlorpromazine (Thorazine) administration.

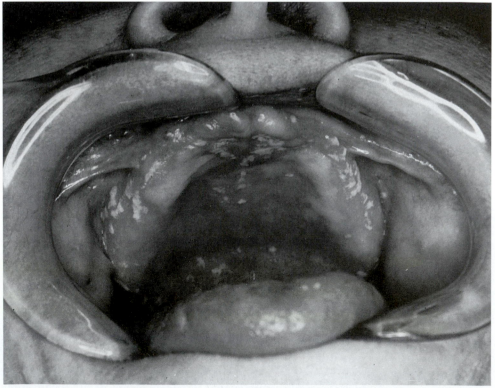

▪ *f* i g u r e **7–29**   Candidiasis in a patient taking prednisone for rheumatoid arthritis.

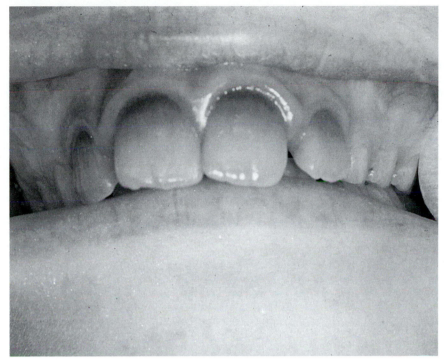

■ *f* i g u r e 7–30   Discoloration of teeth caused by tetracycline ingestion.

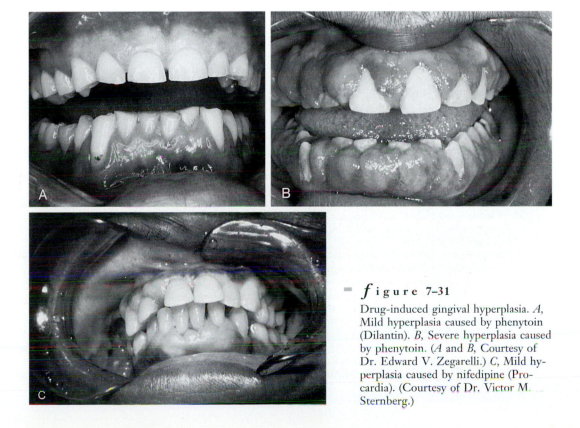

■ *f* i g u r e 7–31

Drug-induced gingival hyperplasia. *A*, Mild hyperplasia caused by phenytoin (Dilantin). *B*, Severe hyperplasia caused by phenytoin. (*A* and *B*, Courtesy of Dr. Edward V. Zegarelli.) *C*, Mild hyperplasia caused by nifedipine (Procardia). (Courtesy of Dr. Victor M. Sternberg.)

SELECTED REFERENCES

BOOKS

Andreoli TE, Carpenter CCJ, Plum F, et al: Cecil Essentials of Medicine, 3rd ed. Philadelphia, WB Saunders, 1993.

Cotran RS, Kumar V, Robbins SL: Robbins Pathologic Basis of Disease, 5th ed. Philadelphia, WB Saunders, 1994.

Cottone JA, Terezhalmy GT, Molinari JA: Practical Infection Control in Dentistry. Philadelphia, Lea & Febiger, 1991.

Halstead CL, Blozis GG, Drinnan AJ, et al: Physical Evaluation of the Dental Patient, St. Louis, CV Mosby, 1982.

Little JW, Falace DA: Dental Management of the Medically Compromised Patient, 4th ed. St. Louis, CV Mosby, 1993.

Neville BW, Damm DD, Allen CM, Bouquot JE: Oral and Maxillofacial Pathology. Philadelphia, WB Saunders, 1995.

Regezi JA, Sciubba JJ: Oral Pathology. Clinical-Pathologic Correlations, 2nd ed. Philadelphia, WB Saunders, 1993.

Rose LF, Kaye D: Internal Medicine for Dentistry. St. Louis, CV Mosby, 1990.

Shafer WG, Hine MK, Levy BL: A Textbook of Oral Pathology, 4th ed. Philadelphia, WB Saunders, 1983.

JOURNAL ARTICLES

Arkel YS: Evaluation of platelet aggregation in disorders of hemostasis. Med Clin North Am 60:881, 1976.

Bainton DF, Finch CA: The diagnosis of iron deficiency anemia. Am J Med 37:62, 1964.

Barone R, Ficarra G, Gaglioti D, et al: Prevalence of oral lesions among HIV infected intravenous drug abusers and other risk groups. Oral Surg Oral Med Oral Pathol 69:169, 1990.

Bessho K, Tagawa T, Murata M, et al: Monostotic fibrous dysplasia with involvement of the mandibular canal. Oral Surg Oral Med Oral Pathol 68:396, 1989.

Carlson ER, Chewning LC: Polycythemia vera in an oral surgical patient: A case report. Oral Surg Oral Med Oral Pathol 67:673, 1989.

Centers for Disease Control and Prevention: 1993 Revised classification system for HIV infection and expanded surveillance case definition for AIDS among adolescents and adults. MMWR 41(RR-17), 1992.

Duffy JH, Driscoll EJ: Oral manifestations of leukemia. Oral Surg Oral Med Oral Pathol 11:484, 1958.

Eisenberg E, Krutchkoff D, Yamase H: Incidental oral hairy leukoplakia in immunocompetent persons. Oral Surg Oral Med Oral Pathol 74:332, 1992.

Epstein JB, Silverman S Jr: Head and neck malignancies associated with HIV infection. Oral Surg Oral Med Oral Pathol 73:193, 1992.

Fletcher PD, Scopp IV, Hersh RA: Oral manifestations of secondary hyperparathyroidism related to long term hemodialysis therapy. Oral Surg Oral Med Oral Pathol 43:218, 1977.

Garraty G, Petz LD: Drug-induced hemolytic anemia. Am J Med 58:398, 1975.

Glick M, Muzyka BC: Alternative therapies for major aphthous ulcers in AIDS patients. J Am Dent Assoc 123:61, 1992.

Green TL, Greenspan JS, Greenspan D, et al: Oral lesions mimicking hairy leukoplakia: A diagnostic dilemma. Oral Surg Oral Med Oral Pathol 67:422, 1989.

Greenspan JS, Barr CE, Sciubba JJ, et al: Oral manifestations of HIV infection: Definitions, diagnostic criteria and principles of therapy. Oral Surg Oral Med Oral Pathol 73:142, 1992.

Greenspan JS, Greenspan D: Oral hairy leukoplakia: Diagnosis and management. Oral Surg Oral Med Oral Pathol 67:396, 1989.

Hernandez YL, Daniels TE: Oral candidiasis in Sjögren's syndrome: Prevalence, clinical correlations, and treatment. Oral Surg Oral Med Oral Pathol 68:324, 1989.

Holmstrup P, Westergaard J: Periodontal diseases in HIV-infected patients. J Clin Periodontol 21:270, 1994.

Inokuchi T, Sano K, Kamingo M: Osteoradionecrosis of the sphenoid and temporal bones in a patient with maxillary sinus carcinoma: A case report. Oral Surg Oral Med Oral Pathol 70:278, 1990.

Johnson WT, Leary JM: Management of dental patients with bleeding disorders: Review and update. Oral Surg Oral Med Oral Pathol 66:297, 1988.

Kanas RJ, Abrams AM, Recher L, et al: Oral hairy leukoplakia: A light microscopic and immunohistochemical study. Oral Surg Oral Med Oral Pathol 66:334, 1988.

Kaugars GE, Burns JC: Non-Hodgkin's lymphoma of the oral cavity associated with AIDS. Oral Surg Oral Med Oral Pathol 67:433, 1989.

Konotey-Ahulu FI: The sickle cell diseases. Arch Intern Med 133:64, 1974.

Leggott PJ: Oral manifestations of HIV infection in children. Oral Surg Oral Med Oral Pathol 73:187, 1992.

Lumerman H, Freedman PD, Kerpel SM, et al: Oral Kaposi's sarcoma: A clinicopathologic study of 23 homosexual and bisexual men from the New York metropolitan area. Oral Surg Oral Med Oral Pathol 65:711, 1988.

McDonough RJ, Nelson CL: Clinical implications of factor XII deficiency. Oral Surg Oral Med Oral Pathol 68:264, 1989.

Miescher PA: Drug-induced thrombocytopenia. Hematology 10:311, 1973.

Murrah VA, Scholtes GA: Antibody testing and counseling of dental patients at risk for human immunodeficiency virus (HIV) infection and associated clinical findings. Oral Surg Oral Med Oral Pathol 66:432, 1988.

Ohishi M, Oobu K, Miyanoshita Y, et al: Acute gingival necrosis caused by drug-induced agranulocytosis. Oral Surg Oral Med Oral Pathol 66:194, 1988.

Park JB, Park N-H: Effect of chlorhexidine on the in vitro and in vivo herpes simplex virus infection. Oral Surg Oral Med Oral Pathol 67:149, 1989.

Pindborg JJ: Classification of oral lesions associated with HIV infection. Oral Surg Oral Med Oral Pathol 67:292, 1989.

Rams TE, Andriolo M Jr, Feik D, et al: Microbiological study of HIV-related periodontitis. J Periodontol 62:74, 1991.

Redding SW, Luce EB, Boren MW: Oral herpes simplex virus infection in patients receiving head and neck radiation. Oral Surg Oral Med Oral Pathol 69:578, 1990.

Samaranayake LP: Oral mycoses in HIV infection. Oral Surg Oral Med Oral Pathol 73:171, 1992.

Schiodt M: HIV-associated salivary gland disease. Oral Surg Oral Med Oral Pathol 37:164, 1992.

Sciubba J, Brandsma J, Schwartz M, et al: Hairy leukoplakia: An AIDS associated opportunistic infection. Oral Surg Oral Med Oral Pathol 67:404, 1989.

Sreebny LM, Valdini A, Yu A: Xerostomia: Part II. Relationship to nonoral symptoms, drugs and diseases. Oral Surg Oral Med Oral Pathol 68:419, 1989.

Swango PA, Kleinman D, Konzelman JL: HIV and periodontal health. J Am Dent Assoc 122:49, 1991.

Wahlin YB: Effects of chlorhexidine mouthrinse on oral health in patients with acute leukemia. Oral Surg Oral Med Oral Pathol 68:279, 1989.

Williams CA, Winkler JR, Grassi M, et al: HIV associated periodontitis complicated by necrotizing stomatitis. Oral Surg Oral Med Oral Pathol 69:351, 1990.

REVIEW QUESTIONS

1. Which one of the following statements is FALSE?
   (A) Primary immunodeficiencies are less common than are secondary immunodeficiencies
   (B) Persons with T-lymphocyte deficiencies are susceptible to viruses and fungi
   (C) Primary immunodeficiencies are all combined B-lymphocyte and T-lymphocyte deficiencies
   (D) Secondary immunodeficiency can result from corticosteroid medication

2. The most severe result of infection with HIV is called
   (A) Candidiasis
   (B) AIDS
   (C) AIDS-related complex
   (D) DiGeorge's syndrome

3. The most commonly used test to determine HIV infection is a test for
   (A) Viral antigen
   (B) T-lymphocyte function
   (C) B-lymphocyte function
   (D) Antibodies

4. The initial infection with HIV can be
   (A) Asymptomatic
   (B) Accompanied by lymphadenopathy
   (C) Accompanied by acute illness
   (D) All of the above

5. Oral candidiasis
   (A) Is an early sign of underlying immunodeficiency
   (B) Is always a white lesion
   (C) Occurs only on the tongue
   (D) Is rarely associated with HIV infection

6. In immunodeficient patients, herpes simplex infection
   (A) Occurs only on keratinized mucosa
   (B) Is diagnosed on the basis of the clinical appearance
   (C) Is painless
   (D) May meet the criteria for the diagnosis of AIDS

7. Hairy leukoplakia is associated with the
   (A) Human papillomavirus
   (B) Herpes simplex virus
   (C) Coxsackievirus
   (D) Epstein-Barr virus

8. In patients infected with HIV, the most common intraoral location of Kaposi's sarcoma is the
   (A) Buccal mucosa and tongue
   (B) Floor of the mouth
   (C) Palate and gingiva
   (D) Lower lip

9. Which one of the following is NOT a characteristic of HIV-associated periodontal disease?
   (A) Pain
   (B) Minimal bone loss
   (C) Spontaneous bleeding
   (D) Interproximal necrosis

10. Hyperpituitarism results from an excessive production of growth hormone. It is most often caused by one of the following, which is a benign tumor:
    (A) Pituitary adenoma
    (B) Pituitary sarcoma
    (C) Carcinoma in situ
    (D) Ameloblastoma

11. Hyperthyroidism in children can lead to
    (A) Partial anodontia
    (B) Amelogenesis imperfecta
    (C) Ankylosis
    (D) Early exfoliation of the deciduous dentition and early eruption of the permanent teeth

12. Hypercalcemia, hypophosphatemia, and abnormal bone metabolism are characteristic of which one of the following conditions?
    (A) Hyperthyroidism
    (B) Hypothyroidism
    (C) Hyperparathyroidism
    (D) Hyperpituitarism

13. Which of the following is characteristic of diabetes mellitus?
    (A) Hyperglycemia
    (B) Lack of insulin
    (C) Vascular changes
    (D) All of the above

14. Polydipsia, polyuria, and polyphagia are all characteristic of which one of the following?
    (A) Fibrous dysplasia
    (B) Hyperthyroidism
    (C) Insulin-dependent diabetes mellitus
    (D) Addison's disease

15. Which one of the following is characterized by precocious puberty in females?
    (A) Monostotic fibrous dysplasia
    (B) Albright's syndrome
    (C) Jaffe-Lichtenstein–type polyostotic fibrous dysplasia
    (D) Paget's disease of bone

16. Bone resorption, osteoblastic repair, loss of the lamina dura, hypercementosis, and "cotton-wool" radiopacities are all characteristic of
    (A) Albright's syndrome
    (B) Letterer-Siwe disease
    (C) Paget's disease of bone
    (D) Polyostotic fibrous dysplasia

17. Which one of the following is NOT a characteristic of type II diabetes mellitus?
    (A) Obesity
    (B) Occurs at 40 years of age or older
    (C) Autoimmunity is the key to its development
    (D) Glucose control can be achieved without daily insulin injections in most cases

18. Which of the following oral complications can occur in diabetes mellitus?
    (A) Candidiasis
    (B) Xerostomia
    (C) Excessive periodontal bone loss
    (D) All of the above

19. Achlorhydria, failure to absorb vitamin B_{12}, and megaloblastic anemia are characteristic features of which one of the following?
    (A) Pernicious anemia
    (B) Thalassemia
    (C) Sickle cell anemia
    (D) Thrombocytopenic purpura

20. Which of the following are characteristic of sickle cell anemia?
    (A) Inherited blood disorder found predominantly in blacks
    (B) Occurs as a result of abnormal hemoglobin and decreased oxygen in the red blood cells
    (C) Patient can experience weakness, fatigue, and joint pain
    (D) All of the above

21. Which one of the following is characterized by a decrease in platelets?
    (A) Celiac sprue
    (B) Thrombocytopenia
    (C) Mediterranean anemia
    (D) Plummer-Vinson syndrome

22. Secondary aplastic anemia can be caused by
    (A) Chemotherapy
    (B) Dental radiographs
    (C) A genetic disorder
    (D) An autoimmune factor

23. Which one of the following is characterized by an abnormal increase in the circulating red blood cells?
    (A) Leukopenia
    (B) Polydipsia
    (C) Thrombocytopenia
    (D) Polycythemia

24. Leukopenia most often involves which cell type?
    (A) Eosinophils
    (B) Neutrophils
    (C) Basophils
    (D) Erythrocytes

25. If a patient's white blood cell count is 1000/mm³, one might suspect
    (A) Leukopenia
    (B) Thrombocytopenia
    (C) Hemophilia
    (D) Cyclic neutropenia

26. Excessive numbers of abnormal white blood cells are characteristic of
    (A) Agranulocytosis
    (B) Leukopenia
    (C) Cyclic neutropenia
    (D) Leukemia

27. Normal bleeding time is usually between
    (A) 1 and 6 minutes
    (B) 2 and 3 minutes
    (C) 15 and 45 seconds
    (D) 15 and 30 minutes

28. The normal prothrombin time is
    (A) 2 to 5 minutes
    (B) 11 to 16 seconds
    (C) 10 to 15 minutes
    (D) 1 to 6 seconds

29. Antibody testing to determine if a person has been infected with HIV includes which of the following specific tests?
    (A) Schilling
    (B) CBC
    (C) PT and PTT
    (D) ELISA and Western blot

30. Which one of the following oral conditions is an early sign of a deficiency in the immune system and is commonly found in patients with HIV infection?
    (A) Geographic tongue
    (B) Advanced periodontitis
    (C) Oral candidiasis
    (D) Histoplasmosis

31. Which one of the following oral conditions is not specifically characteristic of patients with HIV or AIDS?
    (A) Herpes simplex
    (B) Hairy leukoplakia
    (C) Kaposi's sarcoma
    (D) Leukoedema

32. Linear gingival erythema (LGE) has specific characteristics that include spontaneous bleeding, petechiae on the attached gingiva and alveolar mucosa, and a band of erythema at the gingival margin; which one of the following statements is TRUE?
    (A) These tissues respond well to scaling and root planing
    (B) Excellent oral hygiene and home care techniques will eliminate these gingival conditions
    (C) This condition will automatically develop into advanced periodontal disease in all HIV patients
    (D) LGE patients do not respond to scaling or oral hygiene techniques; the gingival condition exists independently of the patient's oral hygiene status

33. Symptoms of leukemia can be similar to those found in
    (A) Hepatitis
    (B) Amelogenesis imperfecta
    (C) Nonthrombocytopenic purpura
    (D) Mononucleosis

34. In treating fibrous dysplasia, which one of the following modalities is the only one recommended?
    (A) Surgery
    (B) Radiation therapy
    (C) Chemotherapy
    (D) Bone marrow depressants

35. Which one of the following is not characteristic of primary hyperparathyroidism?
    (A) Osteoclastic resorption
    (B) Excessive production of parathyroid hormone
    (C) "Cotton-wool" radiographic appearance
    (D) Decreased serum calcium

8

Temporomandibular Disorders and Dental Implants

ANTHONY J. CASINO

·

RICHARD S. TRUHLAR

·

Objectives

After studying this chapter, the student should be able to:

1. Label the following on a diagram of the temporomandibular joint:
   Glenoid fossa of the temporal bone
   Articular disc
   Mandibular condyle
   Joint capsule
   Superior belly of the lateral pterygoid muscle.
2. State the function of the muscles of mastication.
3. State two symptoms of a temporomandibular disorder.
4. List at least two problems that are suggestive of temporomandibular dysfunction.
5. State the function of radiographs in the evaluation of a patient with symptoms suggestive of temporomandibular dysfunction.
6. List and describe the two main categories of treatment of temporomandibular disorders.
7. Describe what is meant by the term **osseointegration.**
8. State the most important clinical parameter used to assess implant health.
9. List four signs of peri-implant disease.
10. Describe the radiographic finding indicative of a failing implant.
11. Explain why plastic instruments are used to remove plaque and debris from the implant–tissue interface.
12. List two causes of implant failure.
13. Describe the role that a dental hygienist might play in the management of a patient with dental implants.

Vocabulary

Abutment (ah-but′mint)   With dental implants, a transmucosal element that screws into the top of an implant fixture and, in turn, can support a single crown or a framework for a fixed or detachable prosthesis; periodontal probing is performed around the abutment to monitor clinical attachment levels

Alloy (al′oi)   The product of a fusion of two or more metals in a liquid state

Arthrography (ar-throg′rah-fē)   Radiography of a joint after injection of opaque contrast material

Arthroscopy (ar-thros′cah-pē)   A method for evaluating a joint involving the insertion of small cannulas along with a camera and instruments into a joint

Articular disc (ar-tik′u-ler disk)   A pad of fibrocartilage or dense fibrous tissue present in some synovial joints—for example, the temporomandibular joint

Articulation (ar-tik-ū-lā′shin)   A joint

Auscultation (aws-kul-tā′shin)   Listening to sounds within the body

440

Blade (blād) An endosseous implant, usually constructed of cast chromium-cobalt alloy or machined of titanium, with a narrow (buccolingual) body that has openings or vents through which tissue grows to obtain retention in the alveolus

Creptitus (krep'i-tus) A dry, crackling sound

Endosseous implant (en-dos'ē-us im'plant) A fixture that is placed into the alveolar or basal bone and that protrudes through the mucoperiosteum, serving to support a prosthodontic abutment

Fibro-osseointegration (fi'brō-os'e-ō-in'ti-grā'shin) An interposition of a ligament (connective tissue) between the implant and the bone causing a possible substantial reduction in load transfer to the bone

Fixture (fiks'tur) A generic term usually denoting a root form implant

Inert (in-ert') Lacking in physical activity, chemical reactivity, or an expected biologic or pharmacologic effect

Osseointegration (os'e-ō-in-ti-grā'shin) Direct apposition of bone to the implant surface when seen by light microscopy

Plasma spray (plas'ma sprā) A method of coating an implant surface by spraying it with a molten material under high pressure

Polymer (pol-i-mer) A long-chain hydrocarbon

Root form implant (root form im'plant) A cylindric endosseous implant

Subperiosteal implant (sub-per-i-os'tē-al im'plant) An appliance made of an open-mesh frame designed to fit over the surface of the bone beneath the periosteum; attached to this frame are one or more struts, which penetrate the mucoperiosteum and serve as prosthodontic abutments

Synovial fluid (si-nō'vē-al floo'id) The transparent, viscous fluid that is secreted by the synovial membrane and found in joint cavities

Synovial membrane (si-nō'vē-al mem'brān) Tissue that forms a portion of the lining of some joints—for example, the temporomandibular joint

*Peri implant mucositis - Inflam.
Changes confined to the soft tissues
surrounding implants; a condition
analogous to gingivitis around
tooth w/ no bone loss

TEMPOROMANDIBULAR DISORDERS

Temporomandibular disorders, also called **TMDs,** are due to abnormalities in the functioning of the **temporomandibular joint** or associated structures. These have been a clinical and diagnostic challenge in dentistry for many years. TMDs and jaw dysfunction problems were written about in the late nineteenth century, and the relationship of these disorders to the muscles of mastication was first published in 1933. An understanding of the anatomy of the temporomandibular joint, the muscles of mastication, and normal joint function is important to the understanding of TMDs.

Temporomandibular Joint Anatomy

The temporomandibular joint is the **articulation** between the condyle of the mandible and the glenoid fossa of the temporal bone (Fig. 8–1). It is a highly specialized joint that differs from other similar joints because of the fibrocartilage that covers the bony articulating surfaces. A disc called the **articular disc** is interposed in the space

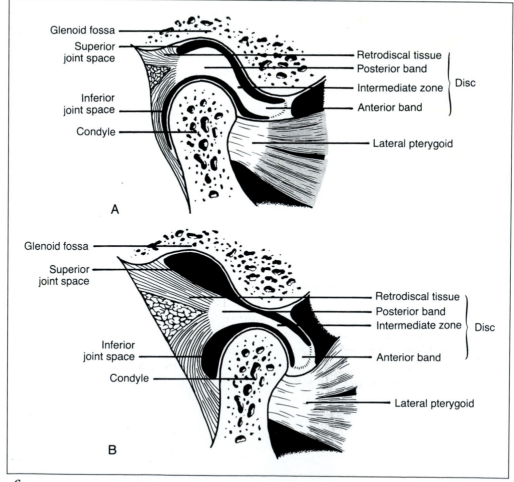

f i g u r e 8–1   Lateral views of the temporomandibular joint. *A,* Jaw closed. *B,* Jaw open. (From Kaplan AS, Assael LA: Temporomandibular Disorders. Philadelphia, WB Saunders, 1991, p 3.)

between the temporal bone and the mandible. This disc divides the space into an upper compartment (superior joint space) and a lower compartment (inferior joint space) (see Fig. 8–1). The joint is also unusual because it is able to assume both a rotational or hinge movement and a gliding movement. Gliding movements occur in the upper compartment, while the lower compartment functions primarily as the hinge component. The temporomandibular joint is often classified as a hinge joint with movable socket.

The articular disc is attached to the lateral and medial aspects of the condyle, to the superior belly of the lateral pterygoid muscle, and to the joint capsule (see Fig. 8–1). The disc and the surfaces of the bone are avascular (i.e., they do not contain blood vessels). The spaces in the joint are filled with fluid called **synovial fluid,** which is produced by the **synovial membrane,** which lines the joint. Nourishment to the avascular structures is provided by the synovial fluid. The joint is protected by the fibrous connective tissue joint capsule.

Muscles of Mastication

Understanding the location and action of the **muscles of mastication** is important in the evaluation of TMDs. **Palpation** of these muscles during a clinical evaluation is used to determine whether muscle spasm or dysfunctional muscle activity is occurring.

The muscles of mastication comprise major muscles about the facial region that govern the movement of the mandible. These muscles include the masseter, temporalis, medial pterygoid, lateral pterygoid, and anterior digastric and mylohyoid (suprahyoids) (Figs. 8–2 to 8–4). The function of these muscles is to create the mandibular envelope of motion. Three of these muscles, the masseter, medial pterygoid, and temporalis, are elevator muscles that, when activated, close the mandible. The opening, or depressor, function is accomplished mainly by the lateral pterygoid muscle with some help from the anterior digastric muscle. Studies have shown that the two components of the lateral pterygoid muscle are active at different times in the functioning of the mandible (see Fig. 8–4). The superior portion of the muscle seats the articular disc on the eminence of the articulating surface. The inferior belly is attached to the mandibular condyle and functions during mouth opening.

Normal Joint Function

The harmonious function of the temporomandibular joint depends on various factors. The anatomic relationship of the condyle-disc complex governs the smooth functioning of the mandible. This articulation, along with the muscles of mastication, provides the movement of the mandible. While the muscles of mastication are the machinery that powers mandibular movement, the anatomic joint structures, such as the condyle, articular eminence, and disc, act as the gears or bearings of the jaw.

In **normal joint function** the jaw begins at a rest position of maximum occlusal contact. In this position the mandibular condyle rests within the glenoid fossa, with the articular disc situated between the condyle, roof of the glenoid fossa, and articular eminence (see Fig. 8–1A). During rotational (hinge) movement the condyle moves anteriorly on the disc, with the disc assuming a more posterior relationship. During hinge movement the condyle moves forward in relationship to the disc. During translation (slide movement) the mandible continues to move anteriorly on the disc and the disc assumes a more posterior relationship, and the entire condyle disc assembly moves anteriorly as a unit. The inferior and superior joint spaces assume different configurations during each of these movements.

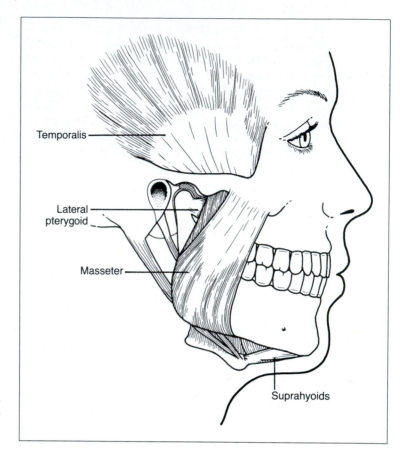

The muscles of mastication. The temporalis, lateral pterygoid, masseter, and suprahyoid muscles are illustrated. (From Kaplan AS, Assael LA: Temporomandibular Disorders. Philadelphia, WB Saunders, 1991, p 5.)

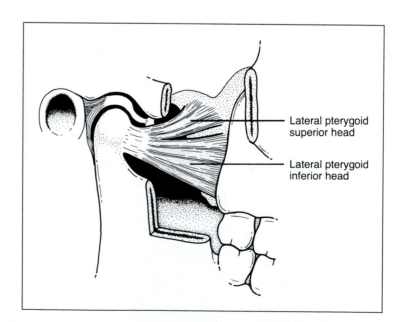

▪ *f* i g u r e 8–3

The muscles of mastication. The two distinct heads of the lateral pterygoid muscle are illustrated. (From Kaplan AS, Assael LA: Temporomandibular Disorders. Philadelphia, WB Saunders, 1991, p 5.)

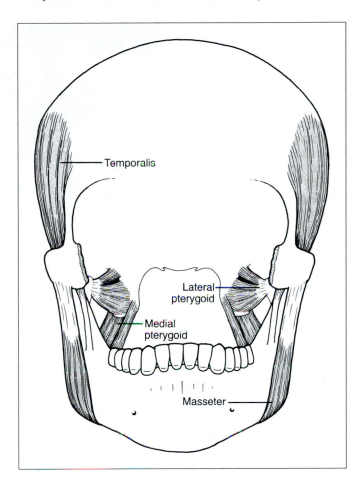

▪ *f* **i g u r e 8–4**

The muscles of mastication. Illustrated are the four paired muscles of mastication: the masseter, temporalis, medial pterygoid, and lateral pterygoid muscles. (From Kaplan AS, Assael LA: Temporomandibular Disorders. Philadelphia, WB Saunders, 1991, p 4.)

Diagnostic Procedures

Temporomandibular dysfunction can be caused by disorders of the muscles of mastication or internal derangements of the components of the joint. Two separate but sometimes related complaints, pain and dysfunction, characterize TMDs, and patients may complain of either or both. Appropriate treatment is based on accurate diagnosis. Accurate diagnosis is based on the evaluation of the history of the presenting complaints and a thorough clinical examination.

A history of aberrant growth, previous injuries, illnesses, joint complaints, muscle complaints, and possible emotional disturbances is important in the evaluation of patients with TMDs. A history of the jaw dysfunction should elicit any

- Problems with chewing
- Malocclusion
- Abusive habits and mannerisms
- Bruxing and clenching
- Problems with the dentition
- Extensive dental or orthodontic treatment
- History of surgical treatment of the jaws

The clinical examination includes locating the source of pain and the presence of restriction of mandibular movement. The pursuit of the pain source begins with a systemic examination of the muscles of mastication, usually by palpation. **Auscultation**

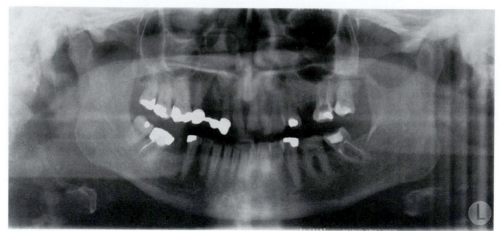

▪ *f* i g u r e 8–5   Panoramic radiograph of a patient with temporomandibular dysfunction and normal anatomy of the mandibular condyles.

(using a stethoscope) and palpation of the joint are included in the examination. The clinician relates joint noises such as clicking, crepitus (crackling), or popping to the mandibular movement cycle. The patient is asked to move the mandible in a normal rotation and also in translatory (forward slide) cycle. Interincisal opening is measured along with any obvious deviation of motion to the right or left side. The patient's ability to go into lateral excursions to the right and left side is noted. The patient is asked to go into protrusive movement to see whether there are any deviations or disc interferences within the joint. Finally, the patient's occlusion is evaluated to determine gross abnormalities and whether the occlusal abnormalities are related to the patient's temporomandibular problem.

Radiographic studies are used in attempting to determine the etiology of the patient's pain or dysfunction. Several different types of radiographs and views are obtained to determine the shape of the condyle and whether there is evidence of degenerative joint disease (Figs. 8–5 and 8–6). Several specialized diagnostic studies have become available over the past several years that are useful in the diagnosis of

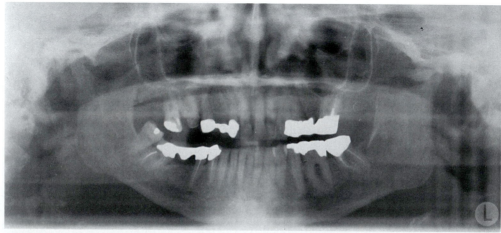

▪ *f* i g u r e 8–6   Panoramic radiograph showing resorption of both the right and the left condyles. In this patient degenerative arthritis followed bilateral surgery of the temporomandibular joint. The left coronoid process was removed during surgery.

TMDs. Temporomandibular joint **arthrography** is used to determine the disc position. This, in conjunction with **magnetic resonance imaging (MRI),** is used to determine the position and condition of the disc and soft tissues (Fig. 8–7). More recently, temporomandibular joint **arthroscopy** (inserting small cannulas with camera and instruments into the joint) has been used to visualize directly both the hard and the soft tissues of the temporomandibular joint.

TMDs can be categorized as disorders of the masticatory muscles, internal derangements or displacement of the disc, and disorders of the joint. Disorders of the joint include inflammation of the soft tissues and arthritis. Many types of arthritis can affect the temporomandibular joint. Some of these are traumatic arthritis, degenerative arthritis, infectious arthritis, and rheumatoid arthritis. Many other conditions may also affect this joint. Some of these are fibrosis of the temporomandibular joint capsule, hyperplasia of the mandibular condyle, and benign and malignant neoplasms of the temporomandibular joint.

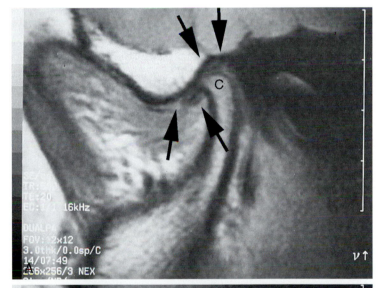

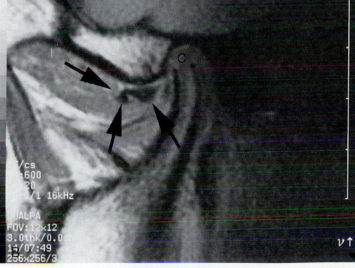

▪ *f* i g u r e 8–7

A, Magnetic resonance imaging (MRI) scan of the right temporomandibular joint showing the normal position of the disc. C = condyle. Arrows point to the disc. *B,* MRI scan of the left temporomandibular joint in the same patient showing displacement of the disc.

Treatment

Appropriate treatment of TMDs follows an accurate diagnosis. Conservative non-surgical approaches to TMDs have provided many patients with relief, while misadventured surgical treatments have caused significant problems to patients and have resulted in permanent dysfunction.

The two major categories of treatment include nonsurgical and surgical modalities. Nonsurgical treatment includes pharmacologic relief of pain (analgesics, muscle relaxants, and pain relievers), physical therapy (ultrasound, warm heat, spraying and stretching of the muscles, and jaw exercises), and mandibular splints that guide the jaw into a new position or provide for an interocclusal separation of the patient's dentition. A variety of surgical modalities are used to treat TMDs, including arthroscopic procedures, disc plication (replacing the disc to its normal anatomic position), and meniscectomy (complete removal of the damaged disc).

DENTAL IMPLANTS

The implantation of natural or synthetic materials for the purpose of replacement of lost human teeth has been attempted for thousands of years. The earliest attempts used naturally occurring minerals and metals such as gemstones or gold. In the past half century or so, tremendous advances in the science of **biomaterials** have resulted in experimentation with the relative purity and strength of new materials.

In the mid-1960s, researchers began to understand the critical relationship between the **inertness** of the surgical implant material and the host tissue response of the patient. The inertness of the surgical implant material is related to both the type and the purity of the material used. To be successful, dental implant material must be **biocompatible.** The ideal properties of a dental implant material are generally considered to be

- High strength
- Maximal inertness
- Ability to bend (ductility)

Of the biomaterials currently available, metals and their alloys and ceramics are most widely used. The metals used for **root form implants** in bone **(endosseous implants)** include titanium and its alloy (titanium-aluminum-vanadium), while subperiosteal frameworks have usually been cast from another alloy (cobalt-chromium-molybdenum) and more recently from titanium. Titanium and its alloys readily form an oxide layer. The process of forming this oxide layer is known as self-passivation. It is believed that this oxide layer serves to isolate the metal from the bone and accounts for its biocompatibility. Several different ceramics are also being used for endosseous implants.

Surgical techniques that create minimal mechanical, chemical, and thermal trauma to the tissue were introduced in the 1970s by Brånemark and co-workers. These techniques, combined with the use of commercially pure titanium implant fixtures and an understanding of the concept of tissue integration **(osseointegration),** have been responsible for the success of dental implants. An understanding of the clinical assessment of implant health is essential to understanding the problems that may be associated with dental implants.

Clinical Assessment of Implant Health

The single most important clinical parameter used to assess implant health is **clinical mobility.** In a healthy, osseointegrated implant, the bone is in close apposition to the implant fixture and the implant demonstrates no mobility (Fig. 8–8). In the past, mobility of up to 1 mm in any direction was considered acceptable. The most recent guidelines based on clinical research allow for *no* clinical mobility in a properly osseointegrated implant fixture.

Implant mobility may be assessed by a number of techniques. Implant fixture mobility is assessed with the prosthesis removed. Prior to checking for implant mobility, the abutment screw is firmly tightened. Force applied to the fixture-abutment complex by the blunt ends of two dental instruments should create no discernible movement. This method of assessment is sometimes referred to as a static determination of mobility.

Two dynamic methods involving percussion of the implant-abutment complex are also used to evaluate osseointegration. In the first dynamic method, the complex is struck by a blunt metallic dental instrument, and the resultant sound is a high-pitched, almost ringing sound if the complex is well integrated. If there has been a failure of integration, the bone-implant interface has been replaced by a zone of connective tissue, resulting in a duller, thud-like sound. The second dynamic method uses an electromagnetic rod to percuss the implant abutment 16 times, and the speed with which the rod decelerates is measured. This gives an indirect assessment of the rigidity of the bone-implant interface. This device is currently the focus of extensive research.

Although detection of implant mobility is a late and absolute diagnostic sign of implant failure, use of other periodontal parameters has failed to predict implant failure satisfactorily. Other methods that have been used to evaluate implants include probing depth and pocket formation. Some clinicians argue that implants should not be probed

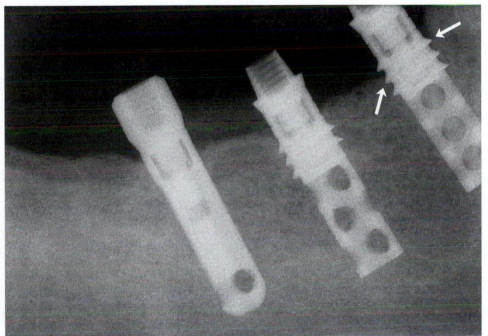

▪ *f* i g u r e **8-8**   Periapical radiograph of a root form implant demonstrating acceptable bone response. Arrows indicate bone loss to the first thread of the implant fixture, a result common in this fixture design.

because the probe penetrates the delicate epithelial cuff attachment, creating a path for bacterial ingress. The rationale for probing, however, is that it allows for detection of changes in bone and soft tissue attachment levels before they are radiographically apparent, especially for detection of changes on the buccal and lingual surfaces. Probing with a plastic probe prevents implant surface contamination by metal transfer (Fig. 8–9). Gentle force or an electronic pressure-sensitive probe prevents undue disruption of the peri-implant soft tissue seal. Probing depths of less than 4 mm are typical. The microbiota associated with healthy implants are similar to those found around healthy natural teeth—specifically, a predominance of gram-positive, nonmotile cocci and rods.

Signs of **peri-implant disease** include

- Bleeding on probing
- Suppuration
- Swelling
- Erythema

The microorganisms associated with failing implants include gram-negative rods, with black-pigmented *Bacteroides* and *Fusobacterium* spp. found regularly. Studies are underway to determine whether the placement of implants in a partially edentulous mouth with periodontally involved teeth puts the implants at increased risk for the development of peri-implantitis due to colonization by bacteria from these dental sources.

Radiographic Assessment of Implant Health

The most recent guidelines for demonstration of an acceptable bony response around endosseous implants allow up to 1 mm of bone loss the first year, followed by

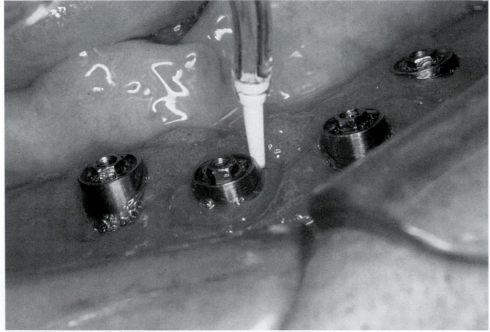

■ *f i g u r e* **8–9**   Healthy peri-implant tissues. Probing depths are less than 3 mm. There is an absence of erythema, bleeding, and suppuration on probing. The probe shown here is pressure sensitive with a nonmetallic tip.

no more than 0.2 mm of bone loss each subsequent year (see Fig. 8–8). It was previously recommended that bone loss not exceeding a third of the vertical height of the implant would be acceptable.

Demonstration of a peri-implant radiolucency is indicative of a failing implant, and the fixture usually has to be removed (Fig. 8–10). Additional diagnostic information that may be obtained radiographically includes a fracture of the implant fixture and incomplete seating of the abutment screw.

Proper radiographic technique for adequate imaging of an implant fixture can be difficult. The objective is to check for peri-implant and periapical radiolucencies. The depth of the vestibule is often very limited because of the loss of alveolar height that accompanied loss of the natural dentition. The limited vestibule interferes with proper placement of the film packet for paralleling technique. For situations such as these, the bisecting angle technique may be used to image the entire implant, albeit in a slightly distorted manner. Combined with this, for a less-distorted image of the coronal area of the bone-implant interface, a horizontal, bite-wing technique may be used.

Maintenance Procedures for Vertical Implants

Maintaining healthy tissue around the dental implant involves prevention of the progression of gingivitis to peri-implantitis and prevention of disruption of the perimu-

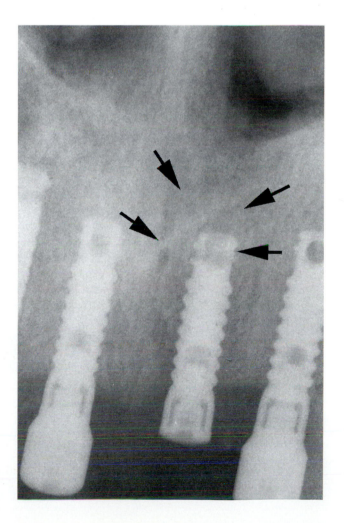

■ *f* i g u r e 8–10
Periapical radiograph showing a perifix-ture radiolucency *(arrows)* indicating prob-able compromise of the labial cortical plate.

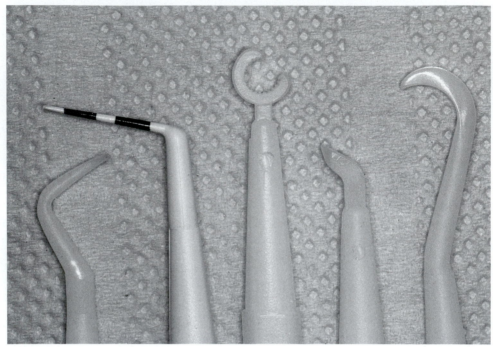

▪ *f i g u r e* **8–11**   Examples of plastic instruments commercially available for maintenance of implant abutment–soft tissue interface.

cosal seal by bacteria or instrumentation. In order to maintain optimum health, the following must be accomplished:

▪ Plaque must be inhibited
▪ Early microbial colonization on the implant surfaces must be stopped
▪ All existing plaque must be removed
▪ The existing plaque must be changed from pathogenic to nonpathogenic

It is widely accepted that a **smooth abutment surface** is more conducive to a plaque-free environment than a roughened surface. Therefore, care must be taken to maintain the smooth nature of the abutment surface. Research has demonstrated that the hardest implant surface currently available is the single-crystal sapphire. Hydroxyapatite is the surface easiest to alter, and pure titanium falls between the two. To prevent scratching of the abutment surface, plastic instruments are used to remove plaque and debris from the implant-tissue interface (Fig. 8–11). Sonic and ultrasonic scalers are the instruments that are harshest on implant surfaces. Titanium-tipped curets produce grooves and surface pitting on implant surfaces. Prophylaxis and polishing pastes can produce random grooving, with small crystals forming at the ends of the grooves. Unitufted brushes in combination with an antimicrobial agent such as chlorhexidine have been shown to be the least abrasive method of polishing the implant. Acidic fluoride preparations have been reported to etch titanium surfaces. If fluoride treatments are to be used for natural teeth adjacent to implants, a neutral sodium fluoride preparation is recommended.

Treatment of Unhealthy Implants

Treatment of unhealthy implants involves identifying the cause of the problem. The two major causes of peri-implant disease and implant failure are

- Mechanical overload
- Bacterial infection

Mechanical Overload

Mechanical overload can be suspected in the following situations:

- The prosthetic framework does not precisely fit the implant abutment
- The patient demonstrates heavy occlusal function or parafunction
- The implant has been placed in poor quality bone or insufficient quantity of bone
- The position and/or number of implants placed does not favor ideal load transmission

Treatment. Correction of these problems may include

- Changes in design of the prosthesis and refabrication of the prosthesis
- Patient retraining
- Occlusal equilibration
- Improving the implant number and position

Surgery may also be used to recontour deep peri-implant soft tissue pockets or to regenerate bone around the implant (Fig. 8–12).

Bacterial Infection

Treatment. Bacterial infection of the tissues surrounding an implant is treated in a similar fashion to bacterial infection in the natural dentition. The first phase focuses on controlling the acute infection and reducing inflammation by

- Local mechanical débridement of the abutment surface with plastic instruments
- Adjunctive use of topical or systemic antimicrobial agents
- Improved patient oral hygiene

The second phase, if necessary, may be surgical treatment of residual peri-implant defects. Treatment of the contaminated implant surface at the time of surgery is advocated by many clinicians in order to promote better wound healing. Three chemo-therapeutic regimens currently in use for this purpose include application of a supersaturated solution of citric acid (pH = 1) for 30 to 60 seconds, a sodium bicarbonate slurry used as an air-powder abrasive, and a paste made of tetracycline or doxycycline and sterile water.

Further treatment of the implant surface at the time of surgery can include smoothing rough implant surfaces, including exposed screw threads, resorbed hydroxyapatite coating, or plasma-sprayed titanium. This is called **implantoplasty** and is accomplished with high-speed finishing burs under copious irrigation. The surface is polished with fine pumice or prophylaxis paste and a rubber cup.

Guided bone regeneration with the use of occlusive membranes either with or without bone grafts is the technique most widely used to attempt to correct bony defects around an implant (see Fig. 8–12). This may be used either at the time of placement or subsequently. If an ailing implant is to be treated with guided bone regeneration, it is most advantageous if the prostheses can be removed, including the abutments, 6 to 8 weeks prior to the surgery to allow the patient to establish optimal oral hygiene and tissue health and to allow the soft tissues to heal over the implant fixture if possible. This creates a fuller soft tissue flap for coverage of the membrane during healing.

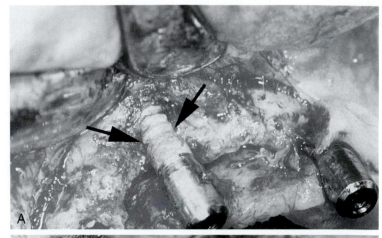

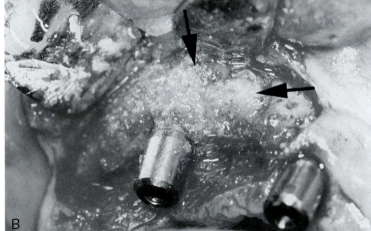

▪ *f* i g u r e **8–12**

A, A labial bony dehiscence *(arrows)* of a hydroxyapatite-coated endosseous implant in the maxillary anterior region. *B*, Regenerative surgical procedure of the dehisced implant *(arrows)* uses a combination of demineralized freeze-dried bone allograft, resorbable hydroxyapatite, and tetracycline hydrochloride. *C*, Placement of an occlusive membrane over the grafted site prior to closure of the flap (GORE-TEX Regenerative Material, WL Gore and Associates, Inc., Flagstaff, AZ). (Courtesy of Dr. Anthony J. Casino.)

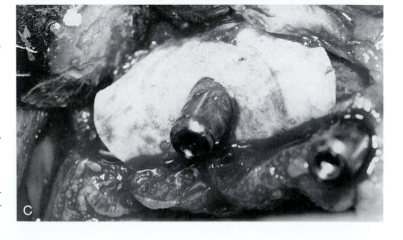

The Role of the Hygienist in the Management of Implants

The dental hygienist may play an important role in the management of patients with dental implants, both in patient education and in periodic maintenance to prevent plaque accumulation, which may result in gingivitis and possible progression to peri-implantitis.

SELECTED REFERENCES

BOOKS

Brånemark P-I, Zarb GA, Albrektsson T (eds): Tissue-integrated Prosthesis. Osseo-integration in Clinical Dentistry. Chicago, Quintessence, 1985.
Kaplan AS, Assael LA: Temporomandibular Disorders. Philadelphia, WB Saunders, 1991.
Meffert RM: Implant therapy. In Nevins M, Becker W, Kornman K (eds): Proceedings of the World Workshop in Clinical Periodontics. American Academy of Periodontology, 1989, Section VIII, pp 1–19.

JOURNAL ARTICLES

Dworkin SF, Huggins KH, LeResche L, et al: Epidemiology of signs and symptoms in temporomandibular disorders: Clinical signs in cases and controls. J Am Dent Assoc 120:273, 1990.
Lekholm U, Ericcson I, Adell R, Slots J: The condition of soft tissues at tooth and fixture abutments supporting fixed bridges: A microbiological and histological study. J Clin Periodontol 13:558, 1986.
McNeill C, Mohl ND, Rugh JD, Tanaka TT: Temporomandibular disorders: Diagnosis, management, education, and research. J Am Dent Assoc 120:253, 1990.
Mombelli A, van Oosten MAC, Schurch E, Lang NP: The microbiota associated with successful or failing osseointegrated titanium implants. Oral Microbiol Immunol 2:145, 1987.
Rapley JW, Swan RH, Hallmon WW, Mills MP: The surface characteristics produced by various oral hygiene instruments and materials on titanium implant abutments. Int J Oral Maxillofac Implant 5:47, 1990.
Schiffman EL, Fricton JR, Haley DP, Shapiro JR: The prevalence and treatment needs of subjects with temporomandibular disorders. J Am Dent Assoc 120:295, 1990.
Smith DE, Zarb GA: Criteria for success of osseointegrated endosseous implants. J Prosthet Dent 62:567, 1989.
Thomson-Neal D, Evans G, Meffert RM, Davenport WD: A SEM evaluation of various prophylactic modalities on different implants. Int J Periodontics Restorative Dent 9:301, 1989.
Zablotsky MH: Chemotherapeutics in implant dentistry. Implant Dent 2:19, 1993.

REVIEW QUESTIONS

1. Disorders of the articulation between the mandible and maxilla are called
    (A) Synovial hyperplasias
    (B) Mandibulomaxillary dysfunction
    (C) Temporomandibular disorders
    (D) Mandibular dysfunction

2. Using a stethoscope to listen to abnormal noises in the temporomandibular joint is called
    (A) Audiology
    (B) Auscultation
    (C) Palpation
    (D) Arthrography

3. Which one of the following is the most important aspect of the management of temporomandibular disorders?
   (A) Palpation of the muscles of mastication
   (B) Establishing an accurate diagnosis
   (C) Using a nonsurgical approach
   (D) Adjusting the occlusion

4. The method of evaluating and treating temporomandibular disorders by inserting small cannulas with camera and instruments into the joint is called
   (A) Arthroscopy
   (B) Magnetic resonance imaging
   (C) Occlusal equilibration
   (D) Meniscectomy

5. Properties considered to be important for a dental implant material include all of the following except
   (A) High strength
   (B) Maximal inertness
   (C) Resorbability
   (D) Biocompatibility

6. Commonly used parameters to monitor implant health include all of the following except
   (A) Probing pocket depth
   (B) Surface smoothness of abutment
   (C) Mobility
   (D) Inflammation

7. Which radiographic finding for implant health is the currently accepted standard?
   (A) Bone loss up to 1 mm the first year and less than 0.2 mm loss each following year
   (B) Bone loss at a rate equal to that of the natural dentition
   (C) Demonstration of a peri-implant radiolucency
   (D) Bone loss not exceeding one third of the vertical height of the implant fixture

8. The most important clinical parameter used to assess implant health is
   (A) Assessment of home care
   (B) Pocket depth
   (C) Mobility
   (D) Absence of pain

9. In a healthy osseointegrated implant, the bone is
   (A) Separated from the implant by a wide band of fibrous connective tissue
   (B) In close apposition to the implant
   (C) Partially replaced by cartilage
   (D) Connected to the implant by a periodontal ligament

10. Plastic instruments are used for removing plaque and debris from implant abutments because they
    (A) Are more efficient
    (B) Are easier to clean
    (C) Prevent scratching of the surface of the implant
    (D) Prevent injury to the surrounding gingival tissue

Glossary

Abutment With dental implants, a transmucosal element that screws into the top of an implant fixture. The abutment, in turn, can support a single crown or a framework for a fixed or detachable prosthesis. Periodontal probing is performed around the abutment to monitor clinical attachment levels.

Acantholysis Dissolution of the intercellular bridges of the prickle cell layer of the epithelium.

Acute Of short duration or of short and relatively severe course.

Agranulocytosis A marked decrease in the number of granulocytes, particularly neutrophils.

Alleles Genes that are located at the same level or locus in the two chromosomes of a pair and that determine the same functions or characteristics.

Allergy A hypersensitive state acquired through exposure to a particular allergen. Re-exposure to the same allergen elicits an exaggerated reaction.

Alloy The product of a fusion of two or more metals in a liquid state.

Amenorrhea Abnormal temporary or permanent cessation of menstrual cycles.

Amino acid An organic compound containing the amino group NH_2. Amino acids are the main component of proteins.

Anaphylaxis A type of hypersensitivity or allergic reaction in which the exaggerated immunologic reaction results from the release of vasoactive substances such as histamine. The reaction occurs on re-exposure to a foreign protein or other substance after sensitization.

Anemia Reduction to less than normal of the number of red blood cells, quantity of hemoglobin, or the volume of packed red blood cells in the blood.

Ankyloglossia Extensive adhesion of the tongue to the floor of the mouth or the lingual aspect of the anterior portion of the mandible caused by a short lingual frenum.

Anodontia Complete or almost complete congenital lack of teeth.

Anomaly Marked deviation from normal, especially as a result of congenital or hereditary defects.

Antibody A protein molecule, also called an immunoglobulin, that is produced by plasma cells and reacts with a specific antigen.

Antigen Any substance that is able to induce a specific immune response.

Aplasia (adjective, aplastic) Lack of development.

Arthralgia Severe pain in a joint.

Arthrography Radiography of a joint after injection of opaque contrast material.

Articular disc A pad of fibrocartilage or dense fibrous tissue present in some synovial joints—for example, the temporomandibular joint.

Articulation (noun) A joint.

Auscultation The act of listening to sounds within the body.

Autoantibody An antibody that reacts against an antigenic constituent of the person's own tissues.

Autoimmune disease A disease characterized by tissue injury caused by a humoral or cell-mediated immune response against constituents of the body's own tissues.

Autoimmunity Immune-mediated destruction of the body's own cells and tissues; immunity against self.

Autosomes (adjective, autosomal) The non-sex chromosomes that are identical for men and women.

Blade An endosseous implant, usually constructed of cast chromium-cobalt alloy or machined of titanium, with a narrow (buccolingual) body that has openings or vents through which tissue grows to obtain retention in the alveolus.

Barr body   Condensed chromatin of the inactivated X chromosome, which is found at the periphery of the nucleus of cells in women.

Benign   Not malignant; favorable for recovery.

B lymphocyte   A lymphoctye, also called a B cell, that matures without passing through the thymus. It matures into plasma cells that produce antibodies.

Brachydactyly   Short fingers or toes, or both.

Bulla (adjective, bullous; plural, bullae)   A circumscribed, elevated, fluid-filled lesion that is larger than 5 mm in diameter and usually contains serous fluid.

Calcitonin   A polypeptide secreted by the C cells of the thyroid gland.

Carcinoma   A malignant tumor of epithelial tissue.

Carrier   In genetics, a heterozygous individual who is clinically normal but who can transmit a recessive trait or characteristic; also, a person who is homozygous for an autosomal dominant condition with low penetrance.

Cell-mediated immunity   Immunity in which the predominant role is played by T lymphocytes.

Centimeter (cm)   One hundredth of a meter. Equivalent to a little less than ½ inch (0.393 of an inch).

Central   In oral pathology, a lesion occurring within bone.

Centromere   The constricted portion of the chromosome that divides the short arms from the long arms.

Chemotaxis   The directed movement of white blood cells to the area of injury along a chemical concentration gradient.

Chiasmata   The intercrossing of chromatids of the same or homologous chromosomes that takes place at metaphase of first meiosis for the purpose of genetic recombination.

Chromatid   Either of the two vertical halves of a chromosome that are joined at the centromere.

Chromatin   A general term used to refer to the material (DNA) that forms the chromosomes.

Chronic   Persisting over a long time.

Coagulation   Formation of a clot.

Coalescing   The process by which parts of a whole join together, or fuse, to make one.

Codominance   The full expression in a heterozygote of both alleles of a pair of chromosomes, with neither influenced by the other. A good example is the AB blood group.

Codon   The vertical sequence of three bases in DNA that codes for an amino acid.

Coloboma   A cleft generally seen on the iris or the eyelids.

Commissure   The site of union of corresponding parts—for example, the corners of the lips.

Concrescence   A condition in dentistry in which two adjacent teeth are united by cementum.

Congenital   Present at and existing from the time of birth.

Consanguinity   Blood relationship. In genetics, the term is generally used to describe matings or marriages among close relatives.

Corrugated   Having a surface that appears wrinkled.

Crepitus   A dry, crackling sound.

Crossing over   The exchange of segments between chromatids of the same or homologous chromosomes that takes place at metaphase of first meiosis. Crossing over is the result of chiasmata.

Cyst   An abnormal pathologic sac or cavity that is lined with epithelium and is enclosed in a connective tissue capsule.

Deletion   In genetics, the loss of part of a chromosome.

Dens in dente   "A tooth within a tooth"; a malformed tooth caused by an invagination of the crown before it is calcified.

Dentinogenesis   The formation of dentin.

Deoxyribonucleic acid (DNA)   A substance composed of a double chain of polynucleotides; both chains coiled around a central axis form a double helix. DNA is the basic genetic code or template for amino acid formation.

Diffuse   In the description of a lesion, the

borders of the lesion are not well defined, and it is not possible to detect the exact parameters of the lesion.

Dilaceration   An abnormal bend or curve, as in the root of a tooth.

Diploid   Having two sets of chromosomes; the normal constitution of somatic cells.

Dominant   In genetics, a trait or characteristic that is manifested when it is carried by only one of a pair of homologous chromosomes.

Dysplasia   Disordered growth.

Ecchymosis   A small, flat, hemorrhagic patch, larger than a petechia, on the skin or mucous membrane.

Emigration   The passage of white blood cells through the endothelium and wall of small blood vessels.

Encapsulated   Surrounded by a capsule of fibrous connective tissue.

Endosseous implant   A fixture that is placed into the alveolar or basal bone and that protrudes through the mucoperiosteum, serving to support a prosthondontic abutment.

Erythema   Redness of the skin or mucosa.

Expressivity   In genetics, the degree of clinical manifestation of a trait or characteristic.

Exudate (inflammatory exudate)   Fluid with a relatively high content of serum proteins and leukocytes formed as a reaction to injury of tissues and blood vessels.

Fever   An elevation of body temperature to greater than the normal of 98.6° F (37° C).

Fibrin   An insoluble protein that is essential to the clotting of blood.

Fibro-osseointegration   In patients with dental implants, an interposition of connective tissue between the implant and the bone causing a possible substantial reduction in load transfer to the bone.

Fissured   Having surface clefting or grooves.

Fixture   A generic term usually denoting a root form implant.

Flare   Redness of the skin or mucosa around an area of an irritant.

Fusion   The union of two adjoining tooth germs.

Gamete   Spermatozoon or ovum.

Gemination   In dentistry, a single tooth germ splits completely or partially, forming separate crowns. The tooth usually has a single root and root canal; also called twinning.

Genetic heterogeneity   Having more than one inheritance pattern.

Granuloma   A tumor-like mass of inflammatory tissue consisting of a central collection of macrophages, often with multinucleated giant cells, surrounded by lymphocytes.

Granulomatous disease   A disease characterized by the formation of granulomas.

Haploid   A cell with a single set of chromosomes. A gamete is haploid.

Hematocrit   The volume percentage of red blood cells in whole blood.

Hemolysis   The release of hemoglobin from red blood cells by destruction of the cells.

Hemostasis   The stoppage or cessation of bleeding.

Hepatomegaly   Enlargement of the liver.

Heterozygote (adjective, heterozygous)   An individual with two different genes at the allele loci.

Homozygote (adjective, homozygous)   An individual having identical genes at the allele loci.

Hormone   A chemical substance produced in the body that has a specific regulatory effect on certain cells or a certain organ or organs.

Humoral immunity   Immunity in which antibodies play the predominant role.

Hypercalcemia   An excess of calcium in the blood.

Hyperchromatic   Staining more intensely than normal.

Hyperemia   An excess of blood in a part of the body.

Hyperglycemia   An excess of glucose in the blood.

Hyperplasia   An abnormal increase in the number of normal cells in normal arrangement in a tissue.

Hypersensitivity   A state of altered reactivity in which the body reacts to a foreign agent with an exaggerated immune response.

Hypertelorism   Abnormally increased distance between two organs or parts. Orbital or ocular hypertelorism— abnormally increased distance between the orbits.

Hyperthermia Increased body temperature.

Hypertrophy An enlargement of a tissue or organ caused by an increase in size but not in number of cells.

Hypochromic Stained less intensely than normal.

Hypodontia Partial anodontia. The lack of one or more teeth.

Hypohidrosis Abnormally diminished secretion of sweat.

Hypophosphatemia Deficiency of phosphates in the blood.

Hypotrichosis Presence of less than the normal amount of hair.

Immune complex A combination of antibody and antigen.

Immunodeficiency A deficiency of the immune response caused by hypoactivity or decreased numbers of lymphoid cells.

Immunoglobulin A protein, also called an antibody, synthesized by plasma cells in response to a specific antigen.

Impacted teeth Teeth that cannot erupt into the oral cavity because of a physical obstruction.

Inert Lacking in physical activity, chemical reactivity, or an expected biologic or pharmacologic effect.

Insulin A peptide hormone produced in the pancreas by the beta cells in the islets of Langerhans. Insulin regulates glucose metabolism and is the major fuel-regulating hormone.

Invasion The infiltration and active destruction of surrounding tissues.

Ketoacidosis An accumulation of acid in the body resulting from the accumulation of ketone bodies.

LE cell A cell that is a characteristic of lupus erythematosus and other autoimmune diseases. It is a mature neutrophil that has phagocytized a spherical inclusion derived from another neutrophil.

Leukocytosis A temporary increase in the number of white blood cells circulating in blood.

Leukoplakia A clinical term used to identify a white, plaque-like lesion of the oral mucosa that cannot be wiped off and cannot be diagnosed as any other disease.

Lobule (adjective, lobulated) A segment or lobe that is part of a whole. Lobules sometimes appear fused together.

Local Confined to a limited part, not general or systemic.

Lymphadenopathy Any disease process that affects lymph nodes such that they become enlarged and palpable.

Lymphoid tissue Tissue composed of lymphocytes supported by a meshwork of connective tissue.

Macrodontia Abnormally large teeth.

Macrophage A large, mononuclear phagocyte derived from monocytes. Macrophages become mobile when stimulated by inflammation and interact with lymphocytes in an immune response.

Macule A flat area on the skin or mucosa, usually distinguished by color, that is different from the surrounding tissue.

Malignant Likely to cause the death of the host.

Malignant tumor Cancer; a tumor that is resistant to treatment and frequently causes death; a tumor that has the potential for uncontrolled growth and dissemination or recurrence, or both.

Margination A phenomenon that occurs during the relatively early phases of inflammation in which white blood cells tend to occupy the periphery of the blood vessels and adhere to endothelial cells that line the vessels.

Metastasis (plural, metastases) The transport of neoplastic cells to parts of the body remote from the primary tumor and the establishment of new tumors in those sites.

Metastatic tumor A tumor formed by cells that have been transported from the primary tumor to a site not connected to the primary tumor.

Microcyte A red blood cell that is smaller than normal.

Microdontia Abnormally small teeth.

Millimeter (mm) One thousandth of a meter (a meter is equivalent to 39.3 inches). The periodontal probe is of great assistance in documenting the size or diameter of a lesion that can be measured in millimeters.

Mitotic figures Dividing cells caught in the process of mitosis.

Mucositis Mucosal inflammation.

Multifactorial conditions Those conditions in which the phenotype results from a combination of genetic factors and environmental influences.

Multilocular A term used to describe a radiographic appearance of multiple, rounded compartments or locules. These can appear "soap bubble–like" or "honeycomb-like."

Myalgia Muscle pain.

Natural killer cell (NK cell) A lymphocyte that circulates in the blood and primarily protects against viral infections.

Necrosis The pathologic death of one or more cells or a portion of tissue or organ, resulting from irreversible damage.

Neoplasia The process of the formation of tumors by the uncontrolled proliferation of cells.

Neoplasm Tumor; a new growth of tissue in which the growth of tissue is uncontrolled and progressive.

Neutropenia A diminished number of neutrophils in the blood.

Nevus (plural, nevi) A benign, localized overgrowth of melanocytes; also, a birthmark.

Nikolsky's sign Seen in some bullous diseases, such as pemphigus vulgaris and bullous pemphigoid; the superficial epithelium separates easily from the basal layer on exertion of firm sliding manual pressure.

Nodule A palpable, solid lesion in soft tissue that is up to 1 cm in diameter and may be above, level with, or beneath the skin or mucosal surface.

Nondysjunction The result of chromosomes that were crossing over and did not separate; therefore, both migrate to the same cell.

Nucleotide A hydrolytic product of nucleic acid formed by a nitrogen-containing base, a five-carbon sugar (deoxyribose), and a phosphate.

Odontogenic Tooth forming.

Oncology The study of tumors or neoplasms.

Opportunistic infection A disease caused by a microorganism that does not ordinarily cause disease but becomes pathogenic under certain circumstances.

Osseointegration Direct apposition of bone to an implant surface when seen by light microscopy.

Osteoporosis A hereditary disease marked by abnormally dense bone.

Ovulum Ovum, the mature female germ cell.

Pallor Paleness.

Palpation The act of feeling with the hand.

Papillary Describing a small nipple-shaped projection or elevation usually found in clusters.

Papule A small circumscribed lesion usually less than 1 cm in diameter that protrudes above the surface of normal surrounding tissue.

Parathormone Parathyroid hormone.

Parenteral Administered by injection.

Pathogenic microorganism A microorganism that causes disease.

Pavementing Adherence of white blood cells to the endothelial cells lining an injured blood vessel.

Pedunculated Attached by a stem-like or stalk-like base.

Penetrance The prevalence of individuals with a given genotype that manifest clinically the phenotype associated with that trait.

Peripheral Located away from the center—indicates that the location of a lesion is in the soft tissue surrounding a bone.

Petechia A minute red spot on the skin or mucous membranes resulting from escape of a small amount of blood.

Phagocytosis A process of ingestion and digestion by cells.

Phenotype The physical and clinical visible characteristics of an individual. Genotype is the genetic composition. Phenotype is its observable appearance.

Plasma spray A method of coating an implant surface by spraying it with a molten material under high pressure.

Platelet A disc-shaped structure, also called a thrombocyte, found in the blood, which plays an important role in blood coagulation.

Pleomorphic Occurs in various forms.

Polycythemia An increase in the total red blood cell mass in the blood.

Polydactyly The presence of extra fingers or toes, or both.

Polymer A long-chain hydrocarbon.

Predilection A disposition in favor of something; preference.

Primary tumor The original tumor; the source of metastasis.

Purpura A group of disorders characterized by purplish or brownish-red discolorations caused by bleeding into the skin or tissues.

Purulent Containing or forming pus.

Pustule Varying-sized circumscribed, pus-filled, elevated lesions.

Radiolucent The black or dark areas in a radiograph that result from the ability of radiant energy to pass through the structure. Less dense structures (e.g., the pulp) are radiolucent.

Radiopaque The white or clear appearance in a radiograph that results from the inability of radiant energy to pass through a structure. The more dense the structure (i.e., amalgam restorations), the whiter it appears in the radiograph.

Receptor A cell surface protein to which a specific hormone can bind; such binding leads to biochemical events.

Recessive In genetics, a trait or characteristic manifested clinically with a double gene dose in autosomic chromosomes or with a single dose in males if the trait is X-linked.

Repair The restoration of damaged or diseased tissues.

Rheumatoid factor A protein, an immunoglobulin M (IgM), found in serum and detectable on laboratory tests. It is associated with rheumatoid arthritis and other autoimmune diseases.

Ribosome The cytoplasmic organelles in which proteins are formed based on the genetic code provided by RNA.

Root form implant A cylindric endosseous implant.

Root resorption Observed radiographically when the apex of the tooth appears shortened or blunted and irregularly shaped. It occurs as a response to stimuli, which can result from a cyst, tumor, or trauma.

Sarcoma A malignant tumor of connective tissue.

Scoliosis Lateral curvature of the spine.

Serous A substance having a watery consistency; relating to serum.

Sessile Broad based.

Somatic cells All the cells of the human body with the exception of the primitive germ cells (oogonia and spermatogonia).

Spermatozoon The mature masculine germ cell.

Spina bifida A defect in the spine caused by a lack of the vertebral arches through which the spinal cord protrudes.

Spina bifida occulta Similar to spina bifida, but with little or no protrusion.

Splenomegaly Enlargement of the spleen.

Stomodeum The embryonic structure that becomes the oral cavity.

Subperiosteal implant An appliance made of an open-mesh frame designed to fit over the surface of the bone beneath the periosteum. Attached to this frame are one or more struts that penetrate the mucoperiosteum and serve as prosthodontic abutments.

Supernumerary In excess of the normal or regular number, as in teeth.

Syndactyly Soft tissue or bone fusion, or both, of fingers and toes.

Synovial The transparent, viscous fluid that is secreted by the synovial membrane and found in joint cavities.

Synovial membrane Tissue that forms a portion of the lining of some joints—for example, the temporomandibular joint.

Systemic Pertaining to or affecting the body as a whole.

Thrombocyte A platelet.

Thrombocytopenia Decrease in the number of platelets in circulating blood.

Thymus A lymphoid organ that is situated in the chest. It reaches maximal development at about puberty and then undergoes gradual involution.

T lymphocyte A lymphocyte that passes through the thymus before migrating to tissues. The T lymphocyte, also called a T cell, is responsible for cell-mediated immunity.

Trisomy A pair of chromosomes with an identical extra chromosome.

Tumor A neoplasm; also, a swelling or enlargement.

Unilocular A term used to describe a radiographic appearance of a single, rounded compartment or locule.

Vesicle A small, elevated, fluid-filled lesion that is less than 1 cm in diameter.

Well circumscribed The borders of the lesion are specifically defined, and one can clearly see the exact margins and extent of the lesion.

Wheal A localized swelling of tissue due to edema during inflammation often accompanied by severe itching.

Whitlow An infection involving the distal phalanx of a finger.

Xerophthalmia Abnormal dryness of the eyes.

Xerostomia Dryness of the mouth caused by a decrease in salivary flow.

ANSWERS TO REVIEW QUESTIONS

CHAPTER 1	2. B	28. A	6. D	32. A
1. C	3. D	29. C	7. D	33. D
2. D	4. B	30. C	8. A	34. C
3. D	5. D	31. B	9. B	35. C
4. B	6. B	32. A	10. C	36. B
5. D	7. D	33. D	11. A	37. C
6. A	8. B	34. B	12. C	38. D
7. C	9. A	35. A	13. B	39. B
8. B	10. B	36. D	14. C	
9. A	11. D	37. C	15. B	**CHAPTER 4**
10. C	12. C	38. B	16. A	1. C
11. A	13. A	39. C	17. C	2. A
12. B	14. C	40. B	18. D	3. D
13. A	15. C	41. B	19. A	4. B
14. B	16. B	42. A	20. D	5. A
15. D	17. C	43. C	21. B	6. D
16. A	18. B	44. B	22. C	7. B
17. D	19. A	45. A	23. B	8. A
18. A	20. A	46. B	24. B	9. D
19. C	21. B	47. D	25. D	10. C
20. A	22. B		26. D	11. A
21. A	23. C	**CHAPTER 3**	27. C	12. B
22. D	24. B	1. C	28. D	13. A
23. B	25. C	2. B	29. B	14. B
	26. D	3. D	30. B	15. D
CHAPTER 2	27. D	4. A	31. D	16. C
1. B		5. D		17. A

18. A
19. C
20. A
21. B
22. B
23. C
24. D
25. C
26. A
27. D
28. A
29. A
30. B
31. B
32. A
33. D
34. A
35. B
36. D
37. C
38. B
39. A
40. B
41. D
42. C
43. B
44. C
45. D

CHAPTER 5
1. D

2. A
3. B
4. C
5. A
6. D
7. C
8. C
9. B
10. D
11. C
12. C
13. D
14. D
15. D
16. B
17. A
18. A
19. D
20. A
21. D
22. A
23. C
24. A
25. B
26. C
27. B
28. C
29. D
30. B
31. C

32. A
33. D
34. B
35. C
36. D
37. B
38. A
39. B
40. C

CHAPTER 6
1. C
2. A
3. B
4. D
5. B
6. C
7. A
8. D
9. B
10. D
11. A
12. D
13. C
14. C
15. B
16. A
17. A
18. B
19. C
20. B

21. D
22. D
23. A
24. B
25. C
26. A
27. D
28. C
29. C
30. A

CHAPTER 7
1. C
2. B
3. D
4. D
5. A
6. D
7. D
8. C
9. B
10. A
11. D
12. C
13. D
14. C
15. B
16. C
17. C
18. D
19. A

20. D
21. B
22. A
23. D
24. B
25. A
26. D
27. A
28. B
29. D
30. C
31. D
32. D
33. D
34. A
35. D

CHAPTER 8
1. C
2. B
3. B
4. A
5. C
6. B
7. A
8. C
9. B
10. C

Index

Index

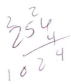

Note: Page numbers set in *italics* refer to illustrations; page numbers followed by t refer to tables. CP stands for color plates.

A

ABO blood group, as phenotype, 346
  inheritance patterns and, 353
Abrasion, of teeth, *75*, 75–76
Abscess(es), in actinomycosis, 173
  incision and drainage of, 60
  periapical, 107–108, *109–110*, CP80
    fistula with, 60
    in hypophosphatemic vitamin D–resistant rickets, 377
  periodontal, *101*
Abutment, of dental implants, surface of, 452
  with dental implant, definition of, 440
Acantholysis, defined, 128
  in pemphigus vulgaris, 163
Acetone, in diabetes mellitus, 391
Acetylsalicylic acid. See *Aspirin*.
Acids, teeth erosion from, 77
Acquired immunodeficiency syndrome (AIDS), 137.
    See also *Human immunodeficiency virus (HIV)*.
  aphthous ulcers and, 139
  clinical manifestations of, 419
  defined, 417–418, 418t
  diagnosis of, 417–418
  HIV infection and, 417
  oral manifestations of, 420–423, 420t, *421–427*, *425*, *427*
Acromegaly, macroglossia in, 389, *389*
Actinomyces israelii, 173
Actinomycosis, *173*, 173–174
Acute necrotizing ulcerative gingivitis (ANUG), 36, *37–38*, 175–176, *176*, CP76, CP78
  in acute leukemia, 410
Acyclovir, 193
Addison's disease, 394
Adenine, in DNA, 344
Adenocarcinomas, salivary gland, 284
Adenoid cystic carcinoma, 284, *285*, *287*, *291*, 291–292
Adenolymphoma, 288, *290*, 291
Adenoma, parathyroid, in hyperparathyroidism, 390
  pituitary, 388–389
  salivary gland, 284, *285–286*
    monomorphic, *286*, 288, *290*
    pleomorphic (benign mixed tumor), *285*, 288, *289*, CP16

Adenomatoid odontogenic tumor, 304, *306*, 306–307
Adrenal cortical insufficiency, primary (Addison's disease), 394
Adrenocorticotropic hormone, in Addison's disease, 394
Agenesis, cleft lip-palate and, 367
  in hypophosphatasia, 376
Aging, lingual varicosities and, 41
Agranulocytosis, defined, 387
  diagnosis and treatment of, 409
  oral manifestations of, 409
AIDS. See *Acquired immunodeficiency syndrome (AIDS)*.
Albright's syndrome, 396
Alcohol, squamous cell carcinoma and, 281
Alkaline phosphatase, in hypophosphatasia, 376
  in Paget's disease, 25, *34*, 400
  units for measuring, 400
Alleles, 346
  defined, 337
Allergy(ies), 135–137. See also *Hypersensitivity*.
  causes of, 145
  defined, 128
  fixed drug eruption as, 145
  to drugs, 136–137
Alloy, defined, 440
Alveolar bone, in hypohidrotic ectodermal dysplasia, 376
Alveolar osteitis (dry socket), 116
Amalgam fragment, *27*
Amalgam restorations, *9*, *28*
Amalgam tattoo, 13, *18*, *27*, 88, *89*, CP83
Ameloblastic fibroma, 304, *305*
Ameloblastoma, 294, *294–296*, 297
  in nevoid basal cell carcinoma syndrome, 362
  peripheral, of gingiva, 311
Ameloblasts, enamel pearl and, 244
Amelogenesis, 214
Amelogenesis imperfecta, 25, *30*, 352, 370–373, *371–372*, CP95
  characteristics of, 371–372, *371–372*
  pitted, 371, *371*
  snow-capped, 372, *372*
  types of, 371–372, *371–372*
Amino acid, defined, 337